BEYOND 100™

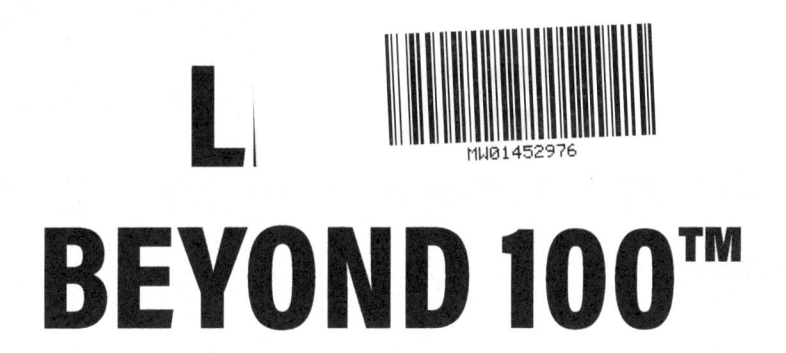

Reverse Your Biological Age Today

Graham Simpson, MD

Foreword by Ryan Smith, founder of Trudiagnostic

Copyright © 2022 Graham Simpson ALL RIGHTS RESERVED

316 Windmill Croft Dr., Las Vegas
Nevada 89148

Dr. Graham Simpson MD asserts the moral right to be identified as the author of this work. All rights reserved. No part of this publication may be adapted or reproduced, stored in a retrieval system, or transmitted, in any form or by any means, electronic, mechanical, photocopying, recording or otherwise, without the prior permission of the author and publisher.

Disclaimer

All information is believed accurate at the time of going to press but is not so warranted. The publisher shall not be responsible for errors or omissions.

All content within this report is commentary or opinion and is protected under Free Speech laws in all the civilized world. The information herein is provided for educational and entertainment purposes only. It is not intended as a substitute for professional medical advice of any kind.

In no event shall Dr. Graham Simpson be liable for any consequential injury, damages or death arising out of any use of, or reliance on any content or materials contained herein, neither shall Dr. Graham Simpson be liable for any content of any external internet sites referenced and services listed.

Always consult your own licensed medical practitioner if you are in any way concerned about your health. You must satisfy yourself of the validity of the professional qualifications of any health care provider you contact as a result of this book.

CONTENTS

Foreword 6
Introduction 9

Era I Medicine: Prepare the Soil (LB5) 19
Chapter 1: Biological Age Versus Chronological Age 20
Chapter 2: The History and Examination 27
Chapter 3: The INTEGRAL Health Analysis 37
Chapter 4: Specialized Diagnostic Tests 81
Chapter 5: Healing The Toxic Triad 128

Era II Medicine: Reduce Mind-Body Stress (LB100) 143
Chapter 6: Deregulated Nutrient Sensing 148
Chapter 7: Microbiome Dysfunction 159
Chapter 8: Mitochondrial Dysfunction 175
Chapter 9: Loss of Proteostasis 188
Chapter 10: Genomic Instability 195
Chapter 11: Altered Intercellular Communication 216
Chapter 12: Epigenetic-Alterations 224
Chapter 13: Cellular Senescence 235
Chapter 14: Stem Cell Exhaustion 248
Chapter 15: Telomere Attrition 261
Chapter 16: Temporal Hierarchy of the Metrics of Aging 268
Chapter 17: What the Blue Zones Tell Us About Longevity? 273

Era III Medicine: Integrate Structures of Consciousness (One Mind) .. 289
Chapter 18: Re-evaluating Monotheistic Religions 290
Chapter 19. The Structures of Consciousness 304
Chapter 20: One Mind 321

Afterword 334
Additional Reading 347

For Larry - friend, colleague , and mentor who helped show me the way.

Foreword
by Ryan Smith

Age is the number one risk factor for almost all disease and death. Thus, we have known that the ability to measure and treat the aging process can have a major impact on the health of everyone in the world. However, treating and managing age is something that has often been difficult to study and apply to human health because of the length of human lifespans and the lack of direct causal features of aging. However, we are on the verge of a longevity revolution as we now are able to measure the aging process with a higher resolution than ever before. And as a result, we are learning new and valuable lessons for aging. This revolution has been led by the usage of DNA methylation.

DNA methylation is a type of epigenetic regulation. Methylation in particular is a chemical tag on your DNA which controls your level of gene expression. In simplistic terms, epigenetics controls are the on and off switches which regulate your DNA. Of all of these epigenetic controls, DNA methylation is one of the most prevalent and currently easiest to measure.

As far back as the late 1960s, there was extensive reporting of strong associations between age and DNA methylation in various organisms and tissues. However, in a major development for aging biomarkers, the early 2010s saw the development of epigenetic clocks, which use mathematical algorithms to derive an estimate of the epigenetic age of a DNA source such as blood.

Central to the development of these clocks has been the assumption that discrepancies between methylation clock age and an individual's chronological age would thus identify instances of accelerated or decelerated aging. This initial hypothesis has been supported strongly as we have seen the difference between biological age and chronological age are highly predictive of negative health outcomes seen with aging.

Since the creation of these clocks, hundreds of associations between DNAm age acceleration and various exposures (for example, traumatic stress, lifetime stress), phenotypes (for example, obesity, fitness) or health outcomes (for example, lung cancer, mortality) have been reported.

These associations continued to get more pronounced as the clocks which have been created have improved. One of the most important improvements has been moving away from so-called 1st generation clocks which are trained to predict chronological age. Instead, 2nd and 3rd generation clocks have been created which focus on predicting phenotypic scores of aging which are defined from age related phenotypic variables such as plasma based proteomics or clinical biomarkers. These clocks have shown to be better at predicting negative health outcomes and at capturing biological signals we know are fundamental in the aging process.

DNA methylation is not the only molecular biomarker which has shown to be predictive and informative of the aging process. Spurred by recent advances in high-throughput omics technologies, a new generation of tools to measure biological aging now enables the quantitative characterization of aging at molecular resolution for proteomic, transcriptomic, metabolomic, and other platforms. This has helped us quantify and measure the aging process in ways we previously haven't before. These developments will signal a major change in how we understand and optimize our aging progress.

In this book, Dr. Graham Simpson explores the leading contributors to the aging process and discusses what we know about the best ways to measure, and treat, age as a primary disease.

Dr Graham Simpson is one of the world's leading experts on Diabesity, reversing 'insulin resistance', anti-aging and longevity and sexual rejuvenation. Dr Simpson MD graduated from the University of Witwatersrand Medical School in Johannesburg, South Africa. He is American Board Certified in Internal Medicine and Emergency Medicine. He is a founding member of the American Holistic Medical Association (AHMA) and is also a licensed homeopath. A passionate doctor, futurist, researcher, scientist, educator, and international best-selling author and Founder of Eternity Medicine, and Live Beyond 100 (LB100) Dr Simpson has written several books.

I first met Dr. Graham Simpson at a hotel in Dubai in 2018. We had arranged the meeting to discuss peptides; a type of new and innovative medication which was just being introduced into the UAE. Dr. Simpson was interested in using the newest science to help treat the epidemic of insulin resistance he was seeing throughout many of his patients in the Middle East. In this book, Dr. Simpson clearly tries to use the same principle of applying the newest science and data to a health problem of incredible proportions; aging.

Whether you are completely new to aging or a seasoned medical provider, this book will breakdown the science behind the aging mechanisms we have identified and show clear concrete examples of how Dr. Simpson has navigated these issues in his own clinical practice. Dr. Simpson recognizes that lifespan is nothing without optimal healthspan as well; making this a great introduction into the aspects of aging and their actionable healthcare solutions.

- Ryan Smith, Founder of TruDiagnostic

INTRODUCTION

"Life can only be understood backwards, but it must be lived forwards."
- Soren Kierkegaard.

My chronological age has exceeded three score years and ten as written in Psalm 90:10 of the King James Bible from the original Hebrew: - The days of our years are three score years and ten; and if by reason of strength they be four score years, yet is their strength labour and sorrow; for it is soon cut off, and we fly away.

Chronological and Biological age correlate with each other, so the signs of aging appear around a similar chronological age in most people. But often people exhibit signs of Biological aging at very different rates. Some 70 year olds run marathons, write great books, surf every day and are as productive as they were in their 40's while many others of the same age can't care for themselves and suffer from serious chronic diseases like diabetes, heart disease, dementia and cancer.

Recently scientists and researches have been able to develop accurate 'Age Clocks' that can measure our Biological Age as compared to our Chronological Age.

More than 20 years ago Gianni Pes and Michael Poulain working for National Geographic, with a grant from the National Institute on Aging, identified and studied the longest-lived people in the world and initially identified 5 Blue Zones where people eluded diabetes, heart disease, dementia and several types of cancer. These Blue Zones were Okinawa (Japan), Sardinia (Italy), Nicoya (Costa Rica), Icaria (Greece) and Loma Linda (California, USA).

Recognizing that only about 20% of the average persons lifespan is dictated by genes, these researches were looking for the common denominators among these long lived populations. I will discuss the 9 common denominators later but suffice is to say that they all involve Metabolic or Psychological Stress.

Elizabeth Blackburn PhD (Nobel Prize winner for the discovery of telomerase) and Elissa Epel PhD wrote, The Telomere Effect in 2017 that showed clearly how we live each day has a profound effect not just on our health and wellbeing, but how we age. They show that the DNA of our cells become progressively damaged causing our cells to become irreversibly aged. These senescent cells leak pro-inflammatory substances that make us more vulnerable to more pain and chronic illness. They describe how telomeres can make you feel old or help you stay young and healthy as they describe in the following: -

"Do you know the protective plastic tips at the ends of shoelaces? These are called aglets. The aglets are there to keep shoelaces from fraying. Now imagine that your shoelaces are your chromosomes, the structures inside your cells that carry your genetic information. Telomeres, which can be measured in units of DNA known as base pairs, are like the aglets; they form little caps at the ends of the chromosomes and keep the genetic material from unraveling. They are the aglets of aging. But telomeres tend to shorten over time.

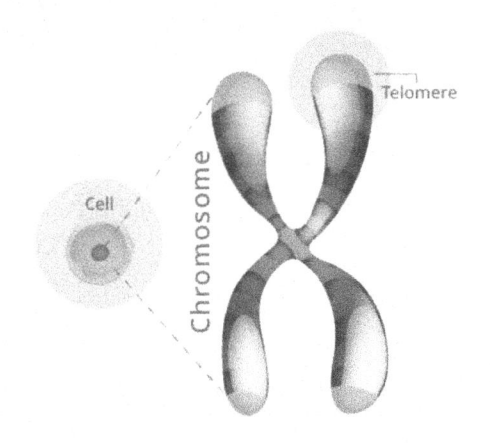

When your shoelace tips wear down too far, the shoelaces become unusable. You may as well throw them away. Something similar happens to cells. When telomeres become too short, the cell stops dividing altogether. Telomere's aren't the only reason a cell can become senescent. There are other stresses on normal cells that we don't yet understand very well. But short telomeres are one of the primary reasons human cells grow old, and they are one mechanism that controls the Hayflick limit.*"

David Sinclair PhD, from Harvard published Lifespan in 2019 and showed that all the Hallmarks of Aging that Carlos Lopez-Otin discussed in the Journal Cell in June 2013 could be explained by his Information Theory of Aging. Sinclair had noticed that yeast cells fed with lower amounts of sugar were not just living longer, but their DNA was exceptionally compact delaying the catastrophic number of DNA breaks, nuclear explosion, sterility and death. If we didn't have a way to repair DNA we wouldn't last long. That's why, way back in the primordium, the ancestors of every living thing on the planet evolved to sense DNA damage; slow cellular growth and divert energy to DNA repair until it was fixed – what he called the survival circuit.

"In animal studies, the key to engaging the sirtuin program appears to be keeping things on the razor's edge through calorie restriction – just enough food to function in healthy ways and no more. This makes sense. It engages the survival circuit, telling longevity genes to do what they have been doing since primordial times: boost cellular defenses, keep organisms alive during times of adversity, ward off diseases and deterioration, minimize epigenetic change, and slowdown aging."

Today, human studies are confirming that a low carb diet and periodic "intermittent fasting" can have tremendous health benefits.

Over the last several years, I have had great success with reversing Diabesity. This was covered in The Metabolic Miracle and my 4 Week Diabesity Cure books. With a high fat, moderate protein, low carb (HFLC) diet and time restricted eating we are able to quickly improve both metabolic and psychological stress the primary drivers of a shorter Healthspan and Lifespan. This is the basis of Era I a necessary prerequisite to Living Beyond 100 outlined in Era II.

Before concluding this introduction I want to introduce you to "First Principles Thinking" which are the Building Blocks of True Health and are the basis for the Living Beyond A Hundred (LB100) program.

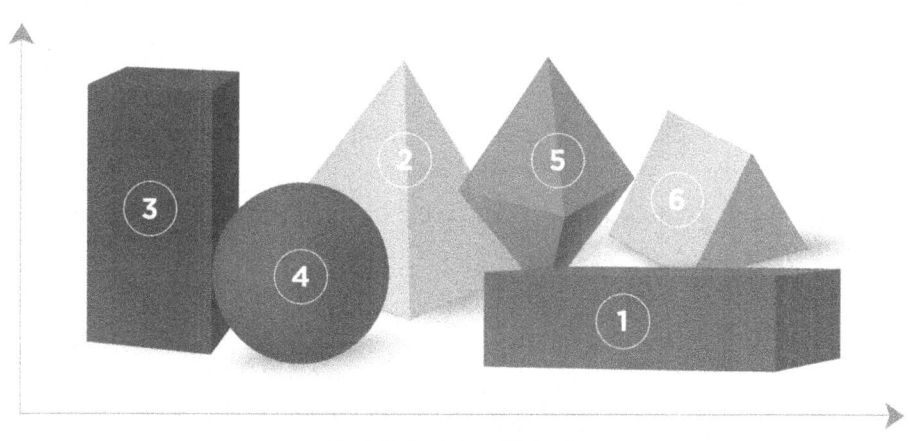

First Principles Thinking

First-principles thinking is one of the best ways to reverse-engineer complicated problems like Healthcare and unleash creative possibility – the idea is to breakdown complicated problems into basic elements and reassemble them from the ground up.

Reasoning by first principles removes the impurity of assumptions and conventions. What remains are the essentials. This thinking clears the clutter from what we've told ourselves and allows us to rebuild our health from the ground-up!

Here are the 6 Key Fundamental First Principles that will help you rebuild your health.

1. The Illness-Wellness Continuum

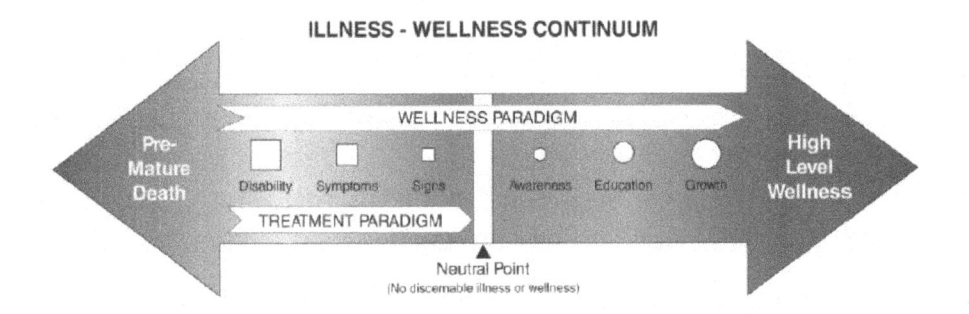

The LB100 Program will first **Measure** you to see where you fall on the wellness-illness continuum. What matters most right now is the direction each of us are facing - is it toward high level wellness or toward premature death? You can't change what you don't measure!

2. The Iceberg Metaphor

In order to see the pattern of your health (disease) we need to look under the surface of the water to assess your lifestyle, culture and behaviour. We are then able to address the 'root cause' of your disease and **Mentor** you using our INTEGRAL Health Model.

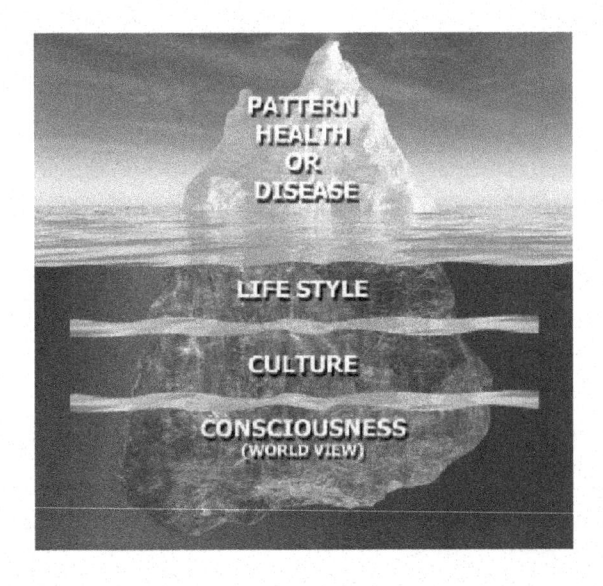

3. Proactive Medicine

The Increments of Chronic Disease

Age	Stage	Atherosclerosis	Cancer	Osteoarthritis	Diabetes	Emphysema	Cirrhosis
20	Start	Elevated Sugar	Carcinogen exposure	Abnormal cartilage staining	Obesity	Smoker	Drinker, Sugar, Grains
30	Discernible	Small Plaques on arteriogram	Cellular metaplasia	Slight joint-space narrowing	Abnormal glucose tolerance	Mild airway obstruction	Fatty liver on biopsy
40	Subclinical	Larger Plaques on arteriogram	Increasing metaplasia	Bone spurs	Elevated fasting-blood sugar	X-ray inflation	Enlarged liver
50	Threshold	Leg pain on exercise	Carcinoma in situ	Mild articular pain	Sugar in wine	Shortness of breath	Upper GI hemorrhage
60	Severe	Angina Pectoris	Clinical Cancer	Moderate articular pain	Hypoglycemic drug requirement Recurrent hospitalization	Recurrent hospitalization	Ascites (swelling in abdomen)
70	End	Stroke, Heart Attack	Metastatic Cancer	Disabled	Blindness, neuropathy, nephropathy	Intractable oxygen debt	Jaundice, hepatic come

4 P Medicine

Personalized

Predictive

Preventive

Participatory

Disease takes a long time to develop as shown above. Using our Proactive approach we reverse "insulin resistance" and then implement a series of Anti-aging remedies. At all times we **Monitor** your progress to reverse your biological age.

4. The "Root Causes" of Disease

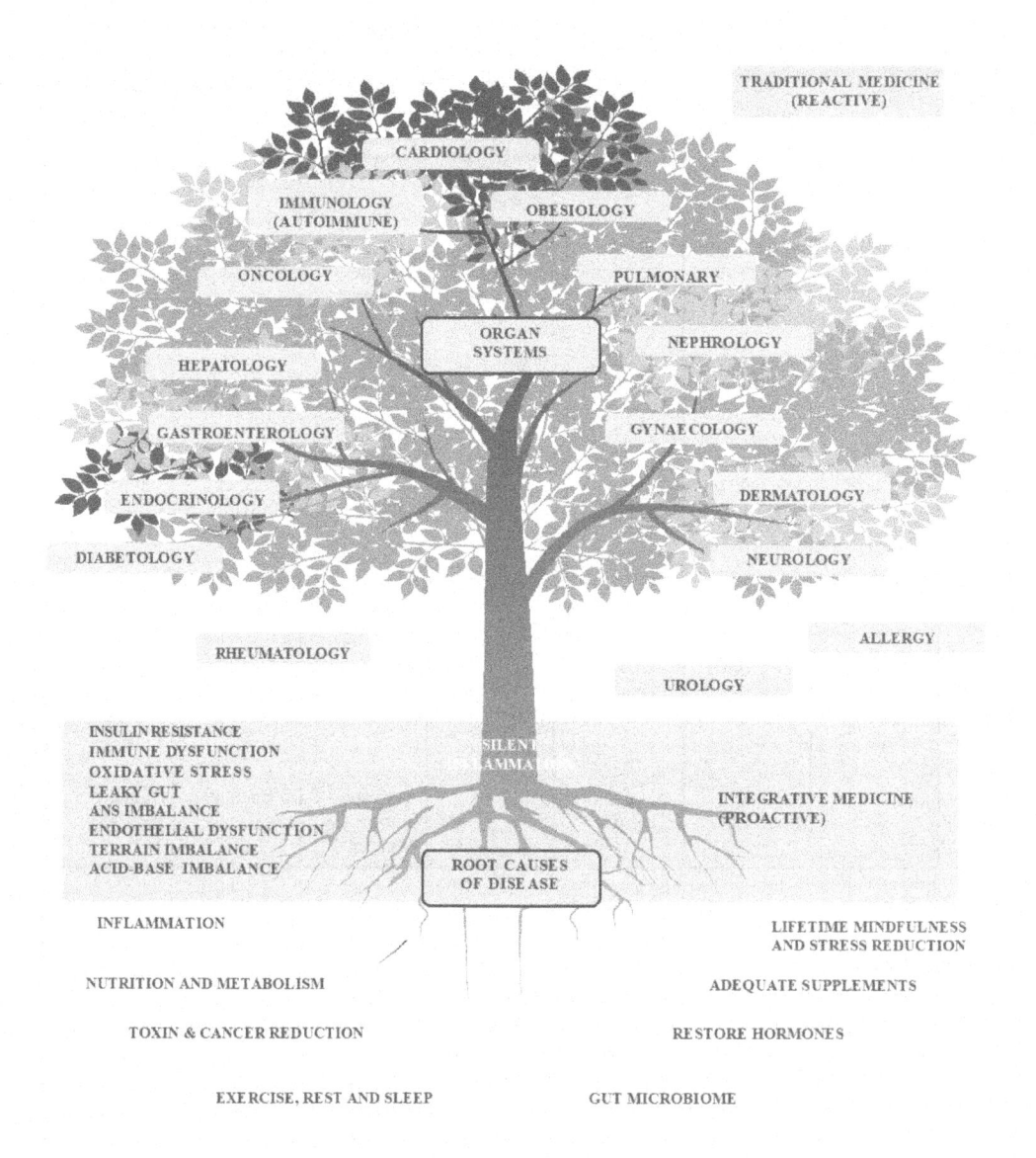

Tree diagram:

Branches/Leaves (TRADITIONAL MEDICINE - REACTIVE):
- CARDIOLOGY
- IMMUNOLOGY (AUTOIMMUNE)
- OBESIOLOGY
- ONCOLOGY
- PULMONARY
- ORGAN SYSTEMS
- NEPHROLOGY
- HEPATOLOGY
- GASTROENTEROLOGY
- GYNAECOLOGY
- ENDOCRINOLOGY
- DERMATOLOGY
- DIABETOLOGY
- NEUROLOGY
- RHEUMATOLOGY
- ALLERGY
- UROLOGY

Roots (ROOT CAUSES OF DISEASE / SILENT INFLAMMATION):
- INSULIN RESISTANCE
- IMMUNE DYSFUNCTION
- OXIDATIVE STRESS
- LEAKY GUT
- ANS IMBALANCE
- ENDOTHELIAL DYSFUNCTION
- TERRAIN IMBALANCE
- ACID-BASE IMBALANCE

INTEGRATIVE MEDICINE (PROACTIVE):
- INFLAMMATION
- LIFETIME MINDFULNESS AND STRESS REDUCTION
- NUTRITION AND METABOLISM
- ADEQUATE SUPPLEMENTS
- TOXIN & CANCER REDUCTION
- RESTORE HORMONES
- EXERCISE, REST AND SLEEP
- GUT MICROBIOME

Proactive Lifestyle Medicine: Research on the human genome has shown that more than 80% of the expression of our genes (phenotype) comes from our lifestyle (environment). **Genes load the gun, but our lifestyle pulls the trigger!** Thus, if our genetic expression can be changed, we are not hardwired for disease. The major factors altering our epigenetics are our lifestyle that lead to the "root causes" of most disease (or health) as shown above. Make sure you understand these first principles that explain the trunk and big branches and especially the "roots" to move you from Reactive traditional medicine to Proactive Health and Longevity.

INTEGRAL MODEL Explains The "Root Causes" of Disease

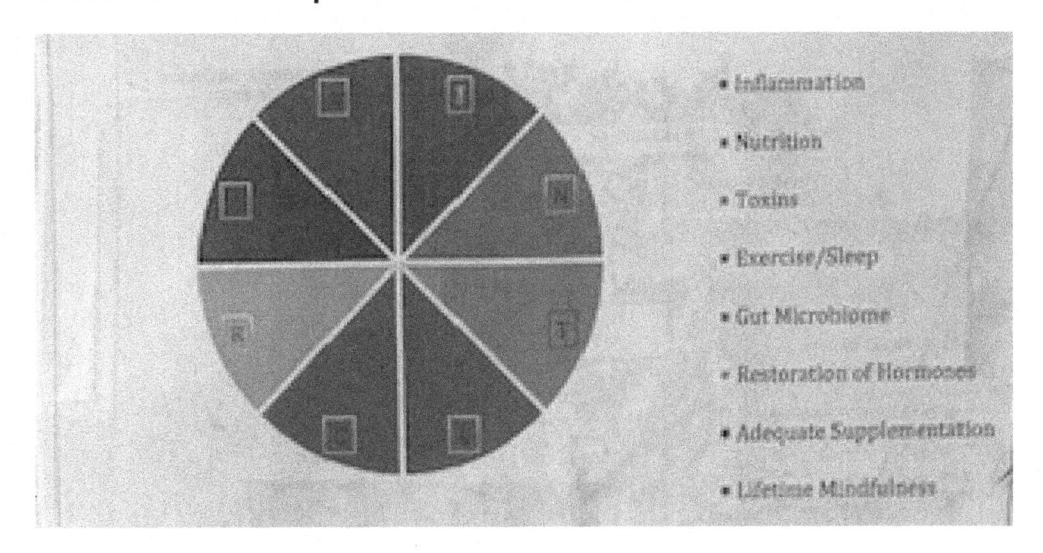

- Inflammation
- Nutrition
- Toxins
- Exercise/Sleep
- Gut Microbiome
- Restoration of Hormones
- Adequate Supplementation
- Lifetime Mindfulness

5. Genetics And Epigenetics Cause Aging

Epigenetics (80%)

Metabolic and Psychological Stress due to lifestyle and environment.

AGING AND IT'S ROOT CAUSES (INTEGRAL HEALTH)

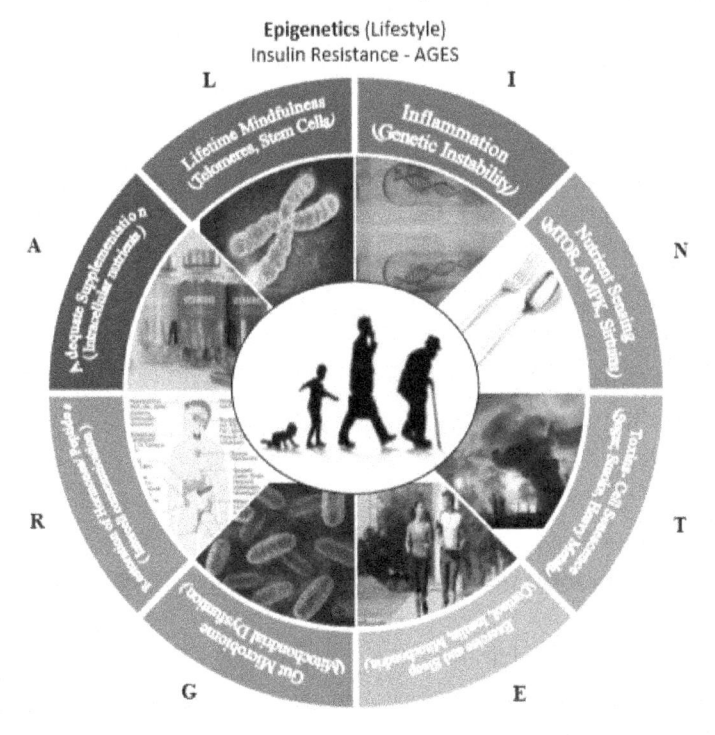

Epigenetics (Lifestyle)
Insulin Resistance - AGES

Genetics (20%)

LB100 includes a persons genetic pattern (Hereditary) together with their epigenetic pattern (Lifestyle) for an integrated approach for increasing both Healthspan and Lifespan.

6. Squaring The Curve

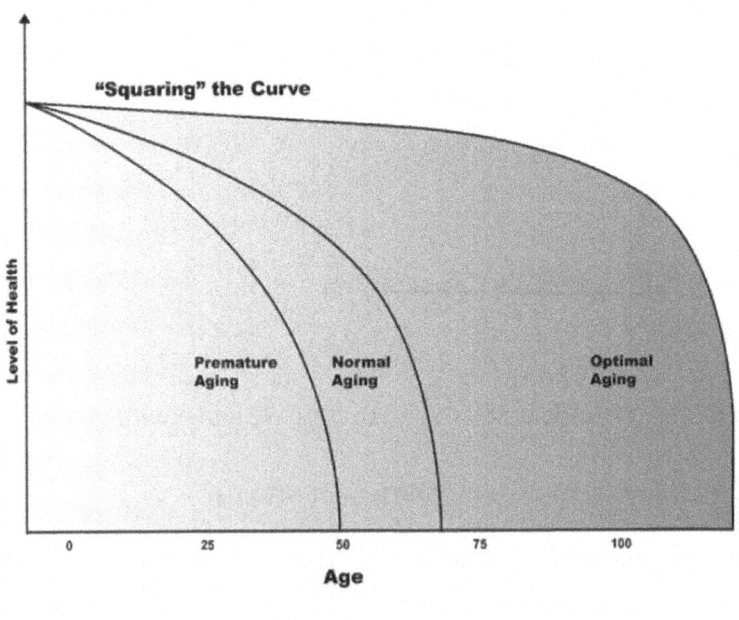

"Squaring" the Curve

Level of Health

Premature Aging | Normal Aging | Optimal Aging

Age

Optimal Lifespan

We employ a "whole person" approach focused on reducing both **Metabolic Stress** (Insulin Resistance) and **Psychological Stress**- both forms of stress shorten our telomeres and our longevity.

The LB100 program provides a simple, practical program that you can implement from the comfort of your home, to not only extend your Healthspan but also your Lifespan.

I have based this on my experience as a practicing physician over the past 40 years, my personal anti-aging journey and the latest longevity science.

What is truly game changing, as we demonstrate, you can now document the improvement in your pace of aging and the lowering of your Biological age. This can be as much as twenty years lower than your chronological age.

Using these methylation "age clocks" can be very motivating and will also help fine tune your personal anti-aging program to help you Live Beyond 100.

My hope to all is that you will Live Beyond 100, Healthy and Happy and not 'fly away' too soon.

Las Vegas, Nevada

2022

ERA I Medicine

Prepare the Soil (LB5)

Recovering Metabolic Flexibility

After twenty-five years of researching aging and having read thousands of scientific papers, if there is one piece of advice I can offer, one surefire way to stay healthy, one thing you can do to maximize your lifespan right now, it's this: **eat less.**

David Sinclair, PhD
Lifespan

CHAPTER 1: BIOLOGICAL AGE VERSUS CHRONOLOGICAL AGE

I am excited to present to you what I consider one of the most important discoveries in longevity research that is going to have a major impact in how you will live your life and how you will age.

Methylation based biological aging clocks have changed the way we look at aging and preventive medicine! Aging is the biggest risk factor for most chronic diseases. Unfortunately, traditional determinants of age (the number of years since birth) don't always match up with how each individual ages. As mentioned earlier, some people in their 70's look and feel like they are 50, and then there are some 70-year-olds that look like they could be 90. This is called **phenotypic variation,** and as a result, people have been searching for objective markers to measure the aging process. Thankfully, a highly accurate one was created by measuring epigenetic biomarkers.

Having an objective biological age measurement has massive implications for preventive health and future investigations. However, if we can combine this with an instantaneous rate of aging, we can learn even more about our aging process, our individual aging biology, and the interventions for better preventive health when we combine these two metrics. My friend Ryan Smith has developed one of the leading labs in the field.

- His report is able to tell you how many years you are aging per year at the precise moment.

- This is good to have in addition to biological age because it separates what you are doing now versus what markers you might have accumulated over the past or through hereditary inheritance from your parents and grandparents.

- You want your rate of aging to be below 1!

- Fastest rate of aging has been 1.4 biological years/1.0 year of chronological aging.

- Slowest rate of aging has been 0.6 biological years/1.0 year of chronological aging.

- The average person will age at a rate of 1.0 biological years/ 1.0 year of chronological aging.

- Dietary interventions like fasting have been shown to decrease the aging rate.

- Many other therapies are now demonstrating an ability to slow Biological aging as I will discuss.

- The Pace of Aging (PoAM) was created by Duke and Columbia via a longitudinal study. This means the researchers followed the same individuals over time which is different from other algorithms of aging.

YOUR PACE OF AGING VALUE:

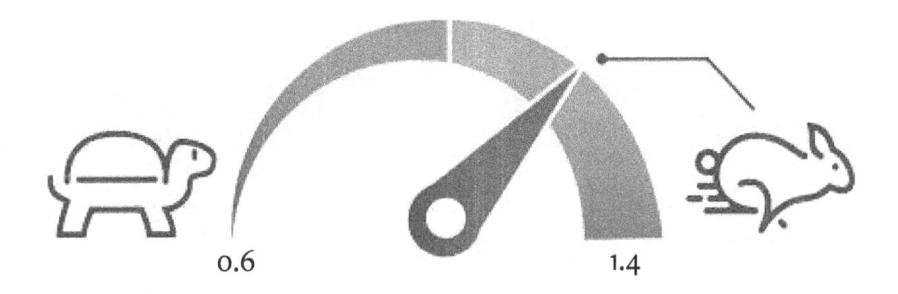

0.6   1.4

PoAM Value: 1.34

Methylation reports combine clinically useful insights for you to understand. Since biological age can clearly show how your lifestyle can change the aging process you now have the keys to your healthspan and lifespan.

Knowing that your choices each day can make measurable, objective differences in how you age is a great motivator for sticking to your LB100.

You only compete with yourself to keep lowering your biological age metrics between tests each year. Let me explain how these methylation clocks work.

What are CpG sites?

They are the locations on your DNA where the team pull methylation information to calculate all your epigenetic metrics. Making up your DNA, there are 4 types of nucleotides. Most of you are familiar with the ATCG pair (Adenine, Thymine, Cytosine and Guanine). A CpG site is where a Cytosine comes right before a Guanine. CpG sites are practically the only place on the genome that allows methyl groups to attach, and most CpG sites are located at the start site of a gene.

This allows the methylation of a CpG site to also change the expression of that gene.

What is a Beta Value?

A Beta Value is the degree of methylation on a CpG site. Basically, how much is the gene associated with that site turned on or off? This is the most common way to measure DNA methylation.

Beta values between 0 and 1 are approximately the percentage of methylation for that CpG site. When a gene is a 100% methylated, then it is off. It can no longer be read by your cells, and is skipped over.

After extracting your DNA and isolating the CpG sites, the laboratory uses a complex, state-of-the-art algorithm to sort through the beta values on your CpG sites to calculate your Biological Age as well as the other trait and risk reports.

Having access to your beta values for these CpG sites gives you the freedom to take that data and use it any way you'd like. The high-tech array technology looks at over 900,000 CpG sites in your DNA.

However, not every single one of them is relevant to biological age. The reason they look at so many is because they want to offer you more than just biological age.

Their R&D team is combing through the data to discover new patterns of methylation that could detect health risks, and personal traits.

By having all of the possible sites already mapped, it means they can retroactively update old results to show the progress of health risks they didn't even know how to test for when you first sent in the sample!

Associated risks and treatment options vary between accelerated aging found in different areas of the body:

Since there is no single, perfect way to measure aging, and we want to offer the most accurate version of your biological age, we breakup different aging metrics into a collection of reports to help you understand your Biological aging process and make educated decisions so as to slow your Biological Age.

Algorithmic Reports

These reports use advanced algorithms to evaluate epigenetic aging from a large collection of different CpG Loci.

Epidemiological Biological Age

You'll find a breakdown of your overall **biological age score**, and the most accurate information currently available about the many **historic and present-day factors that may have impacted it**.

This report acts as an introduction to Epigenetics and an overview into how these markers can be changed.

Immune System Age (Extrinsic and Intrinsic)

These reports look at aging as it relates to **immune cell subsets.** This lets you isolate your baseline aging from the age of your immune system.

By separating these two from your overall biological age, you can find more accurate recommendations on how to change your pace of aging.

DunedinPoAm (Pace of Aging)

Pace of Aging is essentially a speedometer for the **overall biological aging process.**

It is highly predictive of outward signs of aging, and studies have found accelerated aging detected by this algorithm is highly predictive of the development of age-related diseases. This invaluable test is sensitive to short-term changes in lifestyle and interventions.

Telomere Age – Telomere length estimation

Telomere Length has long been a popular biomarker for biological aging. We are able to today to offer Telomere Length detected by methylation as a new Report Expansion.

Telomere Age focuses on aging related to cellular replication and cellular fate.

Specific Loci Reports

These reports show the degree of methylation on specific loci that are thought to be linked to disease, the impact of certain behaviours, or even phenotype traits.

Example:
- Obesity Risk
- Diabetes Risk
- Impact of Alcohol
- Mitotic Clock
- Impact of Smoking
- Empathy Traits
- Hypersexuality Traits
- Skin Aging Report
- Senescence Burden Report
- Stem Cell Depletion Report
- Brain Age Report
- Cancer Risk Report
- Nutrition and Exercise Report
- Pharmaco-epigenetics

In addition to "methylation clocks" we include at no charge the PhenoAge Epigenetic Clock for Biological Age by Morgan Levine.

PhenoAge is a measure of biological age that can also tell you if you are physiologically younger or older than your chronological age. It can predict one's chances of dying in the next 10 years. Chronological age alone is a well known potent predictor of mortality risk and is the basis of actuarial tables used in life insurance to determine premiums.

Health habits such as exercise, smoking, and risk behaviours are added to these actuarial tables to improve risk stratification. Poor health habits, however, do not affect all individuals in the same way. A more powerful way to assess risk of death is to look directly at biomarkers of organ system functioning by measuring the effect of genetic factors and healthy or risky behaviours on a particular individual. It is also useful to assess the effectiveness of therapies and lifestyle changes on biological age, in turn lowering mortality risk.

Morgan Levine, PhD, and her team took this very approach using machine learning algorithms to improve mortality risk assessment in a pool of 9,926 subjects followed for 23 years in the National Health and Nutrition Survey III. Together with chronological age they added nine biomarkers found in routine blood tests to their algorithm and assessed the predictive value of each based on who had died or developed cardiovascular disease, cancer, dementia, diabetes, etc. They found that their algorithm correlated highly with chronological age ($r=0.9$) but also predicted all-cause mortality and death from specific disease better than chronological age alone.

The table below shows the nine blood tests used to calculate the physiological system they measure (i.e., PhenoAge) and the magnitude of effect, or weight, each one has on predicting the overall PhenoAge.

Albumin	Liver	0.0336
Creatinine	Kidney	0.0095
Glucose	Metabolic	0.1953
C-reactive protein	Inflammation	0.0954
Lymphocyte percent	Immune	0.012
Mean cell volume (MCV)	Blood	0.0268
Red cell distribution width (RDW)	Blood	0.3306
Alkaline phosphatase	Liver	0.0019
White blood cell count	Immune	0.0554
Chronological Age		0.0804

The convenient PhenoAge, apart from the fact it is free, can be done from 9 common biomarkers that are included in your LB100 Anti-Aging Panels.

Remember, to ensure an accurate PhenoAge, you must be fasting!

In order for you to get our Methylation Reports, a kit will be sent to your home with instructions. You will provide a couple of drops of blood and mail the kit back to TruAge labs. Results are available in two to three weeks.

CHAPTER 2: THE HISTORY AND EXAMINATION

LB100 uses a simple **3 Step Methodology**:

Step 1: Measure
A. History
B. Examination
C. Diagnostics

Step 2: Mentor
Coaching to reverse Biological Aging

Step 3: Monitor
Using our APP and Dashboard

We embrace Proactive Medicine (4P Medicine) rather than the traditional Reactive Disease model.

Our three goals for Proactive Medicine are:

1. Quantify Wellness

2. Demystify Disease

3. Empower Clients

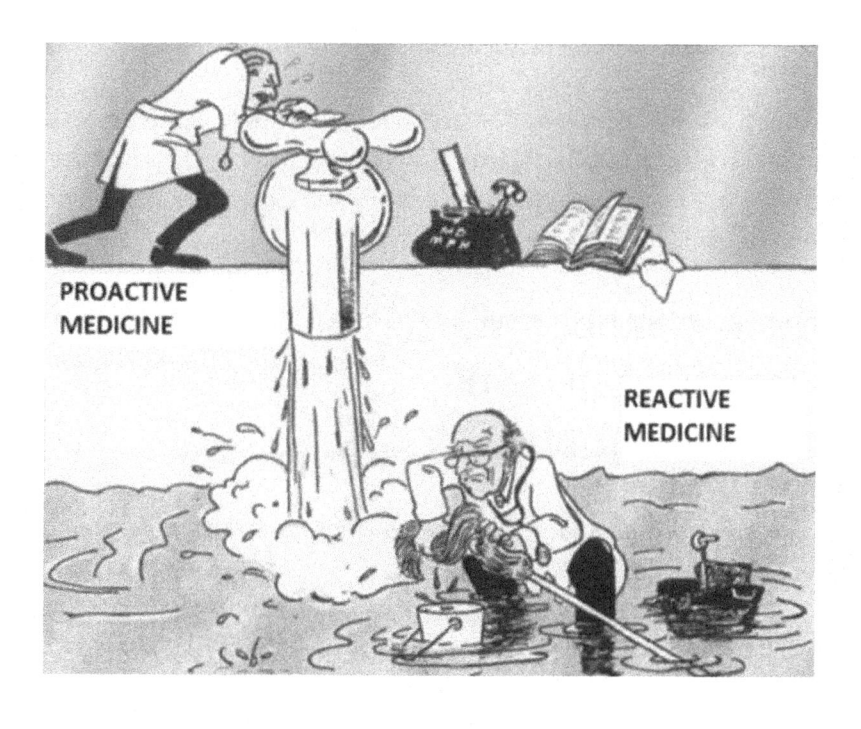

The Illness/Wellness Continuum

As my friend Dr. John Travis has stated, wellness is never a static state. No matter what your current state of health, you can begin to appreciate yourself as a growing, changing person, and allow yourself to move toward a more joyful and positive state of wellbeing.

Illness is often the body-mind's attempt to get us to wake up and become more conscious of our unresolved issues in life. The LB100 Program is an approach to health that encompasses a process of awareness, education and growth. What matters most right now is the direction in which you are facing – is it toward high-level wellness or toward premature death?

The first step in discovering where you are on this continuum is a good History and Examination which I cover in this Chapter. Chapter Three looks at the key Labs we need to track and Chapter Four covers some of the diagnostics we recommend. By integrating your History, Examination, Key Labs and Select Diagnostics you will be ready to Live Beyond A Hundred.

Integral Health is the process through which we humans achieve wellbeing by the ordering of consciousness. This includes the expansion of consciousness (knowledge) and the intensification of consciousness (wisdom).

Graham Simpson, MD

A. The History

It is said that over 80% of diagnoses are made on history alone. In recent times the focus (and the funding) has shifted towards technological advances in investigations, but there is no doubt that the history and examination skills remain the cornerstone of clinical practice.

Our Historical questionnaire is based on the Integral Health Model which I would like to briefly introduce here which is at the heart of the LB100 Program.

The Integral Health Model

Any phenomenon can be approached in an interior and exterior fashion and also as an individual and a member of a collective.

- Ken Wilber

For the past decade or so, it has become obvious to many of us health professionals that a new model of medicine is needed. An understanding of integral health will not only assist us in dealing with the ever-increasing incidence of chronic disease, but it will teach us to acknowledge the multi-dimensional nature of the human being and embrace alternative systems of health delivery that are less invasive and more effective.

With this awareness, the interaction between the physician and client changes. We can no longer adhere to the mechanistic "doctors knows best," fix-it mentality that conventional medicine has upheld throughout much of the last century, treating symptoms of illness instead of getting to the root of a person's problem.

In 1977, George Engel wrote in the journal Science that psychiatry and bio-medicine were in a crisis because they both adhere to a view of disease that was no longer adequate for the scientific tasks and social responsibilities of either medicine or psychiatry. Engel proposed a new biopsychosocial method that treats a person, and not just an illness.

The integral health model we wish to present here extends Engel's idea and is patterned after works of Ken Wilber, Jean Gebser, Larry Dossey and others.

Integral health, here, means integrative, inclusive, comprehensive, and balanced. As Wilber writes, "To understand the whole, it is necessary to understand the parts. To understand the parts, it is necessary to understand the whole. Such is the circle of understanding."

The value of any method lies in how useful it is. I have been applying this integral health model with increasing success and have received positive feedback from other health practitioners engaged in similar practices, as well as clients who have implemented this model. As Wilber points out, any phenomenon can be approached in an interior and exterior fashion, and also as an individual and a member of a collective.

Below I have included a key theorist in each of the 4 quadrants that make up the integral model.

	INTERIOR	**EXTERIOR**
INDIVIDUAL	SUBJECTIVE Psyche (Carl Jung)	OBJECTIVE Biomedicine (Franz Ingelfinger)
COLLECTIVE	INTERSUBJECTIIVE Culture (Jean Gebser)	INTEROBJECTIVE World (Ludwig von Bartalanffy)
	SUBJECTIVE	**OBJECTIVE**

The integral health method I have introduced attempts to deliver a new model for health that honors all four quadrants.

Until recently, most of what we know as medicine was largely confined to the upper right quadrant. In fact, most medicine practiced today is still predominantly from this quadrant. More than 70 years ago, people began to appreciate wellness medicine and mind-body practices (upper left quadrant); though these practices, too, are incomplete. As Aaron Antonovsky wrote, "And yet, the voluminous writing of—shall we call it the holistic approach to health?--- as far as I can tell, shows a near-total absence of reference to, or awareness of, the larger social system in which the mind-body relationship operates." (lower quadrants)

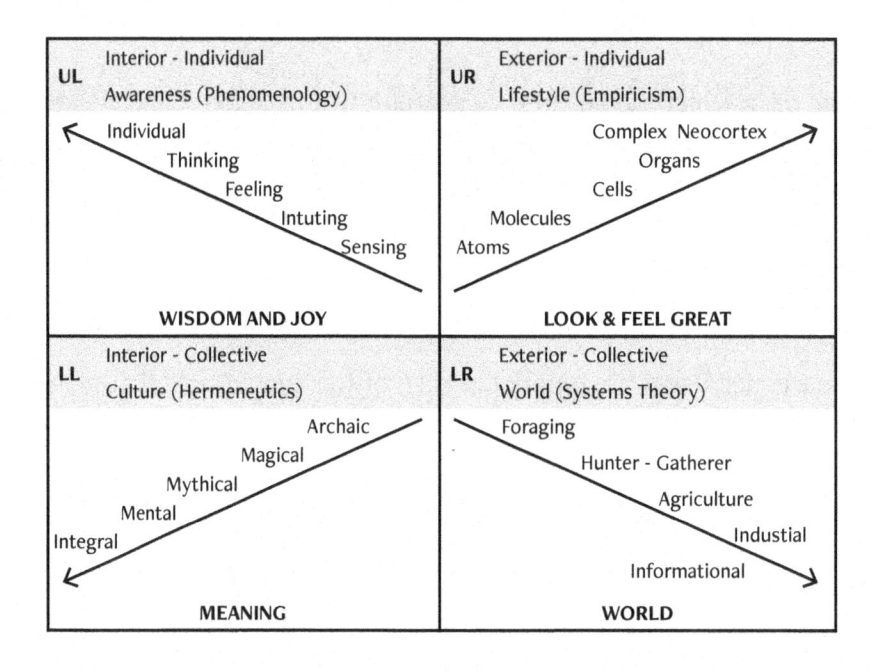

UL	Interior - Individual
	Awareness (Phenomenology)
	Individual
	  Thinking
	    Feeling
	      Intuting
	        Sensing
	WISDOM AND JOY
		UR	Exterior - Individual
			Lifestyle (Empiricism)
			        Complex Neocortex
			      Organs
			    Cells
			  Molecules
			Atoms
			LOOK & FEEL GREAT

LL	Interior - Collective
	Culture (Hermeneutics)
	      Archaic
	    Magical
	   Mythical
	  Mental
	Integral
	MEANING
		LR	Exterior - Collective
			World (Systems Theory)
			Foraging
			  Hunter - Gatherer
			    Agriculture
			      Industial
			        Informational
			WORLD

Culture – shared meaning (social structure) and **World** and its objects (concretized consciousness) are all indispensable (lower quadrants) to understanding the roots of health and wellbeing.

Just as the novel understanding of space gave birth to self-consciousness, (see video link: https://youtu.be/bkNMM8uiMww) a new understanding of time is now giving birth to the integral structure of consciousness. Space-free and time-free mind is unbounded and infinite in space and time, thus is omnipresent, eternal and ultimately one. We have begun to see evidence of the application of this changing worldview in a new spectrum of non-local healing.

It is vital also that the integral physician helps each person reorder their worldview to help realize that they exist within a process of space-time, not as isolated entities adrift in linear time. It is time to impart this knowledge of the interconnectedness of all life and how the spiritual flowing presence can be deeply felt and experienced. To the extent we accomplish this task, we are truly healers. With a single, subtle voice, science, art and the great spiritual traditions all communicate this notion today – that each of us is infinite, immortal, and indestructible.

Note: The easiest way for you to discover these 5 structures is to look in any Art History book. The art objects you see are simply the "concretized consciousness" of man through the ages.

I have also included a video (https://youtu.be/uD472O8-2es) I made 20 years ago that will give you a more dynamic view of these structures of consciousness using several film clips.

THE FOUR QUADRANTS

(UR) **Biomedicine:** (Empiricism) Knowledge comes primarily from sensory experience. It emphasizes the role of empirical evidence in the formation of ideas. Empiricism in the philosophy of science emphasizes evidence, especially as discovered in experiments. **Example: The Hallmarks of Aging**

(UL) **Awareness:** (Phenomenology) Awareness is the ability to directly know and perceive, to feel, or to be cognizant of events. More broadly, it is the state of being conscious of something. Self-awareness is the capacity for introspection and the ability to recognize one-self from the environment and other individuals. While consciousness is a term given to being aware of one's environment and body and lifestyle, self-awareness is the recognition of that awareness. **Example: Integral Consciousness**

(LL) Culture: (Hermeneutics) The art of avoiding misunderstanding. Misunderstanding is to be avoided by means of shared knowledge. This can only be attained by placing human expressions in their historical context. Culture is the social behavior and norms found in human societies. Culture (shared meaning) is the knowledge acquired over time. Multiculturism values the peaceful coexistence and mutual respect between different cultures inhabiting the same planet. **Example: The Structures of Consciousness**

(LR) World: (Systems Thinking) Systems thinking has been defined as an approach to problem solving that attempts to balance holistic thinking and reductionist thinking. By taking the overall system (eg. The Planet) as well as its parts into account systems thinking is designed to avoid potential problems contributing to further development of unintended consequences. **Example: One Mind**

Eternity Medicine is about our awareness of the non-local nature of our mind, that it is infinite, indestructible and immortal. Larry Dossey MD

The LB100 Worldview Wellbeing Questionnaire will ask a series of Yes or No answers that address all 4 quadrants in addition to the more traditional history you may have filled out in the past such as: -

A. The Medical History

Studies have shown how multiple biological processes change early in life and have measurable consequences by midlife that are likely to be important harbingers of later life disability or superior health.

Both important past medical and surgical events should be recorded.

Family History

This gives information about any 'genetic' influences as well as an indication of the environment and lifestyle the client has been exposed to.

Social History

It is important to understand the clients social situation and living conditions, does the individual look after older parents or a handicapped child? Occupations are very relevant to certain disease states and will also indicate the persons level of education.

Drugs

Note all current medications as well as over the counter (OTC) remedies and possible herbal remedies. Note any drug allergies.

Alcohol, caffeine, smoking and other drug use are also important to record.

Nutraceuticals

Many clients involved in a longevity program routinely ingest multiple vitamins and minerals. One needs to note the dose, frequency and time that these nutraceuticals are taken to optimize their program.

Review of Systems

B. The Examination

There is no real dividing line between the history and the examination. The first part of any examination is to observe. Look before you lay on hands.

Examination of the cardiovascular or respiratory system does not start with the stethoscope. You may get valuable information from the facies, skin colouration, gait, handshake and personal hygiene (reflective of physical, psychological and social background). Note the red eye, the freckles on the lips of Peutz-Jeghers syndrome or the white forelock of Waardenberg's syndrome. A number of endocrine disorders may be immediately apparent.

Each doctor has their own protocol when it comes to the examination. I like to start with the Vital Signs and Body Fat Percent.

Blood Pressure

Systolic Blood Pressure (at rest). Systolic blood pressure is the peak blood pressure reached during systole, the part of the cardiac cycle during which the heart contracts and squeezes blood into the peripheral circulation. SBP increases with age and predict strokes and heart attacks in many studies. However, it is not as good a predictor of cardiovascular disease nor your rate of aging as Augmentation Pressure (AP).

Optimal: 80 to 115

Diastolic Blood Pressure (at rest). Diastolic Blood Pressure is the time during the cardiac cycle that the heart muscle is relaxing and filling up with blood. It is often misunderstood to continue to rise with age, when in fact, it reaches a peak in mid-adulthood and then starts to decline because of the decrease in elastic recoil of the aorta and muscular arteries. A decline in DBP in an older adult accompanied by an increase in SBP increases rather than decreases the risk of cardiovascular disease.

Optimal: 65 to 75

Resting Heart Rate. Resting heart rate is the number of times your heart beats per minute. It has been shown to be a good low-tech marker for cardiovascular disease risk. Several studies have shown that resting heart rate predicts cardio-vascular mortality, with the risk decreasing in line with heart rate. The resting heart rate is also an indication of a persons fitness level.

Respiratory Rate: A person's respiratory rate is the number of breaths you take per minute. The normal respiration rate for an adult at rest is **12 to 20 breaths per minute.** A respiration rate under 12 or over 25 breaths per minute while resting is considered abnormal.

Note: Some researchers believe a normal RR is 5-7/min.

Body Temperature. The average normal temperature is generally accepted as 98.6°F (37°C). Some studies have shown that the "normal" body temperature can have a wide range, from 97°F (36.1°C) to 99°F (37.2°C). A temperature over 100.4°F (38°C) most often means you have a fever caused by an infection or illness.

Body Fat Percent. This can be approximated by measuring the RFM knowing just 2 measurements.

Relative Fat Mass (RFM) in Men

RFM = 64 – (20 x height/waist circumference)

Relative Fat Mass (RFM) in Women

RFM = 76 – (20 x height/waist circumference)

The RFM gives a good indication of the fat percent of the person using two simple measurements.

Relative Fat Mass Explained		
Classification	Females (% fat)	Males (% fat)
Athletes	14-20%	6-13%
Fitness	21-24%	14-17%
Average	25-31%	18-24%
Obese	32% and higher	25% and higher

Waist To Height Ratio

In addition, I like to calculate the waist to height ratio which is one of the best anthropomorphic measurements to predict cardio-metabolic risk that shortens our life. Independent of weight, central obesity is highly correlated with metabolic abnormalities. Your waist/height ratio should be less than .5 ie. your waist should always be less than half your height.

Note: I do get a weight on all clients but I find this and the BMI not as helpful as the Percent Body Fat and Waist to Height ratios.

I then proceed with a **Head to Toe Examination** of the client as follows:

- ENT examination.
- Examination of the eye.
- Mental state examination.
- Examination of the cardiovascular system, including auscultation of the heart.
- Examination of the respiratory system.
- Examination of the abdomen.
- Checking for hernia and lumps in the groin and scrotum.
- Examining lumps.
- Neurological history and examination.
- Competence at orthopedic examination, which should include back examination, neurological examination of the lower limbs for knee and hip history and examination purposes, shoulder examination, and assessment of ankle injuries. Examination of tender, hot swollen joints.

- Gynecological history and examination. Breast lumps and breast examination.
- Peripheral pulses.

In the 1980's, handing over a prescription indicated the end of the consultation. Today this is just the beginning of the LB100 program as I will show shortly.

Medicine today has been hijacked by Big Pharma and Big Business.

Living healthy and living long is really very simple. Each of us needs to become the CEO of our own health and recognize that there is a wisdom in our body that has developed over millions (billions) of years. We need to pay attention to the symptoms, both mental and physical, and seek the root cause, not simply cover them up with one or more drugs.

The more you understand about the key elements of optimum health the faster you can return to perfect health. This book I hope, will give you some understanding, to help you avoid chronic illness and live beyond 100!

CHAPTER 3: THE INTEGRAL HEALTH ANALYSIS

The acronym **INTEGRAL** reminds us of the root-cause of disease.

Inflammation

Nutrition and Metabolism

Toxin Reduction

Exercise and Sleep

Gut Microbiome

Restoration of Hormones

Adequate Supplementation

Lifetime Mindfulness and Stress Reduction

Note: Using Key Biomarkers of the root causes of disease we can track a client over a lifetime to predict and prevent chronic disease and rapid aging.

Your **History** and **Examination** discussed in Chapter 2 must be combined with the **labs tests** that are covered here and with select **Diagnostics** covered in Chapter 4.

Inflammation	Optimal Range	Your Results
ESR	Male 0-22mm/___	
	Female 0-29mm	
CRP-hs	<1mg/L	
Ferritin	Male 20-250 ng/ml	
	Female 10-120 ng/ml	
Fibrinogen	200-400mg/dL	
Homocysteine	6-8 mcmol/L	
WBC	3.9-11.4 K/ul	

Granulocyte %	38-75%	
Lymphocyte %	15-49%	
Monocyte %	2-13%	
Eosinophil %	0.0-8%	
Basophil %	0.0-2%	
Granulocyte #	1.6-8.4 K/ul	
Lymphocyte #	1.0-3.6 K/ul	
Monocyte #	0.0-0.9 K/ul	
Eosinophil #	0.0-0.6 K/ul	
Basophil #	0.0-0.2 K/ul	
RBC	4.2-6 M/ul	
Hemoglobin	13.2-18 g/dl	
Hematocrit	43-60%	
MCV	83-103 femtolitres	
MCH	26.0-34 pg	
MCHC	29.5-35.5 g/dl	
RDW	11.0-15.5 K/ul	
Platelet Count	140-400 K/ul	
MPV	7.5-11.6 fL	

Nutrition	Optimal Range	Your Results
Fasting Glucose	70-80 mg/dl	
Fasting Insulin	**<5 mIu/ml**	

HOMA-IR	< 1.2	
HbA1c	<5%	
Uric Acid	**<5mg/dl**	
Triglycerides	<100 mg/dl	
HDL Cholesterol	>40 mg/dl male >50 mg/dl female	
TG/HDL Ration	1	
Total Cholesterol	<200 mg/dl	
Cholesterol/HDL Ratio	<4	
LDL Cholesterol	<100 mg/dl	
LDL/HDL Ratio	<3.5	
Apolipoprotein B (ApoB)	<130 mg/dl	
Lipoprotein (a) (LPa)	5-29 mg/dl	

Toxins	Optimal Range	Your Results
Liver		
Total Protein	5.7-8.2 g/dL	
Albumin	3.2-4.8 g/dL	
Bilirubin Total	0.3-1.2 mg/dL	
Alkaline Phosphase	45-115 u/L	
ALT	0-48 u/L	
AST	0-38 u/L	
Globulin	2.1-3.6 g/dL	

ALB/Glob Ratio (A/G Ratio)	.8-2	
Kidney	**Optimal Range**	**Your Results**
BUN	6-20 mg/dL	
Creatinine	.7-1.3 mg/dL	
BUN/Creatinine Ratio	7.3-21.7	
GFR estimated	+90ml/min	
Electrolyte		
Sodium	136-145 mmol/L	
Potassium	3.5-51. mmol/L	
Chloride	100-110 mmol/L	
CO2	20-31 mmol/L	
Calcium	8.3-10.6 mg/dL	

Exercise	Optimal Range	Your Results
Note: See Specialized Diagnostics (**Chapter 4**) for how to measure your fitness.		

Gut Microbiome	Optimal Range	Your Results
Note: See Specialized Diagnostics (**Chapter 4**) to find out if you have "leaky gut" and food sensitivities.		

Restoration of Hormones	**Optimal Range**	**Your Results**
Thyroid		

Free T3	2.3-4.2 pg/ml		
Free T4	.89-1.76 ng/dl		
Free T3/ Free t4 Ratio	2.4-2.70		
TSH	.5-4.5		
Testosterone			
Total Testosterone	Male 750-1100 ng/dL		
	Female 15-70 ng/dL		
Free Testosterone	Male 5-24 ng/dL		
	Female .7-7.9 ng/dL		
SHBG	60-100 nm/L		
DHEA Sulfate	250-550 ug/dl		
Estrogen	Male 0-34		
	Female cycle		
	Follicular	12.5-166 pg/ml	
	Ovulation	85.8-498 pg/ml	
	Luteal	48.8-211 pg/ml	
	Post-menopause	<6-54 pg/ml	
Hormones	**Optimal Range**		**Your Results**
Progesterone	Male .13-.97 ng/dL		
	Female cycle		
	Follicular	0.1-0.9 pg/ml	
	Luteal	1.8-23.4 pg/ml	
	Ovulation	0.1-12 pg/ml	
	Post-menopause	0-0.1 pg/ml	
FSH	Male 2-12 IU/L		
	Female <30 IU/L		
LH*	Male 1.42-15.4 iu/L		
	Female 1.97-9 iu/L		
Cortisol* 8am	6-23 mcg/dL		

Melatonin*	AM 10pg/ml	PM 60 pg/ml	
Growth Hormone*	IgF1 250-450 mg/ml		

*These hormones are not routinely measured. (FSH/LH are measured to rule out Perimenopause/Menopause).

PSA (in men only)	0-4 ng/ml	

Adequate Supplements	Optimal Range	Your Results
Vit D3	70-80 ng/ml	
Vit B12	550-1,000 pg/ml	

Lifetime Mindfulness and Stress Reduction	Optimal Range	Your Results

Note: See CNS-Vital Signs in **Chapter 4** Specialized Diagnostic tests to assess your brain health.

Step One – **Measure.** If you don't measure you will not be able to improve your Healthspan and Lifespan. These biomarkers together with your Methylation data will help keep you on track with your LB100 program. Remember to measure your Pace Of Aging (POA) you must have at least two separate time points usually a year apart, to calculate the rate of change. Your lab data and expected optimum values will be done frequently during each year of your program.

This chapter will also shed light on what each of these biomarkers mean and why they are important to be included in your longevity program.

Inflammation

Instead of different treatment for heart disease, Alzheimer's, and colon cancer, there might be a single inflammation remedy that would prevent all three.

- Time Magazine Cover Story (February 23, 2004)

Inflammation is now understood to be at the center of a wide range of conditions, from heart disease and hypertension to obesity and diabetes; from Alzheimer's and Parkinson's disease to depression, cancer, and arthritis. In fact, research shows that all chronic disease has a significant inflammatory component. Even aging itself appears to result from the cumulative effects of silent inflammation (what I call Inflam-Aging). When you consider how many of our aging population are affected with one or more chronic diseases (80% of Americans are overweight), you can begin to get an idea of the epidemic of inflammation we face today. I believe that this epidemic of silent inflammation is the single biggest factor responsible for our current healthcare crisis.

Inflammation is caused by the series of immune system responses designed to repair damage to your body by physical agents (trauma and radiation) or infections (bacteria, viruses, parasites), it is an essential part of the healing process. Inflammation can be acute or chronic and is characterized by pain, redness, swelling, and warmth of the tissue as white blood cells (leukocytes) are pulled out of the blood to the site of injury or infection. If the acute inflammatory process fails to fix the problem, then chronic inflammation sets in and can cause long term damage to your tissues.

An erythrocyte sedimentation rate (ESR) is a type of blood test that measures how quickly erythrocytes (red blood cells) settle at the bottom of a test tube that contains a blood sample. Normally, red blood cells settle relatively slowly. A faster-than-normal rate may indicate inflammation in the body. Inflammation is part of your immune response system. It can be a reaction to an infection or injury. Inflammation may also be a sign of a chronic disease, an immune disorder, or other medical conditions.

C-Reactive Protein. C-Reactive Protein is called an acute phase reactant because it is released from the liver during an acute infection to help fight off microbial invaders. In the absence of infection, however, a C-reactive protein level greater than 3mg/L has been associated with an increased risk of CVD in large number of studies. This is thought to be a result of the low level of inflammation (immune system activation) produced by atherosclerotic plaques. A level of 1-3mg/L is normal, but ideally it should be less than 1 (the lower the better).

Ferritin is a blood protein that contains iron. A ferritin test helps you understand how much iron your body stores. If a ferritin test reveals that your blood ferritin level is lower than normal, it indicates your body's iron stores are low and you have iron deficiency. As a result, you could be anemic.

A ferritin level above 300ng/ml may be due to Hemochromatosis an iron overload disorder. This can be genetic or acquired.

Fibrinogen is also one of several blood factors that are called acute phase reactants that rise sharply with conditions causing acute tissue inflammation or damage. Tests for these acute phase reactants, including fibrinogen, may be performed to determine the extent of inflammation in the body.

Optimum value for the fibrinogen is between **200 and 400mg/dl**. A fibrinogen value of less than 50mg/dl may mean you're in danger of bleeding after surgery. A fibrinogen value of more than 700mg/dl may mean you're in danger of forming clots that could harm your heart or brain.

Homocysteine. Homocysteine is an intermediary metabolite produced during the conversion of the amino acid methionine (commonly found in dietary meat protein) into cysteine. This conversion requires adequate levels of vitamin B12 and folic acid. High levels of homocysteine act like free radicals and can damage arteries in the same way as oxidized LDL. Studies have associated levels of homocysteine greater than 9 micromol/L with an increase risk of CVD. While more recent studies have called this association into question, the preponderance of evidence suggests that maintaining a normal to low homocysteine level by ensuring adequate intake of B-vitamin is likely to benefit your cardiovascular health.

The CBC.

WBC's are the cells that guard the body against infection and other foreign material. The white blood cell count can increase significantly when you have an infection; but under normal conditions it represents only about 2% of the total number of white blood cells in your body. The rest are in your lymph glands, gastrointestinal tract, spleen, and other tissues. While there are numerous sophisticated immune function tests, much can be learned about the state of the immune system simply by measuring the number and relative proportions of WBC subsets. WBCs can be divided up into two main types, granulocytes and lymphocytes.

The first three cell types (**neutrophils, eosinophils, and basophils**) are called 'granulocytes' because of fine granules in their cytoplasm that appear after being stained for microscopic examination. These cells make up the largest part of the **innate immune system**, the earliest responders to microbial and parasitic infections. They fight infection by releasing their granules of enzymes and free radical generators which destroy the invading organisms. They recognized the invaders as foreign by molecular structures that appear on most infectious agents. They also release the mediators of inflammation which cause blood to flow to the site of infection.

Lymphocytes do not have granules and are the mediators of the more precise and later responding **adaptive immune system**. Sometimes infections are wiped out by the immediate innate immune system response. But if the infection persists, the body recruits the adaptive immune system, its next wave of defense, which can recognize the particular molecular structure of the invader to more effectively target it. An acute bacterial or parasitic infection usually causes an increase in granulocytes, particularly neutrophils, whereas a viral infection most often increases the proportion of lymphocytes. Once the adaptive immune system has contained the infection, a small number of memory cells are left behind. These cells can persist in the body for decades and then promptly respond when the same infection is confronted which then allows it to mount a faster and brisker response than the first time. This memory feature of the adaptive immune system is the basis for vaccinations.

White Blood Cells. White blood cells can be increased in a number of disease states including bacterial or viral infection, autoimmune disorders, and leukemias in which the number is often above 20,000. Low WBC counts (<3,000) can be found in conditions of bone marrow failure, cancer, acute drug toxicity, certain viral infections, and congenital disorders of decreased bone marrow function. It helps to examine the subsets of the WBC count, such as neutrophils, lymphocytes, and eosinophils for clues to what is causing the change in the WBC count.

Neutrophils. Neutrophils are the most abundant immune cell in the blood stream, accounting for 40-75% of the total WBC; they do the majority of the work of the innate immune system. Their main function is phagocytosis (eating cells) and releasing their granules to destroy the engulfed bacteria and parasites. The ability of neutrophils to secrete bactericidal enzymes declines with age, increasing the severity of common bacterial infections in older adults. At the same time, their ability to turn off the inflammatory signals after the infection clears also declines, leaving the body in a chronic inflammatory state. Interestingly, their number increases with age in healthy adults, probably as a compensatory mechanism to offset the decline in per-cell functional activity.

Lymphocytes. Lymphocytes are the next most abundant white blood cell in the blood stream and can be divided into subsets that have specific functions and characteristic changes with age and disease stage.

Monocytes. Monocytes are released from the bone marrow, circulate in the blood for about 8 hours, and then enter the bone, brain, liver, lung, and skin to differentiate into specialized cells called macrophages. There they function as phagocytes which break down and process invading cells so that parts of them can be "presented" to the adaptive immune system. These cells are very important in controlling inflammation and the function of the other main white blood cell type, lymphocytes.

Basophils. Basophils are found in very low numbers in the blood stream and body (less than 2%). They are recruited to a site of infection and release histamine, a substance that causes capillaries to dilate and become permeable. This allows other important infection-fighting substances to move from the bloodstream into the site of infection. Currently available data indicates that there is no change in basophil number with age.

Eosinophils. Eosinophils circulate in lower numbers, 0-8% of WBC, and their main function is to defend against infection by parasites. An increase in the number of eosinophils above 500 is often indicative of a parasite infection or an allergic reaction to drugs, pollen or other allergen. There is some evidence that eosinophils function decreases with age, but the data is currently limited.

Red Blood Cells and Platelets

Now that you have an idea of the WBC this section will cover the two other components of the common Complete Blood Count the RBC and Platelets.

The WBC tells us about the state of the immune system. The RBC tells us about the state of the oxygen carrying capacity of our blood. The Platelet count is a measure of our ability to form a 'plug' when a blood vessel has been damaged.

Red Blood Cells. Anemia is defined as an RBC below the normal range. It can be caused by acute blood loss from trauma or bleeding of an internal organ. If the blood loss is more gradual, then it can go on undetected until the body's stores of the nutrients necessary to make red blood cells are depleted. An RBC above the normal range is called 'erythrocytosis'.

Hemoglobin. Hemoglobin is the oxygen carrying protein found in the red blood cells of all human and other vertebrate organisms. Low hemoglobin is most often indicative of blood loss and/or iron deficiency, but also can result from a genetic disorder of hemoglobin production such as thalassemia. An elevated hemoglobin level occurs with erythrocytosis.

Hematocrit. Hematocrit is a term similar to the RBC but is the concentration of red blood cells in the blood rather than the number. These two measures of the oxygen carrying capacity of the blood usually track together. They can diverge when you are in a state of dehydration (in which case the number of cells stays the same, but the concentration increases). The hematocrit is the more often used parameter.

Mean Corpuscular Volume. Mean Corpuscular Volume is a measure of the average size of your red blood cells and when it is above or below the normal range can be indicative of particular disease state or nutrient deficiencies. For example, in vitamin B12 and/or folate deficiency, the size of the red blood cells increases. In iron deficiency anemia, the size of the red blood cells decreases.

Mean Corpuscular Hemoglobin. Mean Corpuscular Hemoglobin is the average amount of hemoglobin in each red blood cell (aka 'corpuscle') and can help your doctor understand the type and the cause of anemia you may be exhibiting. It is calculated by dividing the total amount of hemoglobin by the RBC. It is reduced in iron-deficiency anemia.

Mean Corpuscular Hemoglobin Concentration. Mean Corpuscular Hemoglobin Concentration is similar to the MCH, but is calculated by dividing the hemoglobin by the hematocrit. It is the most sensitive indicator of iron deficiency anemia.

Red Cell Distribution Width. Red Cell Distribution Width (RDW or RDW-CV, for cell volume), measures the variation of sizes of red cells. If your cells tend to be about the same size, your value will be lower. If you have a larger variety of sizes of red blood cells, your value will be higher. This value is routinely reported during standard blood tests. B12/folate deficiency (causes RBC to be larger than normal while iron deficiency causes them to be smaller. Thus if there is a mixed iron and B12 folate deficiency), there will be both an increased number of small and large cells and the RDW increases. During active blood loss, the bone marrow steps up the production of red blood cells to replace them and maintain oxygen carrying capacity. These new red blood cells (called reticulocytes), are larger than mature red blood cells and can increase the RDW. The RDW has been shown to be a predictor of mortality in older populations, possibly because it is a marker for vitamin/nutrient deficiencies.

Platelets. Platelets are fragments of bone marrow precursor cells called 'megakaryocytes' and are the critical component in thrombus (clot) formation. In addition to maintaining homeostasis (controlling bleeding), platelets release growth factors that play significant roles in wound healing and repair/regeneration of connective tissue. There are disorders of abnormally low and high platelet count called thrombocytopenia and thrombocytosis, respectively. Ninety five percent of people have a platelet count between 150,000 and 400,000 per microliter. A level 100,000-150,000 may be physiologically insignificant in a small percentage of people, but is more likely to be the early stages of a gradually worsening thrombocytopenia. Platelet levels below 25,000 can lead to an increase in life-threatening hemorrhages from minor trauma. Thrombocytosis above 500,000 can lead to an increase risk of strokes and heart attacks.

Mean Platelet Volume. Mean Platelet Volume is a measure of the average size of your platelets. It is used to determine if a low platelet count is the result of clumping together of individual platelets or an actual decrease in platelet number. Higher MPVs mean the platelets are larger, which could put an individual at risk for a heart attack or stroke. Lower MPVs indicate smaller platelets, meaning the person is at risk for a bleeding disorder.

Information on the CBC is adapted from PhysioAge by Joseph Raffaele, MD

Nutrition

This section I believe holds the key to Longevity as metabolic stress (insulin resistance) can impact all 10 of the Hallmarks of Aging.

No one lives long if you are obese and diabetic – "diabesity". This is why recovering metabolic flexibility is the initial part of the program. You want to be sure you are "insulin sensitive" and have metabolic flexibility before you embark on LB100.

Remember only 5% of diabetics are type 1 – 95% are type 2 and the majority have an increased body fat and insulin resistance with high blood sugar.

A prediabetes state of "glucose intolerance" often occurs 10 or more years before a diagnosis of diabetes is made. A fasting blood sugar (glucose) is 70-80 mg/dl.

Insulin helps blood sugar enter the body's cells so it can be used for energy. Insulin also signals the liver to store blood sugar (glycogen) for later use. Blood sugar enter cells and levels of insulin in the bloodstream decrease, signaling insulin to decrease too.

Living with chronically high levels of insulin (hyperinsulinemia) can lead to weight gain and serious health problems. A fasting insulin should be less than 5 ulu/ml.

HOMA-IR. This stands for Homeostatic Model Assessment of Insulin Resistance. The HOMA-IR test is also one of my favorites and is simple and inexpensive. This calculation works for both the presence and extent of any insulin resistance that you might currently have.

HOMA-IR = Fasting Blood Sugar X Fasting Insulin / 405

- **Insulin Sensitive < 1.2 – Optimum**
- Moderate Insulin Resistance 1.2-2.9
- Severe Insulin Resistance >2.9

Note: Only 12% of the Americans have a HOMA-IR <1.2.

HbA1c. The term HbA1c refers to glycosylated hemoglobin. It develops when hemoglobin, a protein within red blood cells that carries oxygen throughout your body, joins with glucose in the blood, becoming glycated. By measuring HbA1c we are able to get an overall picture of what your average blood sugar levels are over a period of weeks up to 3 months. The higher your HbA1c, the more health complications.

Note: The HbA1c correlates very closely with waist-height ratio (i.e. diabesity) both driven by insulin resistance. Our goal is to have your HbA1c <5 which is optimum.

- Normal <5.7
- Prediabetes 5.7-6.4
- Diabetes >6.4

An optimum HbA1c should be less than 5%.

A Norfolk Cancer Study that measured HbA1c levels and risk of cancer revealed very interesting results not just for cancer but the risk of other chronic diseases and all-cause mortality as the tables below show.

Coronary Vascular Disease (CVD) Rates (per 100 people)

Men	6-7	9	12.1	15.2	25	34
HbA1c	<5.0%	5.0% to 5.4%	5.5% to 5.9%	6.0% to 6.4%	6.5% to 6.9%	>7.0%

As you can see, men and women who Live Below 5.0 have the lowest risk of heart disease. While those with HbA1c of 7 have a 5x risk of dying from CVD.

All Cause Death Rates (per 100 people)

Men	3.8	5.5	7.5	9.9	19	18.5
HbA1c	<5.0%	5.0% to 5.4%	5.5% to 5.9%	6.0% to 6.4%	6.5% to 6.9%	>7.0%

What was even more revealing was that as your HbA1c rose above 7, the mortality from all cardio-metabolic disease, heart disease, cancer, diabetes, mental disease, infections and respiratory disorders etc. all increased.

If your HbA1c is high, you die early!

Measuring the Insulin Resistance

Increased insulin makes us fat and keeps us fat. Increased insulin comes primarily from sugar and grains (and most processed food) that are the cause of high blood sugar levels.

When the blood sugar rises, insulin is released from the pancreas, repeated over and over again, the cells of the body fail to respond to the insulin – they become "insulin resistant". This leads to further rises in blood sugar, insulin and inflammation of your 60,000 miles of blood vessels throughout your body and the growth of visceral deep abdominal fat.

Obesity and most chronic disease seen today throughout the world is due to this "insulin resistance"; for example, if you do not correct your diet, the beta cells of your pancreas become exhausted and burn-out. That results in diabetes and other metabolic-diseases. A second major problem is when the high sugar reacts with protein in your body. It causes "glycation" and rusts important organs like your blood vessels (heart disease), skin (age spots and wrinkles), eye (cataracts), cartilage (arthritis), kidneys (renal failure), brain (dementia) – all signs of increased aging reflected in the advance glycation end-products or the AGE theory of aging.

Joseph Kraft, MD, and other researchers believe that 100% of people having heart disease have "insulin resistance" – cardiologists acknowledge that 75% have diabetes or prediabetes – Kraft showed that the other 25% are not properly diagnosed as you need to load the client with 75gm of glucose and measure 3-5hr insulin levels or Insulin Tolerance Test (ITT) not the usual GTT wrong in 50% of cases. Sugar, not cholesterol, causes heart disease.

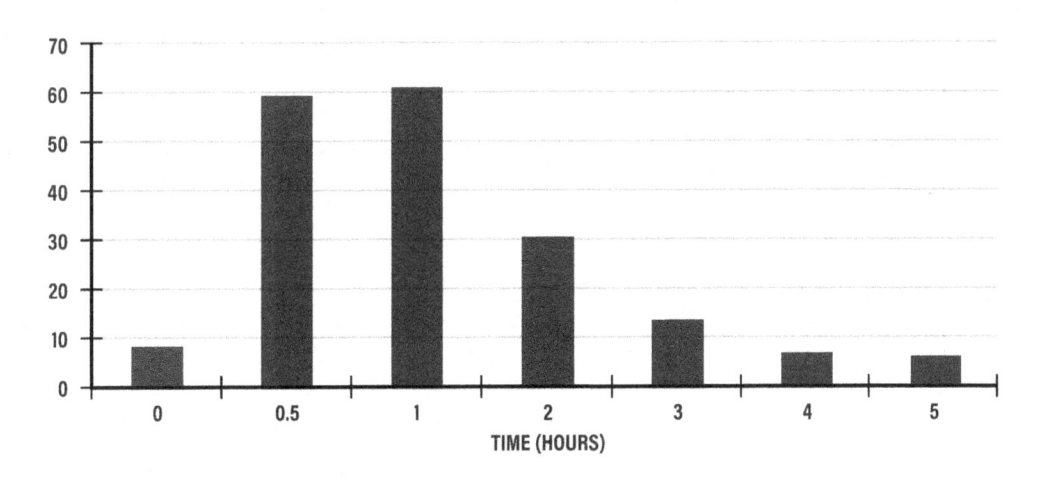

DYNAMIC INSULIN PATTERNS
PATTERN I

Dr. Kraft over a period of 25 years did many glucose/insulin tolerance tests on himself. They would vary between normal sugar with high insulin and normal sugar with normal insulin. The variations were directly related to weight fluctuations of often just 5 or 10 pounds.

Dr. Stout, in 1977, identified the pathology of type 2 diabetes as vascular (arterial), directly related to hyperinsulinemia and not to hyperglycemia. This includes all major arteries, all minor arteries, and all capillaries. All are lined by the endothelium (60,000 miles). By this widespread arterial distribution, every organ has a potential for pathology (insulin causes endothelial dysfunction).

Those with cardiovascular disease not identified with diabetes are simply undiagnosed.

The same is true for high blood pressure (those with systolic BP 120-139 and diastolic of 80-89 can be considered pre-hypertensive) and means you have hyperinsulinemia and probably type 2 diabetes until proven otherwise by insulin assays.

Note: Above graph shows: The 2hr + 3hr sum must = less than 60 microunits/ ml the only normal insulin pattern which is **optimal**.

Dr. Reaven, already in 2011, conducted a study on 208 apparently healthy middle-age people. None were obese (BMI <30) and used a research method (SSPG) to accurately measure insulin levels. The group is split into 3 depending if their insulin levels were low, medium or high and all were followed for 6 years or more as shown in the table below: Note the increased morbidity and mortality in those with higher insulin levels.

	Low Insulin Resistance	Medium Insulin Resistance	High Insulin Resistance
Disease	0	10	24
Death	0	2	4
Total Tragedy	0	12	28

Uric Acid

The first enzyme in fructose metabolism consumes ATP while metabolizing fructose. This generates not only AMP but also activates AMPD and intracellular uric acid accumulates, damaging the mitochondria. Uric acid is much more related to sugar than purines and is a powerful biological signaling molecule. Uric acid was a secondary marker of Metabolic Syndrome described by Dr. Gerald Reaven:

- Normal Uric Acid in Male <4.
- Normal Uric Acid in Female <3.5.
- Fructose elevates Intracellular Uric Acid.
- Uric Acid stimulates the Accumulation of Fat.

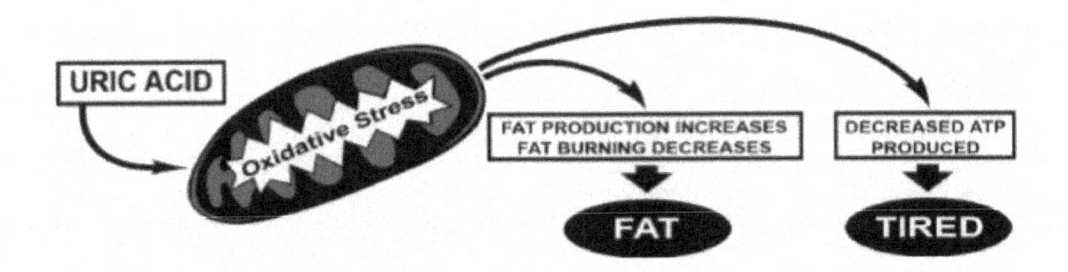

Uric acid affects mitochondria, causing oxidative stress. This results in stimulating fat synthesis, blocking fatty acid oxidation and reducing ATP production. The net effect is to preferentially shunt the energy from food to fat stores.

Uric acid levels directly lead to increased fat storage, and there's a reason for that, dating back millions of years, which you'll soon come to grasp (and appreciate). Our primate ancestors needed high levels of uric acid in order to build fat stores that would ensure their survival during times of environmental challenges, such as food and water scarcity.

Long before any symptoms develop, **asymptomatic hyperuricemia** may well be fomenting an unending, irreversible storm and subtly stoking biological processes that ultimately result in elevated blood sugar and blood pressure, bad cholesterol, excess body fat, and systemic inflammation, which opens the door for any number of chronic degenerative conditions. Put simply, hyperuricemia precedes these debilitating ailments that become difficult to manage once they take root. And, incredibly, in our distant evolutionary past, elevated uric acid served as a survival mechanism.

It bears reiterating: the risk increase was clearly evident at levels considered normal. Other studies have confirmed these findings, showing that uric acid levels mirror levels of systemic inflammation and can actually serve not only as surrogate marker of inflammation but also an amplifier of that inflammation. Which means that uric acid levels are directly tied to every malady under the inflammatory sun. This is what places high uric acid at the heart of any conversation about risk of disease.

Q: What do obesity, insulin resistance, diabetes, nonalcoholic fatty liver disease, hypertension, coronary artery disease, stroke, neurological disorders including Alzheimer's disease, and premature death have in common?

A: High uric acid levels.

Without adequate NO, insulin cannot do its job – the insulin glucose correspondence, or activity, is disrupted. Loss of nitric oxide also triggers hypertension and a loss of vascular compliance, which refers to the ability of blood vessels to respond appropriately to changes in blood pressure.

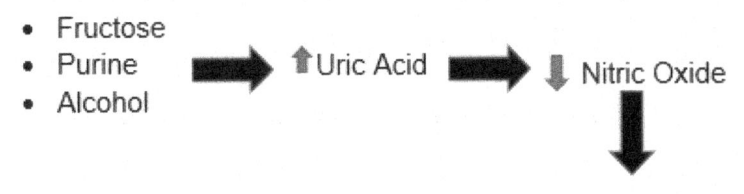

The Uric Acid-Nitric Oxide Connection

The Uric Acid-Nitric Oxide Connection

- Fructose
- Purine
- Alcohol

➡ ↑Uric Acid ➡ ↓Nitric Oxide
⬇
- Insulin Resistance
- Hypertension
- Reduced blood flow to organs

Adapted from David Perlmutter, MD
Drop Acid

Routinely testing your uric acid and blood glucose is among the most powerful strategies for managing your health and knowing when to take action through interventions such as reducing your intake of certain foods and timing your workouts to streamline your metabolism.

Just as brain degeneration begins at a hemoglobin A1c of 5.5 percent, which doctors deem a normal value, so too do uric acid levels above 5 considered as "asymptomatic hyperuricemia" fan the flames of inflammation and chronic disease.

Finally, uric acid suppresses autophagy and diminishes the anti-inflammatory capacity of cells. Put another way, uric acid prevents your cells from clearing out dangerous senescent cells and calming down inflammatory reactions and hasten the aging process.

What is Metabolic Syndrome?

Metabolic Syndrome affects more than one third of the adult population of the USA and was first described by Gerald Reaven from Stanford University in 1988, a percentage that increases to around 50 among people over the age of 60. He noticed a group of risk factors that have a common origin: hypertension, central obesity, high triglycerides, low HDL, and diabetes.

The common cause is "insulin resistance" due primarily from sugar and grains. Insulin and fructose are the two main activators of de novo lipogenesis (DNL).

High triglycerides (increase the risk of heart disease by 61 percent) and low levels of HDL both result from increased VDRL which comes from hyperinsulinemia from too much glucose and fructose.

The liver tries to release the fatty congestion by exporting T.G. and blood levels increase – a classic sign of metabolic syndrome (uric acid is also elevated). Ectopic fat accumulates in other organs such as the pancreas, kidneys, heart and muscle. The predominance of fat around the abdomen becomes noticeable as an increase in waist size (wheat belly). This visceral fat is the most important predictor of metabolic syndrome and heart disease.

Overweight (Waist Size)	Male >40" (100cm)	Female >35" (89cm)
High Blood Sugar	>100	>100
High Blood Pressure	>130/85	>130/85
High Triglycerides	>150	>150
Low HDL Cholesterol	<40	<50

Do you have Metabolic Syndrome?

If you have 3 or more of the above, you have Metabolic Syndrome and have Cardio-Metabolic disease (insulin resistance).

Lipoprotein Tests

Cholesterol – A Weapon of Mass Distraction

The cholesterol story has dominated modern medicine for the last 40 years based on faulty science and Big Pharma and is an important cause of our current Diabesity Pandemic and obscures the true cause of cardio-metabolic disease. The cat is now out of the bag. We now know that the higher your cholesterol is after age 50 the longer you will live. Cholesterol is in fact one of the most important molecules that evolution evolved to keep us healthy. Not only do we now recognize the myriad health effects that cholesterol provides, but we now know that saturated fats are also healthy and do not promote cardiovascular disease.

Cholesterol and Triglycerides are carried in the blood on particles called lipoproteins. Both LDL and HDL carry that exact same cholesterol inside so it is more accurate to call LDL – a "bad" lipoprotein and HDL a "good" lipoprotein.

Dr. William Castelli who led the Framingham Study said "Unless LDL levels are very high (300mg/dl) or higher, they have no value, in isolation, in predicting those individuals at risk for coronary heart disease."

Castelli also recognized that the "ratios" of various lipids were more important than just the isolated number. While the HDL lipoprotein is somewhat unique the LDL belongs to a "family" of LDL lipoproteins. I am indebted to Ivor Cummings for reminding me that the more important food driving this LDL-family is CARBOHYDRATES.

VLDL – is the largest of the LDLs made up of TG (+++) and cholesterol. This very low-density lipoprotein (VLDL) is the mother of LDL.

LDL – is formed from VLDL when it gives up its TG and shrinks. LDL thus is mostly cholesterol with a small about of TG. As people age and eat a Standard American Diet (SAD diet) the VLDL's turn into smaller and denser LDL's that carry less cholesterol. With less cholesterol carried per particle, you need more particles in circulation and this means more particles exposed to oxidation which damages the endothelium. Insulin resistance is the primary driver of both oxidized LDL and sdLDL.

sdLDL – small dense LDL (sdLDL) is what results when LDL becomes distorted in an "inflammatory environment". The primary way to make your LDL go bad is to become insulin resistant from excess carbs, grains, vegetable oils. These sdLDL's can't get taken up by the liver; instead the immune system tries to clean this up. These damaged particles are what ends up on the inside of your inflamed arterial walls that ultimately lead to the arterial plaque, blockage and heart attacks.

Note: The LDL – family of lipoproteins associate with Beta Apolipoprotein (ApoB) while the HDL particles are associated with A1 Apolipoprotein (ApoA1).

Insulin resistance also promotes damage and weakness in the arteries due to high blood pressure, high sugar and other mechanisms.

A study in 2007 looking at the Framingham data showed that both cholesterol and LDL did not predict CHD at all, but the cholesterol ratios predicted CHD very well.

What Castelli did not know at this time was that these ratios reflected insulin resistance status (as Ivor Cummins mentions in his excellent book *Eat Rich Live Long*) rather than "cholesterol" issues per se.

TG/HDL Ratio – to calculate your TG/HDL ratio you simply obtain a fasting lipid panel and divide the triglyceride level by the HDL cholesterol. The closer to 1 the better. If your level is above 2 you are at increased risk for diabetes, heart attack and stroke. The ideal ratio is 1.

Those people who are in the top quartile with the highest TG/HDL ratio are 16x at risk for heart attacks compared to those with lowest ratios.

Not only do the TG/HDL levels correlate with the severity of atherosclerosis but TG/HDL are also related to all-cause mortality.

Total Cholesterol/HDL Ratio – the total cholesterol/HDL ratio is closely related to the TG/HDL ratio. You should be below 5 – an optimum level is <4. As the following table by Ivor Cummins shows the Total Cholesterol/HDL ratio accounts for most of the increased risk. LDL is irrelevant.

The Total/HDL ratio accounts for pretty much **all** of the increase in risk. LDL is irrelevant in comparison.

Coronary Artery Disease Hazard Ratios

LDL <130 (Average LDL=109)		LDL >130 (Average LDL=175)	
Total/HDL <5	Total/HDL >5	Total/HDL <5	Total/HDL >5
1.00	2.49	0.97	2.15

HDL Cholesterol. High-density lipoprotein (HDL cholesterol, HDL-C) is a type of protein that removes excess cholesterol from tissues and carries it to the liver for removal. For this reason it also called the "good" cholesterol. Insufficient levels of HLD-C will result in elevated blood levels of cholesterol which may be deposited in arterial walls and can lead to plaques and wall hardening along with inflammation. A higher level of HDL is thus associated with a lower risk of heart attack or stroke. Exercise has been shown to improve the functionality of HDL and a healthy diet of high fiber and low carbs has a beneficial effect globally on cholesterol levels.

LDL/HDL Ratio – data shows that people with a lower HDL are at very high risk of CAD even if their LDL is nice and low but even more dangerous are those people with a low HDL but also a high LDL. Ideally your LDL/HDL ratio should be <3.5.

Apo A/ Apo A1 – The Master Ratio

This is a more sophisticated test but has become increasingly important in the last decade as a risk factor of insulin resistance and cardio-metabolic disease.

Remember LDL particles have B lipoprotein (ApoB) while HDL particles have A1 lipoprotein (Apo A1). So, the Apo B/Apo A1 ratio tells you the ratio of LDL to HDL. People with insulin resistance tend to have fewer HDL particles and more LDL particles.

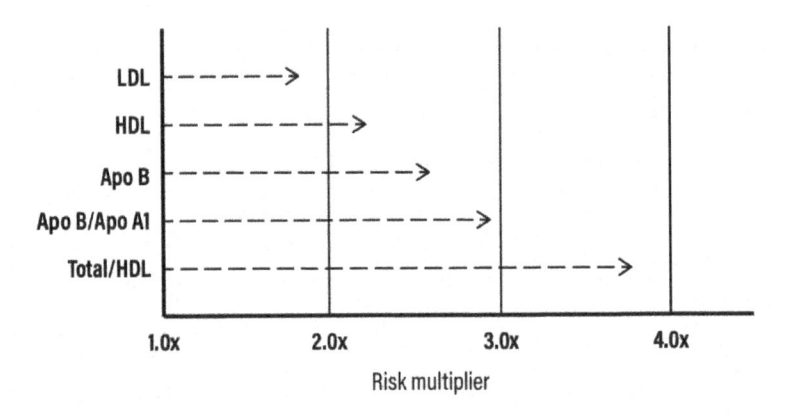

	Risk multiplier
LDL	~2.0x
HDL	~2.25x
Apo B	~2.5x
Apo B/Apo A1	~2.75x
Total/HDL	~3.5x

In addition, if a large percent of your LDL particles are the "small dense" (sdLDL) this is a bad sign. Thus, it is not only the number of LDL particles but their size as well. You have a low risk of disease if you have an LDL-P # less than 750. You have a lower risk of disease if your LDL-particle size is large (beach balls) Pattern A – rather than smaller (baseball) sized particles (Pattern B).

Lipoprotein – a LP(a) – a lipoprotein consisting of an LDL particle to which a large glycoprotein, apolipoprotein (a), is covalently bonded. Elevation of its concentration in serum has been identified as a risk factor for coronary artery disease.

Elevation of plasma lipoprotein LP (a) above 30mg/dL is a strong independent risk factor for coronary artery disease and possibly for stroke. A unique feature for lipoprotein Lp(a) is the structural similarity of its nonlipid moiety, apolipoprotein Lp(a), to plasminogen. This similarity allows it to bond to endothelium and to proteins of cellular membranes. It inhibit fibrinolysis by competing for plasminogen binding sites and also favors lipid deposition and stimulates smooth muscle cell proliferation. Niacin and estrogen lower lipoprotein Lp(a), but HMG CoA reductase inhibitors, fibrates, and bile acid sequestrants do not.

Lp(a) has a strong genetic component. Most people have a level between 5-29mg/dL.

If levels are very high plasma phoresis can help.

Toxin Reduction

There are 6 organs of detoxification. Here we measure the two most important the liver and kidney. The other 4 are the skin, lung, colon and lymphatic system.

The Liver

The liver makes most of the proteins that are found in your blood. A normal range for total protein is 60-80gms. It also measures the amounts of two major groups of proteins in the blood albumin and globulin.

Albumin. Albumin is the most abundant protein in human serum. It is important for maintaining normal osmotic pressure (the force keeping the fluid in the blood vessels), carrying certain hormones, and neutralizing free radicals. It is produced in the liver, and a decreased level can indicate reduced liver function or liver disease. The serum level of albumin decreases with age even in the absence of disease. An increased level is generally the result of dehydration. In the absence of dehydration, a higher serum level is generally a sign of good health.

Globulin. Globulin is the term used for the non-albumin proteins circulating in the blood. These include many proteins but can roughly be divided into two groups. The gamma globulins are mostly composed of circulating antibodies made by mature B-cells called plasma cells. The other groups contains SHBG, transferrin, ferritin, thyroid binding globulin, etc. Elevation of the serum globulins of the gamma variety can occur in lymphoma, multiple myeloma, and monoclonal gammopathy of undetermined significance.

Bilirubin, Direct Bilirubin, Direct is the fraction of the total bilirubin that has been attached to a molecule (glucuronide) to prepare it for excretion. The indirect bilirubin is that fraction of the total that is free and unattached. The total bilirubin is the sum of the indirect and the direct bilirubin. In Gilbert's syndrome, it is the indirect bilirubin that is increased because of a low level of the enzyme that attaches the glucuronide molecule to bilirubin to prepare it for excretion. Gilbert's syndrome causes indirect bilirubin to rise during illness and can lead to a mild case of jaundice.

It is relatively abundant in the blood stream of mammals and may have evolved as a potent antioxidant system to protect against the oxidation of lipids (cholesterol) in cell membranes. Increased levels of bilirubin are an indication of blockage of the bile duct (by gallstones or inflammation), or increased destruction of red blood cells that overwhelms the ability of the liver to process the bilirubin into its water-soluble form for elimination in the urine. Interestingly, levels in the higher end of the normal range are associated with a decreased incidence of heart attack. Chronic slightly elevated levels of bilirubin, in the absence of bile duct blockage, are most often caused by a benign genetic disorder called Gilbert's syndrome (found in about 5-10% of the population). When total bilirubin levels rise above 3mg/dl, a yellowing of the skin called "jaundice" occurs.

Alkaline Phosphatase. Alkaline phosphatase is an enzyme that takes phosphates groups off of molecules and works best in an alkaline (high pH) environment. It is present throughout the body, but particularly in liver, bile duct and bones. The level of alkaline phosphatase is measured as a biomarker for damage to one of the organ system where it is produced. Alkaline phosphatase serum level can be elevated when the bile duct is blocked or inflamed. A healing fracture can cause an increase in alkaline phosphatase. Low levels of alkaline phosphatase can be associated with low thyroid function, but for the most part, a level lower than the low end of normal is of no clinical significance.

Alanine Aminotransferase (ALT). Alanine Aminotransferase is an enzyme that transfers the amino group from alanine during certain energy producing reactions. It is found in liver tissue, but also in skeletal and heart muscle. It is often used as an indicator of liver inflammation because its serum level can increase markedly when liver cells are damaged and leak the enzyme into the circulation, as occurs during hepatitis. Minor elevations can be seen after intense exercise, alcohol consumption, or when taking certain drugs, particularly cholesterol-lowering drugs of the statin family such as Lipitor.

Aspartate Aminotransferase (AST). Aminotransferase is an enzyme similar to ALT except it transfers the amino group of aspartate. It is used as an indicator of liver and cardiac muscle damage. When both ALT and AST are elevated, there is an increased risk of liver damage. The ratio of AST to ALT <2 is often indicative of chronic liver disease from Wilson's disease and alcoholic liver disease. An AST/ALT

<1 is indicative of acute liver disease or that caused by fatty deposits in the liver, as occur in obesity and diabetes.

Albumin/Globulin Ratio. Albumin/Globulin ratio can serve as a more sensitive flag for disorders of high or low production of albumin or globulins because the individual levels can fluctuate according to hydration status. A low ratio can be caused by increased production of gamma globulins, as occurs in multiple myeloma. A high ratio is usually a sign of good health unless it is associated with a very low globulin, in which case it may signal hypogammaglobulinemia, which can be caused by kidney disease.

Urea Nitrogen in Blood. Urea Nitrogen in Blood is produced when your body breaks nitrogen containing protein down into its constituent amino acids and the liver combines the nitrogen into the waste product urea. There is a relatively constant production of BUN, which the kidneys then filter out and excrete into the urine. Diseases that affect the kidneys or the liver can raise BUN. Other causes include heart failure, dehydration, and or gastrointestinal bleeding. Low BUN is not very common and if present is usually not a cause for concern. The most common cause of an elevated BUN in an otherwise healthy individual is mild dehydration.

Creatinine. Creatinine is a product of the breakdown of creatine, compound produce by your muscles when they are actively contracting. Because creatinine is produced at a relatively constant rate and is excreted almost exclusively by your kidneys, its serum level is a good indicator of kidney filtration rate (health). However, an increased serum level can be found in people with higher muscle mass or who have been exercising vigorously prior to the test. Cystatin C is a newer measure of kidney function that is not affected by these factors. Low levels of creatinine are usually found in people with relatively low muscle mass and higher levels can indicate kidney function decline. A level above 2 is usually an indication that some impairment of kidney function is present. In most individuals, creatinine slowly increases (0.5-1% per year) with age, making it a biomarker of kidney function aging.

BUN/Creatinine Ratio. BUN/Creatinine Ratio is used to differentiate dehydration or excess BUN production from kidney problems. In kidney failure, both creatinine and BUN rise, so the ratio will not increase. When there is excess BUN production only (from e.g. gastrointestinal bleeding) you will see an increased BUN/Creatinine. A mildly elevated ratio (22-25) can occur in people with low muscle mass (which causes a low creatinine level) and slight dehydration, but is usually not a cause for concern.

Glomerular Filtration Rate (GFR). Your kidneys filter your blood by removing waste and extra water to make urine. The kidney's filtration rate, called the glomerular filtration rate (GFR), shows how well the kidneys are filtering. The standard way to estimate GFR is with a simple blood test that measures your creatinine level. Creatinine is a waste product from the digestion of protein and the normal breakdown of muscle tissue.

STAGES OF CHRONIC KIDNEY DISEASE		GFR*	% OF KIDNEY FUNCTION
Stage 1	Kidney damage with **normal** kidney function	90 or higher	90-100%
Stage 2	Kidney damage with **mild loss** of kidney function	89 to 60	89-60%
Stage 3a	**Mild to moderate** loss of kidney function	59 to 45	59-45%
Stage 3b	**Moderate to severe** loss of kidney function	44 to 30	44-30%
Stage 4	**Severe** loss of kidney function	29 to 15	29-15%
Stage 5	Kidney **failure**	Less than 15	Less than 15%

*Your GFR number tells you how much kidney function you have. As kidney disease gets worse, the GFR number goes down.

Cystatin C. Cystatin C is a protein produced by cells in the body which is later filtered by the kidney. Measuring Cystatin C gives an indication of the filtration rate of the kidney, a marker of kidney health or injury. It is more sensitive to the small changes in early kidney injury than other proteins such as creatinine. And unlike other kidney function tests, Cystatin-C is less affected by age, gender, protein intake, muscle mass, or ethnicity. Cystatin-C identifies patients with early kidney injury and is also good predictor of the development of cardiovascular disease.

Electrolytes are the positively and negatively charged small molecules (called 'ions') found in your cells, blood stream, and extracellular fluids. They are maintained in a delicate balance by your kidney, lungs, and endocrine system. They are critical in the electrical signaling between and within cells, the acid-base balance (pH), and the maintenance of the fluid balance between different body compartments. Small fluctuations in their relative levels can be due to serious disease processes. Cations and anions (negatively and positively charge ions) travel together as salts to balance the overall charge of a fluid. They are usually measured together in a serum sample because interpretation of one requires knowledge of the levels of most of the others.

Sodium. Sodium is the principal positively charged ion (called a "cation") of the extracellular space. It is the same as the sodium found in most foods and table salt (sodium chloride). The body responds to changes in the serum sodium level in three main ways: 1. Modulating thirst: as little as 1% increase in serum sodium can make you thirsty so you consume water to decrease the level to normal. 2. Producing sodium-regulating hormones: certain hormones (natriuretic peptide) cause the kidneys to lose sodium while others (aldosterone) cause them to retain sodium. 3. Producing water regulating hormones: antidiuretic hormone (ADH) causes the kidneys to hold onto free water. Water follows sodium. When you eat a salty meal, you become thirsty and drink water. The extra fluid is retained (causing the characteristics post-Chinese food bloating and edema) until it can be excreted as the hormonal sodium excretion pathways kick in. ADH is inhibited by alcohol causing the excessive urination of clear water noted after drinking a lot of beer or other alcoholic beverages. When these mechanisms are not functioning well or are overwhelmed, a state of hypernatremia (high serum sodium), or hyponatremia (low serum sodium) can ensue. The most common cause of hypernatremia is dehydration from decreased water intake. Hyponatremia is most commonly from sodium loss through sweat that is replaced only with water. Other causes include diuretics, Addison's disease, diarrhea and kidney disease.

Potassium. Potassium is the principal intracellular cation, and only about 2% of your total body potassium is located in your body fluids and blood stream. Increased serum potassium (hyperkalemia) is most commonly caused by kidney disease, but other medications, such as ACE inhibitors, potassium-sparing diuretics, and NSAIDs, can cause it. Hyperkalemia can cause abnormal heart rhythms and respiratory failure. Low serum potassium (hypokalemia) can be caused by dehydration, vomiting, diarrhea and inadequate repletion when taking diuretics.

Chloride. Chloride is the anion that travels with sodium in and out of cells to help regulate body fluids and acid-base balance. When a problem arises with the serum sodium level, the chloride can diverge from sodium to buffer the pH of the blood temporarily. Chloride is ingested as sodium chloride in food and table salt. Increased chloride levels most commonly indicate dehydration, and a decreased level can be caused by vomiting, chronic lung disease or with a loss of acid from the body.

Carbon Dioxide. Carbon dioxide should really be called bicarbonate or HCO_3 because CO_2 is actually the gas that your lungs exhale. When it is dissolve in water, CO_2 associates with a hydrogen ion to become HCO_3 and acts as a buffer for acid in the blood. A low serum bicarbonate level indicates that your body is in an acidic state and the bicarbonate is being used up to buffer it. This can be caused by diabetes, kidney disease, and chronic diarrhea. A high bicarbonate level indicates alkaline pH of the blood due to acid loss from vomiting, lung disease, or Cushing's syndrome. While it is technically not a mineral but a molecule, it is one of the electrolytes so it is included in this section.

Calcium. Calcium is a mineral cation in your blood that is essential for the healthy functioning of your muscles, nervous system, and heart. Its serum concentration is very tightly regulated by your kidneys and endocrine system because deviations from the normal level can have serious consequences. If there is a mild elevation (less than 10.5), the first thing to do is to repeat the blood test to make sure it is not a lab error. Persistently high calcium (hypercalcemia) is commonly caused by either hyperparathyroidism (benign tumors of the parathyroid gland secreting too much parathyroid hormone) or cancer that has spread to the bones. Low serum calcium is most commonly caused by a low serum protein level (from malnutrition) because the calcium is bound to protein. A follow-up ionized serum calcium level will be normal if this is the only cause. Other causes of hypocalcemia are low vitamin D level, underactive parathyroids (hypoparathyroidism), magnesium deficiency, and kidney failure.

Adapted from PhysioAge
by Joseph Raffaele, MD

Restoration of Hormones

As we age, there is a decline in the levels of several of our hormones. Since the endocrine system is one of the key regulators of integrated biological function, altered hormone secretion and actions are important in the development of diabetes, metabolic syndrome, obesity, osteoporosis, depression, impaired cognition, erectile dysfunction, and loss of energy and strength. More than 40 million men and women are going through andropause and menopause (the hormonal changes associated with aging).

Hormone release is controlled by the hypothalamus in the brain. The hypothalamus, which is located at the base of the brain, communicates directly with the pituitary gland via special nerves and blood vessels. Pituitary hormones then work on target glands like the thyroid, adrenal, pancreas, and testicles. Different hormones are then released from these endocrine glands that have widespread effects throughout the entire body.

For example, testosterone levels decrease in many men during their late thirties. Low testosterone levels have been shown to increase your chances of dying from heart disease and are associated with all causes of death. Older men with low levels of circulating total testosterone had a 40 percent increased risk of dying over the following twenty years compared to men with normal testosterone, independent of age, obesity, and lifestyle.

Hormones are the juice of life. Men and women are revitalized in as little as six to eight weeks after beginning hormonal replacement therapy. One of the problems I frequently see due to the excessive use of statins is low cholesterol levels. This is important when you realize that hormones are derived from cholesterol. Our evidence-based wellness approach uses hormone modulation to help men and women regain and maintain healthy metabolic and endocrine function, adjusted for the client's age – creating the best opportunity for a healthier and more vigorous life. Let's review the major hormones.

Thyroid Hormone Therapy

Synthroid is the most commonly prescribed hormone for hypothyroidism, but it only contains T4. The physiologically active form in the body is T3, but with age and certain chronic disease states, many people have a problem converting T4 to T3. Thus, we have found it is very difficult to provide adequate thyroid supplementation with Synthroid without causing patients to develop a toxicity to thyroid hormone. Natural thyroid hormone, such as Armour, is a desiccated preparation of porcine thyroid glands and contains all thyroid hormone factors (T2, T3 and T4). Unfortunately, many physicians have been bamboozled by the manufacturers of synthetic thyroid hormones into thinking that the natural thyroid products are an inferior, nonstandardized drug. Nothing could be further from the truth.

Most of our clients who switch from Synthroid to Armour or similar compounded T3/T4 report that they feel much better with the natural product. The dramatic improvements that many of them have achieved on natural thyroid therapy often appear miraculous. Often, they are able to lose weight for the first time in many years. Raising the body temperature by just 1°F (which can happen when taking compounded thyroid hormones) equates to fifty-pound weight loss in one year.

Occasionally, it may be necessary to take as much as 5 grains of thyroid daily (full replacement therapy) to obtain complete relief of symptoms. It is not really necessary to receive periodic blood tests, as it is more important to treat the client than to treat the blood test, but performing the test is wise from a medical/legal perspective. Using natural thyroid hormone is very safe. There is little risk of excessive thyroid dosage as long as:

- You feel well
- Your temperature remains below 98.2°F
- Your pulse is less than 75 beats per minute
- Your thyroid function tests remain normal (don't be fooled because many hypothyroid people feel best with TSH levels that are below normal). In fact, as a result of recent research, the upper limit of TSH of 5.5 ulU/mL has been decreased to 2.0-2.5ulU/mL. People feel much better when their TSH is decreased to less than 2 by supplementing with a natural compounded thyroid preparation or Armour rather than Synthroid.

Benefits of thyroid hormone therapy may include:
- Improves energy
- Increases body temperature
- Better skin, hair, nails
- Fewer colds
- Increased libido
- Better mood and improved memory
- Better circulation
- Less pain and joint stiffness

Side effects may include a "wired" feeling (like having too much coffee), fast resting pulse, and insomnia.

Thyroid Stimulating Hormone. Thyroid Stimulating Hormone is produced in the pituitary gland and controls the production and release of thyroid hormones from the thyroid gland. T4, and to a greater degree. T3, inhibit the release of TSH in a negative feedback fashion. Therefore, a higher TSH indicates that the pituitary gland senses there is inadequate circulating thyroid hormone and tries to stimulate further production and release by secreting more TSH. In contrast, a TSH below the normal range – particularly if it is undetectable – indicates the state of hyperthyroidism where excess thyroid hormone is causing the suppression TSH.

Thyroxine. Thyroxine essentially functions as a precursor hormone reservoir (80% of circulating thyroid hormones) of T3. It is released into the circulation and then is converted into T3, either in the liver or target cells such as the heart and subcutaneous fat. IGF-1 is important for the conversion of T4 into T3.

Free T3. Free T3 is the fraction of the total T3 that is not bound to its binding protein and is able to get into cells. Free T3 decreases with age because T4 is less efficiently converted to it by the liver and other tissues. This results in decreased thyroid activity at the tissue level and has been associated with decreased cognitive function, depression, cardiovascular disease, and increased cholesterol.

Testosterone Therapy

In 1889, British neurologists Charles-Edouard Brown-Sequard (1817-1894), thought to be an inspiration for Robert Louise Stevenson's character of Dr. Jekyll, gave himself crushed animal testicles and claimed he became stronger, developed more stamina, and had a better memory. This is one of the earliest examples of a cell therapy treatment.

There are at least five common method used to replace testosterone: creams or gels, lozenges by mouth, injections (SQ or IM), patches and implantation of pellets. Our preference is to use injections in men and creams in women. There are several forms of injectable testosterone approved for use in the U.S., both short-acting (aqueous testosterone, testosterone cyprionate, and testosterone propionate) and long-acting (testosterone enanthate and deca durabolin) forms. Testosterone undecanoate is a new injectable testosterone that needs only four or five injections per year.

Another option is to use human chorionic gonadotropin (HCG). In men their thirties and forties, the pituitary gland slows down or stop producing the stimulating luteinizing hormone (LH). The testicles are not receiving a signal from LH, so they don't produce testosterone. HCG given twice a week will increase testosterone production by the Leydig cells. And unlike with using exogenous testosterone, the testicles will not shrink. HCG should be used if fertility is an issue.

Of note, testosterone replacement is key for diabetic men and women, as their testosterone levels are significantly lower. Testosterone treatment improves insulin resistance, glycemic control, visceral fat burning and blood fats. Testosterone improves the transport of glucose from the blood into the cell and enhances insulin sensitivity. Many people with diabetes are carbohydrate sensitive with an exaggerated insulin response, so a drop in blood sugar triggers constant hunger and they need to eat more simple carbohydrates. Wheat and milk are the most frequent hypersensitivity foods and should be eliminated.

Testosterone benefits may include:

- Improves blood sugar control
- Benefits cardiac health (improves high blood pressure, reduces sugar and cholesterol)
- Builds muscle mass and strength; decreases body fat
- Increases bone density
- Improves mood and sense of well-being
- Boosts energy levels
- Improves verbal and working memory and clarity of thought
- Improves erectile performance and quality of orgasms

Side effects of androgen therapy in men may include water retention, polycythemia (excessive red blood cell mass), hepatotoxicity (highest risk with oral preparations), sleep apnea, adverse lipid profile, gynecomastia (breast growth, nipple sensitivity), acne, hair loss, infertility due to a decrease in pituitary gonadotropin causing decrease spermatogenesis, and benign prostatic hypertrophy (BPH).

Contraindications to testosterone replacement include these absolute contraindications:

- The suspicion of, or already existing, prostate cancer or breast cancer (although most consider men who have had treatment for prostate cancer and no occurrence to be low risk)
- Obstructive uropathy
- Desire to reproduce (change to HCG)
- Hematocrit (HCT) above 55%

Relative contraindications include elevated HCT (52-55 percent); pre-existing cardiac, renal, or hepatic disease; sleep apnea or high risk for sleep apnea (chronic obstructive pulmonary disease in overweight persons or heavy smokers), and gynecomastia. Men with HCT >52% should consult with their doctor and have 500ml of their blood taken out.

Men on testosterone therapy should at least take the herb saw palmetto (Serenoa repens) (160mg) with pygeum twice daily, which blocks the conversion of testosterone to DHT. This helps prevent any complications involving the prostate.

On a final note it is important to measure dihydrotestosterone (DHT) because high levels can elevate PSA levels and should usually remain below 4 nanograms per milliliter (ng/ml).

As men reach their forties, the balance starts shifting from a less androgenic state to one that includes more estrogen. We don't advise treating this elevation in estrogen. There is also an increase in sex hormone binding globulin (SHBG) secreted by the liver that prevents testosterone from working properly.

Free Testosterone. This a test of unattached or "free" testosterone. Most of the testosterone circulates in your body tightly attached to a protein called sex hormone binding globulin (SHBG) and to a lesser extent, the protein albumin. Free testosterone is the portion that is not attached to proteins, and is therefore free to be easily used by your body. If the binding proteins are high, specifically SHBG, there will be less free testosterone that your body can utilize. SHBG increases under certain conditions and thus higher levels of estrogen, thyroid hormones, and weight loss can result in lower free testosterone whereas higher levels of androgens result in increased free testosterone. Therefore, while knowing a total testosterone level is important, the amount of testosterone that is metabolically active will give a clearer picture of any excess or deficiencies that may gave a clinical impact.

Sex Hormone Binding Globulin. Sex Hormone Binding Globulin (SHBG) is a protein made in the liver with the primary function of transporting sex steroid hormones (e.g. testosterone, estradiol) through the blood stream to their target tissues. Once the hormone is released from SHBG, it is free to act at the level of the receptor. Higher levels of SHBG results in lower free, bioactive levels of hormones and can manifests in clinical symptoms of deficiency related to that hormone. Conversely, lower levels of SHBG results in highest levels of the free hormone. Factors such as sex, age, nutritional status affects the levels of SHBG. They are lower in the presence of obesity, insulin resistance, liver disease, and hyperthyroidism and are decreased by a higher protein intake diet, androgens (e.g. testosterone), and growth hormone. SHBG is increased by estrogens, thyroid hormones, contraceptives, a lean body mass, and in calorie restriction or anorexia. Understanding the levels of SHBG in relation to your hormones help us assess your hormone status and make the necessary adjustments to your treatment program.

PSA. For men in their 40's and 50's a PSA greater than 2.5ng/ml is considered abnormal (medium PSA usually 0.6-0.7 ng/ml).

For men in their 60's a PSA greater than 4ng/ml is considered abnormal (medium PSA usually 1-1.5 ng/ml).

Caution: If your PSA rises more than 0.35ng/ml in single year!

Dehydroepiandrosterone (DHEA) Therapy
DHEA Therapy

I typically use doses of 25-50 mg of DHEA daily in men but only 5-10mg in women. Some clinicians will use 1,600-2,000 mg daily for those with serious immune disorders or human immunodeficiency virus (HIV). Smaller doses are effective if DHEA is take sublingually or transdermally. DHEA cream appears to convert readily and to be 2.5 times more potent; this form (7-Keto) of DHEA will also not convert to testosterone.

DHEA benefits may include:
- Improves mental and physical function
- Increases bone density
- Increases lean body mass
- Elevates mood
- Lowers cortisol (the "stress hormone") levels
- Provides protection against cancer
- Protects the brain from Alzheimer's disease
- Decreases heart disease (reduced plaque and sticky platelets)
- Increased insulin sensitivity
- Increases testosterone levels and sexual arousal
- Potent anti-viral effects

Side effects of DHEA may include increased facial hair and size of the liver (due to testosterone increase), and increased levels of estrogen hormone estradiol (except 7-Keto DHEA, which does not convert to testosterone and thus to estradiol).

Women should use a smaller dose 5-10mg per day as testosterone can be raised with higher doses of DHEA.

Note: Dihydrotestosterone is directly created form testosterone by the activity of the important enzyme, 5-alpha reductase. Dihydrotestosterone (DHT) is responsible for the androgenic effects of testosterone such as increased libido, mood, and skin oil production. Inhibitors of 5-alpha reductase like finasteride (Propecia/Proscar) or dutasteride (Avodart), are potent blockers of DHT production.

Estradiol. Estradiol is just as important in men as it is in women, but circulates in a more steady range and at about one-fifth the level of a premenopausal woman. In women, it is the most potent estrogen of the ovaries. It is metabolized into estrone and estriol, both active, but weaker estrogens. In addition to causing the build-up of the lining of the uterus (endometrium) characteristics of a menstrual cycle, estradiol is important for maintaining the health of the arteries, bone, brain, skin, and immune system. Similar to FSH, the estradiol level needs to be interpreted in the context of the timing of the menstrual cycle. It is lowest in the first few days of the period (30-50 pg/ml) and gradually rises (100-150 pg/ml) during the 12 or so days prior to the pre-ovulatory spike (350-700 pg/ml). In the second half of the menstrual cycle (days 15-28), it averages between 150-200 and declines just prior to the onset of the next cycle. In the perimenopause, the levels can fluctuate widely from very low (less than 20 pg/ml) to very high (greater than 700 pg/ml), depending on whether a healthy follicle is recruited. In the post-menopause, the level is less than 20, but can be almost undetectable (less than 5 pg/ml). A minimum level of 30 pg/ml is about what is needed to eradicate hot flushes and maintain healthy bones and skin. A somewhat higher level of 50-100 pg/ml is needed to maintain arterial and brain health. In men, it is important for maintaining the health of the arteries, bone, brain, skin, and immune system. The bulk of estradiol circulating in a man is derived from the direct conversion of testosterone into estradiol by the enzyme called aromatase. The average estradiol level of a man runs between 20 and 50 pg/ml, but gradually increases from the low to the high end of this range as men get older. DHEA also serves as a source of estradiol. Estradiol is metabolized into estrone and then sulfated by the liver into estrone sulfate.

Progesterone. In females, progesterone is the "progestational" hormone because it aids in maintaining a pregnancy (gestation). There is essentially no progesterone (<0.7 ng/ml) circulating in the first half of the menstrual cycle. Once an egg ovulated, the part of the ovary that released it (called the corpus luteum) starts to produce progesterone for about two weeks. A healthy luteal-phase progesterone level runs between 13 and 25 ng/ml. Progesterone transforms and stabilizes the lining of the uterus that has build up in the previous two weeks so that it is ready for a fertilized egg to implant. If no egg is implanted, then the corpus luteum shrivels up and the progesterone declines after 14 days causing the lining to destabilize and shred off.

One of the first signs of perimenopause is the decrease in the amount of progesterone the corpus luteum produces (<9 ng/ml). These lower levels cannot adequate stabilize the lining and can cause the shorter cycle lengths characteristics of perimenopause. Progesterone receptors occur in the breast as well as in the uterus. There they can modulate the effect of estrogens. Progesterone also has bone and central nervous system enhancing effects.

Follicle Stimulating Hormone (FSH). Follicle Stimulating Hormone is a protein hormone secreted from the pituitary gland whose function is to recruit one of the follicles in the ovaries to undergo the final stages of maturation before becoming an egg and being ovulated. At the beginning of a new menstrual cycle, the FSH level begins to rise. Once a follicle is selected, the hormone inhibin is released from the surrounding cells into the circulation and inhibits further secretion of FSH from the pituitary gland. As a woman approaches menopause, the number of follicles declines and it becomes more difficult to find one to recruit. This causes the FSH level to rise (decreased inhibin production) and can help to indicate how far into the perimenopause a woman is. The best time to draw FSH level is the third to fifth day after the first day of the period. If the FSH is above 10-15, then she is most likely in early perimenopause. An FSH level of 15-25 is usually found in the mid-perimenopause, and late-perimenopause and post-menopause usually are associated with levels above 25. Once a woman has not had a period for 12 months, the FSH is usually in the 60-100 range.

Luteinizing Hormone (LH). Luteinizing hormone is a hormone produced by gonadotropic cells in the anterior pituitary gland. The production of LH is regulated by gonadotropin-releasing hormone from the hypothalamus. In females, an acute rise of LH triggers ovulation and development of the corpus luteum. Usually LH is highest in mid-cycle 6.17-17.2 IU/L.

Cortisol Therapy

Cortisol is one hormone that increases as we age. We know that excess levels are associated with difficulty in losing weight and that high levels can also damage the brain. An extreme form of excess cortisol is Cushing's disease, which usually results from a tumor in the pituitary or adrenal gland. Far more common is Cushing syndrome, which results from someone receiving too much cortisone (prednisone). What I would like to mention here is the other side of the spectrum – adrenal fatigue. Many traditional doctors do not give much credence to this disease. In my clinical experience, this is not uncommon. (It is more frequent in women).

Exposure to prolonged excessive stress (physical, mental and emotional) can manifest with adrenal fatigue. Some common symptoms include:

- Difficulty getting up in the morning
- Continuing fatigue not relieved by sleep
- Craving for salt or salty foods
- Lack of energy
- Increased effort to do everyday tasks
- Decreased sex drive
- Decreased ability to handle stress
- Increased time to recover from injury
- Light-headed when standing up quickly
- Mild depression
- Less enjoyment in life
- Memory is less accurate
- Symptoms worse if meals are skipped
- Thoughts are less focused

Adrenal fatigue can be treated, provided you are diagnosed. Besides lifestyle changes (only moderate exercise), you need to improve your diet and add adrenal extracts, nutritional supplements, and balance all your hormones, especially thyroid. Hydrocortisone (Cortef, 5mg) used in the mid-morning and mid-afternoon is often very helpful in the right client.

Note: Best to measure cortisol at 8am.

Melatonin Therapy

Melatonin is a hormone produced during the night from the pineal gland, located in the brain. It is made from amino acid tryptophan, which is converted into serotonin and then melatonin.

Walter Pierpaoli, M.D., Ph.D., author of *The Melatonin Miracle*, has shown that the life span of mice can be extended by at least 25 percent when given melatonin. His research also showed that old mice can be rejuvenated by transplanting their pineal glands with those of young mice. He believes that pineal gland senses that we are too old to produce around age forty-five and begins to produce less melatonin. This signals all other body systems that the aging process has begun. Some scientists believe that a woman's larger pineal gland is the reason women tend to age more slowly and live longer than men.

Dr. Pierpaoli has found that by supplementing with melatonin, one can mimic a more youthful state. Melatonin will help the immune system by preserving the thymus, reducing levels of the stress hormone cortisol, and raising levels of the sex hormones. In addition, it is a potent antioxidant and can also prolong the lives of people with solid tumors.

Melatonin supplementation appears to be very safe. I recommend using 3mg (slow release form) at bedtime. The slow-release form of melatonin helps you get to sleep and will also keep you asleep. Some people need much more than 3mg, often up to 12-18 mg per day, an amount that should be used only under medical supervision. Vitamin D3 (5,000-10,000 IU) and 500 mg magnesium, when added to melatonin, relieves insomnia. Remember, insomnia increases the risk of dying in the next five years by 400 percent. A few individuals will become excessively drowsy within an hour of taking melatonin, thus I recommend taking melatonin only before bedtime.

Melatonin's benefits may include:
- Protects against cancer
- May slow the aging process
- Improves symptoms of seasonal affective disorder (SAD)
- Preserves circadian rhythm; fights jet lag; helps sleep disorders
- Absorbs free radicals as a broad-spectrum antioxidant

Side effects may include drowsiness ("hangover" effect) and vivid dreams.

Growth Hormone Therapy

Human growth hormone (hGH) consists of 191 amino acids and is secreted from the anterior pituitary. The hGH acts on the liver and almost every other tissue in the body. It stimulates insulin growth factor (IgF-1) (Somatomedin C) production and this in turn has numerous metabolic effects throughout the body. More than 40,000 clinical studies from around the world document the benefits of hGH therapy. GH declines with age in every animal species that has been evaluated. Growth Hormone peaks in late puberty and begins to fall after age twenty; obese men produce less than lean mean.

Growth hormone changes in aging

Function	Change with age	Growth hormone treatment
Adipose tissue	Increases	Decreases
Bone density	Decreases	Increases
Bone mass	Decreases	Increases
Cardiac index	Decreases	Increases
Glomerular filtration rate	Decreases	Increases
Maximal breathing capacity	Decreases	Increases
Muscle mass	Decreases	Increases
Muscle Strength	Decreases	Increases
Renal blood flow	Decreases	Increases

Daniel Rudman, M.D., studied twenty-one healthy men who had low IgF-1 level (a good measure of growth hormone deficiency). Twelve of these men received growth hormone injections over a six-month period, which produced remarkable results. Dr. Rudman showed that signs of aging and those of growth hormone deficiency has a wide range of potent effects on adipose tissue, bones, liver, muscle, the nervous system and more. The broad spectrum of favorable effects helps us understand how different symptoms of growth hormone deficiency appear in adults.

The majority of the effects of hGH work through the IgF-1 pathway. Until recently, hGH was considered a useful therapy only in children suffering from growth hormone deficiency, but in 1996, the U.S. Food and Drug Administration (FDA) approved hGH for use in adult patients.

We only prescribe hGH if our comprehensive evaluation reveals an adult growth hormone deficiency. Prescribing is based on multiple controlled studies in peer-reviewed journals in adherence with FDA regulations regarding the indicated use of growth hormone. An IgF-1 level under 250 ng/ml is generally considered evidence of a deficiency of growth hormone. We like to keep the IgF-1 between 250 and 325 ng/ml.

Insulin-Like Growth Factor 1. Insulin-Like Growth Factor 1 is a large, protein hormone that has a similar structure to insulin. It is the hormone used to assess your level of growth hormone (GH) secretion. Because GH is secreted from the pituitary gland in short bursts throughout the day (particularly during the deep stages of sleep, fasting, and after intense exercise), a random GH level doesn't impart much information about your body's total GH production. In contrast, IGF-1, which is produced in most tissues after stimulation by GH, circulates in relatively steady state throughout the day. Therefore, it is a good measure of your total 24 hour GH production. IGF-1 has potent anabolic (muscle and bone building), immune enhancing, and cardiovascular health-promoting effects. It is a good biomarker of aging because the average IGF-1 declines 15% per decade (in both men and women) starting in the mid-twenties. The normal range shown above is age adjusted i.e., because IGF-1 levels decline with age, it is considered "normal for your age" to have a level considerably lower than the optimal range which we believe is the range that is normal for a 25 years old.

Since hGH is a protein, it cannot withstand a trip through the digestive tract because stomach acid and enzymes will break it down. Thus, hGH needs to be injected, generally subcutaneously every day in the morning. Growth hormone is made by the body mostly at night when we sleep, so we do not want to interfere with this production. We have not had much success using different sprays, creams, and other hGH look-alikes.

There are several factors that can help stimulate growth hormone naturally. First, dehydroepiandrosterone (DHEA) is a precursor and can help elevate growth hormone. Melatonin and Vitamin D3 at bedtime can help improve the quality of sleep and will therefore increase the levels of growth hormone. Better nutrition and resistance exercise can also help optimize growth hormone levels.

Growth hormone benefits may include:

- Fewer wrinkles
- Decreases body fat and increases lean mass
- Increases bone density
- Increases aerobic capacity
- Improves recovery from exercise
- Promotes faster wound healing
- Promotes better sleep
- Increases libido
- Improves cognition and memory
- Elevates mood and sense of well-being
- Stimulates immune function
- Improves cholesterol profile

Side effects of growth hormone therapy include mild fluid retention, joint stiffness/discomfort, may worsen insulin resistance, carpal tunnel syndrome (resolves with lower dose), and hypertension (uncommon). Absolute contraindications for use include anyone with a history of cancer (except skin cancer). Relative contraindications include diabetes mellitus.

There is increasing research that seems to indicate that increasing growth hormone use as one ages might shorten the length of our lives (this does not include use over just a few months). I have recently relied on two substitutes in clients who want growth hormone and prefer to use MK677 or Sermorelin.

MK-677 (Ibutamoren)

Ibutamoren Mesylate (MK677) is a non-peptide growth hormone secretagogue (GHS). A GHS is a compound that can help in promoting growth hormone levels. GHS's can replicate the action of ghrelin, a hunger hormone associated with the body's natural circadian rhythm. In clinical tests, Ibutamoren Mesylate has been proven to increase the release of growth hormone and insulin like growth factor-1.

This all mean that healthy users of Ibutamoren Mesylate can increase lean body mass while lowering the body's LDL cholesterol.

Ibutamoren has been studied for its ability to stimulate the brain activity associated with metabolic action, including the pituitary gland and hypothalamus. Because of its ability to trigger growth hormone, Ibutamoren is a promising therapy for osteoporosis and other aging-related conditions.

MK677 is prescribed for oral use (in tablet or capsule form) in 10 mg or 25 mg dosages. Men suffering from low levels of growth hormone can use MK677 to restore growth hormone levels. Healthy levels of growth hormone are necessary for protein synthesis, body mass growth, body fat management, and healthy sleep.

Three Main Pathways of Action:
1. It indirectly increases GH secretion by inducing GHRH from the hypothalamus.
2. Bind to the GHS receptors in the pituitary and signals GH release.
3. Indirectly increases GH secretion by decreasing somatostatin (the GH inhibiting hormone) from the hypothalamus.

Low growth hormone can be measured by a doctor or recognized by signs you see yourself. Muscle atrophy and onset of obesity are possible signs of low growth hormone, as are low energy and decreased sexual desire. If you are seeing these symptoms, a doctor can help diagnose low growth hormone.

MK677 helps to stimulate growth in virtually all tissues including both bone and muscle. By releasing insulin-like growth factor, MK677 creates the conditions necessary for all growth in the human body. The benefits reported by users of Ibutamoren include:

- Increase tendon repair
- Longer REM sleep and shorter sleep latency
- Increase lean muscle mass
- Stronger bones
- Lower body fat
- Improve endurance and stamina
- Increased IGF-1 levels
- Enhances psychological well-being
- High nitrogen levels in the body
- Increase Free T3 levels

Multiple controlled studies have revealed that long term use of MK677 shows significant improvements in bone mineral density. Bone density is critical for bone health in men, the elderly, and the obese. In repeated studies, Ibutamoren consistently increased and maintained bone density.

Since growth hormone has been proven to support healthy sleep patterns, Ibutamoren is believed to be improve sleep because it increases growth hormone. Studies have shown that MK677 not only improves overall sleep quality but also extends the duration of REM (deep) sleep.

Sermorelin Acetate

As mentioned, hGH replacement therapy has been popular for anti-aging and performance since the 1990's, but use of hGH does not come without risks. Sermorelin is a great alternative as it enables you to obtain the benefits of hGH therapy without the associated risks.

Sermorelin is a growth hormone releasing factor (GHRF) – it is a peptide that contains the first 29 amino acids that make up the growth hormone (191 amino acids) in our body. Sermorelin is known as a "secretagogue" whose substance secreted here is growth hormone – thus is it a hGH stimulator and promotes healthy function of the pituitary gland. Beside the cost savings (hGH costs more than $1,000/month) Sermorelin costs about $225 per month and is safe.

Benefits of Sermorelin
- Improves muscle mass and strength
- Decreases fat
- Improves bone density and joint health
- Improves exercise performance
- Greater heart health
- Increases metabolism and improves carbohydrate metabolism
- Improves skin thickness
- Helps regulate the immune system
- Improves energy and libido

Adequate Supplements

Vitamin D. Vitamin D can be synthesized in the skin from a precursor molecule upon exposure to ultraviolet B light. This is an important source because there is not much vitamin D in the typical diet, although it is found in some fish and eggs as well as vitamin-D fortified foods (e.g. dairy products). As a result, vitamin D deficiency is common in Northern latitudes and in the elderly who often get little sun exposure and have poor diets. Vitamin D is critical for maintaining normal calcium metabolism, bone health, and immune system function. Severe vitamin D deficiency in childhood causes rickets (malformed long bones), but lesser levels of deficiency have been demonstrated to adversely affect the cardiovascular and immune systems and cause osteoporosis. Values in the deficient range and below are associated with an increase in hypertension, general joints and muscle aches, and poor immune system function. Vitamin D exists in two forms, D2 and D3. Some studies have suggested that repletion with vitamin D3 more efficiently raises vitamin D levels than repletion with D2. To raise the level of a person with vitamin D insufficiency to sufficiency, it takes a three month course of 5,000 IU of vitamin D3. A number of studies have suggested that higher levels of serum vitamin D are associated with lower rates of common cancers.

Vitamin B12. Vitamin B12 is a water-soluble vitamin found in animal products such as fish, meat, eggs, fowl, and dairy but not generally in plant foods. As a result, vegetarians are at risk for B12 deficiency unless they eat B12-fortified cereals or supplements. There are several forms of B12, but all contain the mineral cobalt and are called cobalamins. In food, B12 is bound to proteins and must be released by stomach acid, whereas the form in supplements and fortified foods is free and doesn't require acid for release. Therefore, people on stomach acid-suppressing medications (proton pump inhibitors, antacids) can have low B12 levels. B12 is important for red blood cell production, nerve cell health, and DNA synthesis. The anemia of B12 deficiency can be corrected or avoided by a high folate level, but this is a dangerous situation because folate will not prevent the neuropathy that results from B12 deficiency. Therefore, these levels should always be assessed together. People in the lower end (200-400) of the "normal" range can be effectively suffering from B12 deficiency. Pernicious anemia is the autoimmune disorder in which the lining of the stomach does not produce intrinsic factor, the molecule necessary for absorption of B12 from the small intestine once it is released in the stomach. B12 deficiency can raise homocysteine.

Note: In Chapter 4 **Spectracell Labs** can measure more than 31 micronutrients if clients want a more comprehensive picture to better tailor their nutritional needs.

CHAPTER 4: SPECIALIZED DIAGNOSTIC TESTS

1. Fitness Testing
2. Body Fat Percent
3. Functional Tests
4. CNS-VS
5. Keto-Mojo
6. Libra-Pro (CGM)
7. Heavy Metal Testing
8. Omega 3 Test
9. Advanced Immune Testing
10. Vitamin and Mineral Testing
11. Leaky-Gut Test
12. Food Sensitivity Testing
13. Cancer Screening
14. Genomic Sequencing
15. Brain Scan (BrainTap)
16. Advanced Lipid Testing
17. Biotoxin Testing
18. Periodontal Testing
19. CIMT
20. CAC
21. DEXA
22. Sphygmocor
23. Endopat
24. Endothelix
25. Ultrasound
26. CT
27. MRI
28. PET
29. Spect Scan
30. TruDiagnostic

#1-16 are non-invasive, easy to get, inexpensive and can provide additional information to your lab tests.

#17-30 are more difficult to get and are often more expensive but may also be required.

1. Fitness Testing

"When you gain control of your body, you will gain control of your life."

Bill Phillips, Body for Life

Fitness, in its simplest use, means capability. Applied then to the human body, physical fitness refers to the capability of the human body. But capability to do what? Generally, it is capability to maintain a state of health and well-being. Specifically, it refers to aptness for certain tasks. In terms of optimum wellness, physical fitness means the capability to do anything you set your mind to:

- Perform day to day tasks with ease
- Have the capacity to handle any stress
- Have a vigorous sex life
- Play with children and grandchildren
- Run a marathon or triathlon
- Have positive self esteem
- Sleep soundly
- Live without chronic disease

Physical fitness means having capability with utmost integrity; it means you have total control of your body. Originally, physical fitness was simply defined as the capacity to carry out the day's activities without undue fatigue. However, this definition has been insufficient since the industrial revolution because automation and computers have drastically reduced the amount of energy expended on a daily basis while leisure time has increased remarkably. Now, physical fitness is more accurately considered a measure of the body's capability to function efficiently and effectively in work *and* leisure. When you are physically fit, your body is an efficient tool that can be and is used to facilitate completion of your goals — and not just in terms of getting things done, but getting things done well.

Before we got on to the health benefits of exercise, here is a fitness test evaluation you should consider. Remember exercise is perhaps the least used but most effective and studied therapy against chronic disease and age.

Fitness Testing

1. Body Fat

You can get your body fat from an impendence fat machine Omron (model #HBF-514C) or you can calculate your relative fat mass using a simple formula.

2. Relative Fat Mass (RFM)

The RFM correlates well with the percent body fat. A good RFM should be 18–24% for a male and 25-31s for a female.

2. Strength

a. Push Ups

Outline form as true military: hands parallel to shoulders, at a width that feels comfortable (Women can do push ups on knees). Client is to execute slow, controlled, full-range pushups (2-count on the way down and on the way up), lead with the chest, and exhale as they push up.

Perform as many as they can until the fatigue results in poor form or patient fails.

Physically demonstrate both form and pace, if necessary.

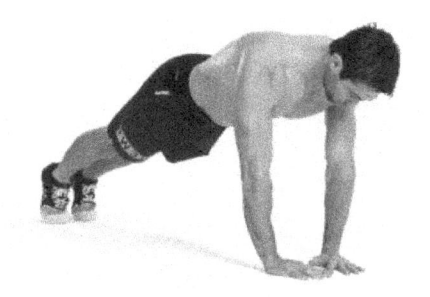

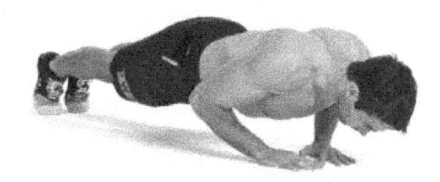

b. Curl Ups

Position client on mat with knees bent, feet flat on the floor, and arms at their sides, palms down. Turn on metronome.

Instruct client to curl up until shoulder blades are up off the floor, with hands sliding forward and fingertips reaching.

Client should use only abdominal muscles, concentrating on shortening the space between their ribcage and pelvis and following the rhythm of the metronome (up on one beat; down on the second). Physically demonstrate if necessary.

Client will perform as many curl-ups as possible until fatigue results in poor form or failure.

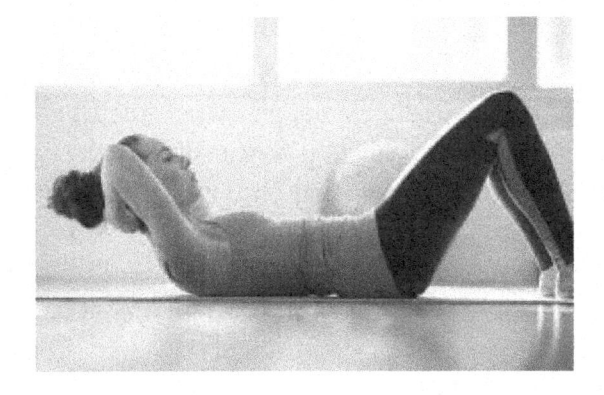

3. Flexibility

a. Flexibility: the capacity of a joint to move through its full range of motion.

b. Absolute flexibility cannot be determined while relative flexibility can be

c. Best methods are subjective visual

d. Flexibility Assessments assess individual flexibility for functional interpretation.

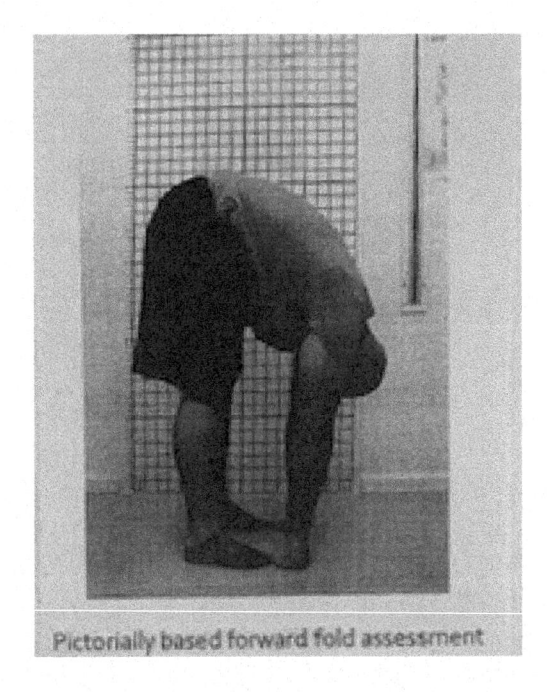

Pictorially based forward fold assessment

e. Flexibility is one of the most essential components of fitness especially in the older client.

4. Posture

a. Maintaining functionality and mobility require the ability to properly load and move the body, which is established through correct posture.

b. Subjective visual is best method.

c. Assessments are performed standing using a central based plumb line

d. Have client stand in front of the Align-a-Bod

e. Instruct client to step forward just enough so they are not leaning on the wall, and to stand with feet hip width, weight equally balanced on both feet, and arms relaxed at their sides. Take anterior and lateral photos.

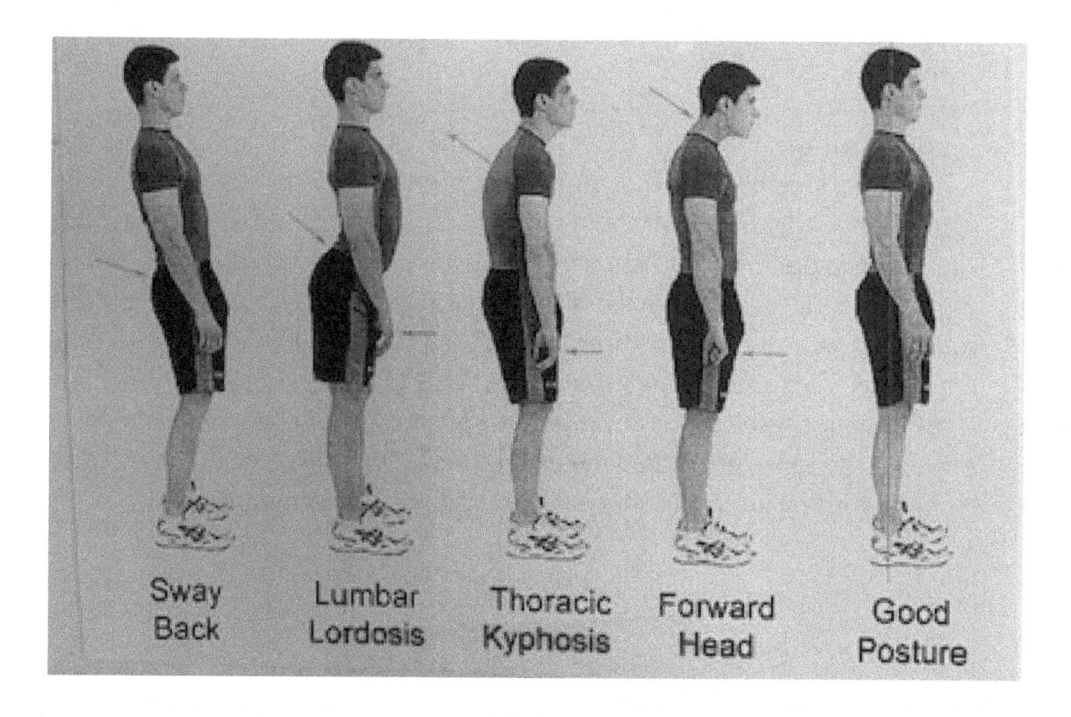

Sway Back | Lumbar Lordosis | Thoracic Kyphosis | Forward Head | Good Posture

5. Balance

a. Stand with your feet 6" apart.

b. Lift one leg and balance with arms outstretched.

c. Now do the same with eyes closed.

d. Record the time in seconds.

6. 3-Minute Step Test

a. **Purpose:** a step test provides a submaximal measure of cardio-respiratory or endurance fitness

b. **Equipment required:** 12-inch (30 cm) step, stopwatch, metronome, stethoscope.

c. Set the metronome to 96 beats (24 steps) per minute and the stopwatch to 3 minutes. (www.webmetronome.com)

d. Demonstrate the following technique to the client: keeping pace with the metronome, step up with your right foot, up with your left, down with your right and down with your left. Allow the client to practice by stepping in time. You can keep track of the client's heart rate in one of two ways—either locate your client's radial pulse (mark with a felt tip) and take it manually, or have your client wear a heart monitor during the test. Advise your client that he should feel free to stop stepping anytime he feels dizziness, light-headedness, chest pain, or nausea or for any other reason. Have your client begin stepping and start the timer, after the time expires, have your client sit down and take his pulse for 1 minute. His score is his resting pulse after 1 minute.

Norms for 3-Minute Step Test
(1-minute Recovery Heart Rate)

		Men			Women		
		15-35	36-55	56-85	18-35	36-55	56-85
Fit (1)	Excellent	70-82	72-88	72-88	72-90	74-95	74-
	Good	83-88	89-98	89-96	91-102	96-105	83-103
	Above average	89-100	99-108	97-103	103-111	106-116	104-116
Average (2)	Average	101-108	109-117	104-113	112-120	117-120	117-122
	Below average	109-117	118-123	114-121	121-128	121-126	123-128
Low Fitness (3)	Fair	118-129	124-134	122-132	129-135	127-137	129-134
	Poor	130-164	135-158	133-152	136-154	138-152	135-151

VO2 Max – The 5th Vital Sign

It provides data on aerobic fitness. VO2 Max is the max rate (V) of oxygen your body can use during exercise. Clients with a VO2 max <16ml/kg/min are in the highest cardio-metabolic risk group. The units used to express VO2 Max are METS.

1 MET=3.5 mlO2/Kg/min

Improvement in VO2 max can occur with weight loss and improved muscle strength.

Scoring Your Fitness Level

	MARKER		FIT (1)	AVERAGE (2)	LOW FITNESS (3)
1	Body Fat	Male	15-20	20-26	>26
		Female	22-28	28-36	>36
2	Strength	Push Up	>12	8-12	<8
		Curl Up	>30	18-30	<18
3	Flexibility		Good	Average	Poor
4	Posture		Good	Average	Poor
5	Balance		>16	10-16	<10
6	Step test (1 min recovery)		depends on age		
	Total:				

Scoring Fitness	Total Points
Low Fitness	>14
Average Fitness	10-14
Fit	<10

2. Body fat Percentage

The body fat percent is more important than body weight. The Relative Fat Mass calculation mentioned earlier correlates well with the body fat percent.

I have a particular gripe about this issue. Most of the doctors I visit in different countries do not measure body fat but simply weight (lbs/kgs) or BMI.

I don't believe you can practice Metabolic Medicine without having some idea of a persons body fat percent.

IDEAL BODY FAT PERCENTAGE AGE CHART

Age (years)	Body fat % Men	Body fat % Women
20	8.5%	17.7%
25	10.5%	18.4%
30	12.7%	19.3%
35	13.7%	21.5%
40	15.3%	22.2%
45	16.4%	22.9%
50	18.9%	25.2%
55	20.9%	26.3%

After thousands of body fat measurements, I can say if a male has a body fat of less than 20% and the female is less than 28%, they are often metabolically relatively healthy. This is not always the case, but it is a pretty good screening test.

Make sure you know your body fat percent. You can buy an inexpensive (4 limb measurements are best) impedance device or get it done at a local gym.

A skilled trainer can also use a caliper measurements to assess your body fat. The 'visceral fat' is the most dangerous, and is the central feature of 'Metabolic Syndrome.'

The gold standard for body fat percent measurement is Underwater Weighing, but if is difficult to locate and inconvenient.

DeXA-Scans – In addition, to body fat and lean mass, it also measure bone mass, it is quick reliable and accurate but more costly than impendence.

Air Plethysmography – or Bod Pod. This is similar to underwater weighing but uses air instead of water.

Waist-Height (Stature) Ratio – This measurements gives an excellent prediction of visceral fat and risk for cardio-metabolic disease.

Although many physical fitness tests can be performed in a physical performance lab most of the tests mentioned below can be done at home.

3. Functional Aging

Functional Aging is the age-associated decline in physical, cognitive, emotional and social functions that may be either so subtle as to be only evident under challenge or so severe to impact daily living.

There are a variety of Functional Aging tests that can give you a good idea of your general vitality and how you are aging. Here are some examples: Many involve the muskulo-skeletal system.

1. Strength and Endurance – 30 sec chair stand and pushups
2. Grip Strength – Dyna monitor
3. Static Balance – 4 stage balance test
4. Flexibility – Alignabod
5. Fitness Recovery – 3 min step test
6. Neurocognitive Function – Walking speed test
7. Functional Mobility – Tug Test
8. Longevity Prediction –
    a. Sit down/Stand up test
    b. General self rated health (GSRH)
9. Cognitive Function – CNS-VS

You can do some of these tests easily at home that can give you important insight into your current health.

5 Home Tests to Check Your Functional Age

1. Walking Speed Test
a. Find a 20-meter long, flat stretch of floor or ground; ideally a finished floor without any obstructions or a flat outdoor paved area.

b. Place some sort of marker at 5 meters, and another at 15 meters from your starting line. This will give you a 5-meter "acceleration zone," a 10-meter zone for the actual test, and a 5-meter "deceleration zone" so you don't subconsciously slow down before the full 10 meters is up.

c. Get a stopwatch, watch with a second hand, or use the stopwatch functionality on your smartphone.

d. At the starting line, start walking as fast as you safely can. Imagine you are trying to reach a bus that is about to pull out.

e. As soon as you cross the first 5-meter marker, start your stopwatch.

f. Keep walking as fast as you safely can.

g. When you cross the 15-meter mark, stop your stopwatch.

h. Slow to a stop in the final 5 meters.

i. Calculate your walking speed by dividing 10 by the number of seconds your stopwatch recorded to get your walking speed in meter/second.

j. Repeat this test another 2-3 times and take the average of the results for a more accurate WS m/s reading.

How to Interpret Your Walking Pace

A 2011 study found that, "In our data, predicted life expectancy at the median for age and sex occurs at about 0.8 m/s; faster gait speeds predict life expectancy beyond the median. Perhaps a gait speed faster than 1.0 m/s suggests better than average life expectancy and above 1.2 m/s suggests exceptional life expectancy."

Age	Exceptional	Healthy	Okay	Worrisome	Poor
20	2.17+	2.02-2.16	1.88-2.15	1.72-1.87	<1.71
20-25	2.05+	1.87-2.04	1.71-2.03	1.58-1.70	<1.59
26-30	2.18+	1.86-2.17	1.66-2.16	1.52-1.65	<1.51
31-35	2.10+	1.77-2.09	1.65-2.08	1.51-1.66	<1.50
36-39	2.02+	1.68-2.01	1.63-2.00	1.50-1.64	<1.49
40-49	1.94+	1.78-1.93	1.58-1.92	1.45-1.57	<1.44
50-59	1.89+	1.72-1.88	1.47-1.46	1.37-1.46	<1.36
60-69	1.75+	1.56-1.74	1.46-1.73	1.26-1.45	<1.25

| 70-80 | 1.61+ | 1.43-1.60 | 1.28-1.59 | 1.12-1.27 | <1.11 |

Additionally, according to a 2013 study, "Each additional minute per mile in walking pace was associated with an increased risk of mortality due to all causes" of 1.8% and, "Those reporting a pace slower than a 24-minute mile [about 1.1 m/s] were at increased risk for mortality due to all-causes (44.3% increased risk)."

2. Strength – Push Ups

The overall fitness of your chest, shoulders, triceps and core is an excellent proxy for your body's function and vitality.

Find a flat space on the floor to do push ups.

(Optional): Set up a metronome or download a metronome app to your phone or computer and set it to 80 beats per minute.

(Alternately) Get a stopwatch, watch with a second hand, or use the stopwatch functionality on your smartphone and place it on the floor where you will see it while doing your push ups.

Get in a push up position (hands on the floor shoulder-width apart, body flat like a plank, elbows at a 45-degree angle to your body).

In time to the beat of the metronome or the count of the seconds on your stopwatch, try to do as many good-form push ups as you can, counting them as you go (lower yourself until your chest touches the ground or your elbows are in line with your shoulders, and remember to keep your lower back flat, not sagging or rounded!).

Keep going until you either reach 80, miss 3 or more beats, or are simply too exhausted to continue.

Record your total number of push ups.

Number of push ups	Likelihood of a Cardiovascular event in the Next 10 years	Rough equivalent age (Men)*	Rough equivalent age (Women)*
0-10	14%	90.5	71
11-20	6%	53	58
21-30	3%	33	45

| 31-40 | 4% | 48 | 53 |
| 40+ | <1% | 17 | 28 |

3. Sit Down-Stand Up Test for Longevity

It is well known that aerobic fitness is strongly related to survival. Claudio Gil Soares de Araujo, a Professor in Rio de Janeiro, has shown also that maintaining high levels of flexibility, muscle strength and coordination also has a favorable influence on longevity.

The test is simple to do. Just sit on the floor from a standing position without using your hands, arms or knees to slow your descent.

Then stand back up—without using your hands, arms, or knees to help boost you back up, if possible. (Hint: Crossing your legs on the way down and the way up seems to help, and loosely holding your arms out to your sides can help with balance.) In the Brazilian study, 2002 men and women ages 51 to 80 were followed for an average of 6.3 years, and those who needed to use both hands and knees to get up and down (whether they were middle-aged or elderly) were almost seven times more likely to die within six years than those who could spring up and down without support. Their musculoskeletal fitness, as measured by the test, was lacking. And musculoskeletal fitness, it turns out, is very important.

- People can score a maximum of 10 points, with 1 point deducted for putting a hand or leg for stability, and half a point docked for wobbling.

- Patients who scored fewer than eight points, were twice as likely to die within the next six years, compared with people with more perfect scores.

- Study claims that musculoskeletal fitness, as assessed by the simple test, can be used to predict death in 51–80 year olds.

Men begin to have trouble doing this test in their early 30s. If you did poorly with this test, all is not lost. These 4 exercises will help fix your endurance, strength and flexibility needed for this longevity test:

1. The squat
2. The glute activation lunge
3. The push up
4. Contralateral limb raises

4. Hand Grip (Dynamometer)

A powerful handshake is often believed to be an indicator of physical vigor. Decades of research have demonstrated that there is more than a grain of truth to this commonly held belief. Standardized handgrip strength, as measured by an instrument called a dynamometer, has been shown in many studies to be a powerful biomarker of aging after the age of 40. (You may have noticed it starts to decline 15 years later than the other biomarkers). In a large study of middle-aged men, those with lower than average handgrip strength were considerably more likely to be dead 25 years later than those with a stronger grip. This is probably because it is a measure not just of the muscular strength of the hand and the forearm muscles, but also the degree of degenerative joint disease and the ability of the central nervous system to exert force.

Hand Grip Strength

Rating*	(lbs)	(kg)
Above average optimum	114-122	30-33
Average	105-113	26-29
Below average	96-104	23-25
Poor	88-95	20-22

5. Peak Flow Meter

FEV1 is a powerful biomarker of aging hiding in the guise of a lung disease test. But both the forced expiratory volume (FEV1) and the forced vital capacity (FVC) tests you take are also important screening tests for lung disease.

Screen for potential lung disease: if your FEV1/ FVC is less than 0.70 then you may have some element of obstructive pulmonary disease like asthma, bronchitis, or COPD. Your provider will ask you to repeat the test if the value is abnormal. From that point, you may move on to more extensive tests or be referred to a pulmonary specialist.

If your FVC is below the normal range for your age, then you may have some element of restrictive lung disease such as emphysema or pulmonary fibrosis.

6. Cognitive Testing (CNS-Vital Signs)

You can perform this simple accurate test at home and complete it in less than 30 mins. On the following page you can see the broad spectrum of domains used to assess Brain function.

Like most neuropsychological or psychological tests, clinicians will recognize, over time, which domains reveal the clinical conditions of their patients. The profiles below may help clinicians evaluate the results. The profiles are based on thousands of well-characterized patients, as well as review of published literature and data.

The Nature of Pattern can vary based on many intrinsic and extrinsic factors: "Over the past century, the syndrome currently referred to as attention-deficit hyperactivity disorder (AD/FHHhHdsasdadaHD) has been conceptualized in relation to varying cognitive problems including attention, reward response, executive functioning, and other cognitive processes. More recently, it has become clear that whereas ADHD is associated at the group level with a range of cognitive impairments, no single cognitive dysfunction characterizes all children with ADHD. In other words, ADHD is not a one-size-fits-all phenomenon. Patients with this syndrome do not fit into any one category and present with widely differing co-occurring disorders – including varying cognitive profiles."

CNS Vital Signs Clinical Domain Description

Neurocognitive Index (NCI)	**Measure:** An average score derived from the domain scores or general assessment of the overall neurocognitive status of the patient. **Relevance:** Summary views tend to be most informative when evaluating a population, a condition category, and outcomes.
Composite Memory	**Measure:** How well subject can recognize, remember and retrieve words and geometric figures. **Relevance:** Remembering a scheduled tests, recalling an appointment, taking medication, and attending class.
Verbal Memory	**Measure:** How well subject can recognize, remember and retrieve words. **Relevance:** Remembering a scheduled tests, recalling an appointment, taking medication, and attending class.

Visual Memory	**Measure**: How well subject can recognize, remember and retrieve geometric figures. **Relevance**: Remembering graphic instructions, navigating, operating machines, recalling images and/or remember a calendar of events.
Psychomotor Speed	**Measure**: How well subject perceives, attends, responds to visual perception information, and performs motor speed coordination. **Relevance**: Ability perform simple motor skills and dexterity through cognitive functions i.e. use of precision instruments or tools, performing mental and physical condition i.e. driving a car, playing a musical instrument.
Reaction Time*	**Measure**: How quickly the subject can react, in milliseconds, to a simple and increasingly complex direction set. **Relevance**: Driving a car, attending to conversation, tracking and responding to a set of simple instructions, taking longer to decide what response to make.
Complex Attention	**Measure**: Ability to track and respond to a variety of stimuli over lengthy periods of time and/or perform mental tasks requiring vigilance quickly and accurately. **Relevance**: Self-regulation and behavioral control.
Cognitive Flexibility	**Measure**: How well subject is able to adopt to rapidly changing and increasingly complex set of directions and/or to manipulate the information. **Relevance**: Reasoning, switching task, decision-making, impulse control, strategy formation, attending to conversation.

Processing Speed	**Measure**: How well subject recognizes and processes information i.e. perceiving, attending/responding to incoming information, motor speed, fine motor coordination, and visual-perceptual ability. **Relevance**: Ability to recognize and respond/react i.e. fitness to drive, occupation issues, possible danger/risk signs or issues with accuracy and detail.
Executive Function	**Measure**: How well subject recognize rules, categories and manages or navigates rapid decision making. **Relevance**: Ability to sequence task and manage multiple tasks simultaneously as well as tracking and responding to a set of questions.
Simple Attention	**Measure**: Ability to track and respond to a single defined stimulus over lengthy period of time while performing vigilance and response inhibition quickly and accurately. **Relevance**: Self-regulation and simple attention control.
Motor Speed	**Measure**: Ability to perform movements to produce and satisfy an intention towards a manual action and goal. **Relevance**: Preparation and production of simple manual motor actions e.g. manipulate and maneuver objects.
Social Acuity	**Measure**: How well subject can perceive, process, and respond to emotional cues. **Relevance**: Spectrum screen, ability to recognize social cues or read facial expressions. Provides insight into inappropriate behavior, decreased inhibition, insensitivity to social standards, and social behavioral regulation.

Reasoning	**Measure:** How well subject able to recognize, reason and respond to non-verbal visual-abstract stimuli. **Relevance:** Problem solving skills, ability to forge insights, discern meaning, and ability to perceive relationships.
Sustained Attention	**Measure:** How well subject can direct and focus cognitive activity or specific stimuli. **Relevance:** How well a subject can focus and complete task or activity, sequence action, and focus during complex thought.
Working Memory	**Measure:** How well subject can perceive and attend to symbols using short-term memory processes (4PCPT). **Relevance:** Ability to carry out short-term memory tasks that support decision making, problem solving, planning, and execution. Enables "right now" responses.

Note: Two of these tests – the Stroop and Symbol Digit Coding are the most age sensitive and helps calculate your brains processing speed and reaction time.

5. What Does The Keto-Mojo Measure?

Glucose and Ketones are primary fuels for the body!

Fatty acids go to the liver that make 3 Ketones.

1. Acetoacetate – small molecule –excreted in **urine**.

2. Acetone – comes as by product from acetoacetate – found in **breath**.

3. BHB – most important – over 10.4 gm/DL in **blood**.

Each person has unique "individual biochemistry" - thus each person has personal data relevant for him/her. The Keto-Mojo can help us test individual foods to assess their effects on our body.

The body will burn either glucose (sugar) or ketones (fat) depending on what's most available.

The GKI – Glucose Ketone Index – allows us to see the ratio between glucose and ketones at any given movement.

Ideal Ketone Level .5-3

If <.5 **not** in ketosis

If .5 to 1.5 in **mild** ketosis – perhaps increase protein or decrease fat

If >3 perhaps not eating enough

Ideal Glucose level 80-90

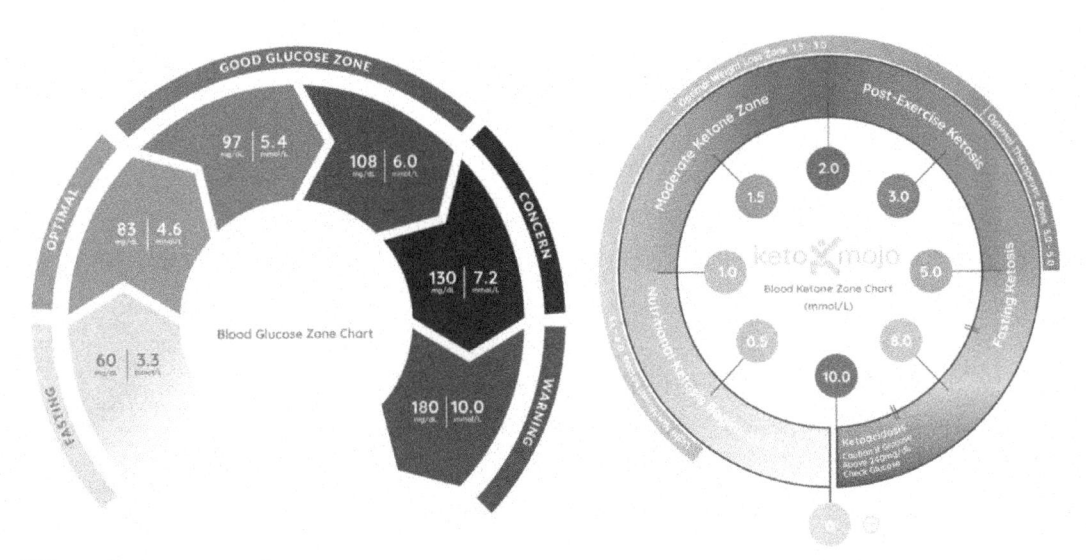

When to measure?
- **In am (Resting)** – same time best.
- Best to wait hr/two after waking due to Dawn Phenomenon especially in diabetics.
- **Just before lunch**
- **1 hour after lunch** – If more than 30mg/dl rise in glucose check for 'bad' food.
- **Just before dinner** – Ketone levels usually highest just before dinner.
- **1 hour after dinner** - Look for excessive rise in blood sugar.

↑ glucose readings	↓ Glucose	↑ Ketones	↓ Ketones
1. X's carbs/sugar	Fasting	Fats (HFLC)	HCLF
2. HCLF diets	HFLC	Exercise (aerobic)	X's protein
3. Rx's (steroids)	Rx's (metformin)	Keto salts	Too little fat
4. Lack of sleep		Keto esters	Resistance Exercise
5. Stress			Stress
6. Resistance exercise			

Note: Glucose and Ketone levels **change throughout the day!**

Fat Adaption

When you become fat adapted your body is able to burn fatty acids without converting them in the liver to ketones.

Resistance exercise happens to increase glucose + decrease ketones.

Aerobic exercise tends to increase ketones.

(1-2 hour after either ketones will often increase)

6. Libra-Pro and Libra-Freestyle (CGM)

A. Libra-Pro (Health Professionals)

- Small and discreet
  The FreeStyle Libre Pro sensor is applied on the back of the upper arm. The sensor is water resistant.

- Very thin filament
  Filament is <0.4 mm thick and inserted 5mm beneath the skin surface to measure glucose levels.

- Up to 14 days of data
  Automatically records glucose level every 15 minutes to provide more insightful patterns.

- Data is blinded from the patient
  No patient interaction with the sensor is required – designed to integrate with patients daily lives.

Daily Patterns with Ambulatory Glucose Profile

AGP offers a standardized visualization of glucose data that is reliable, predictive and actionable. The glucose data, generated by Flash Glucose Monitoring over several days or weeks, are collapsed into a single 24-hour period, creating a view of a modal day.

The view reveals underlying patterns in glucose variability to a greater extent than using HbA1c by itself.

AGP allows healthcare professionals to more effectively visualize and utilize glucose data in the clinical management of diabetes. AGP identifies areas of hyperglycemia, hypoglycemia and glucose variability.

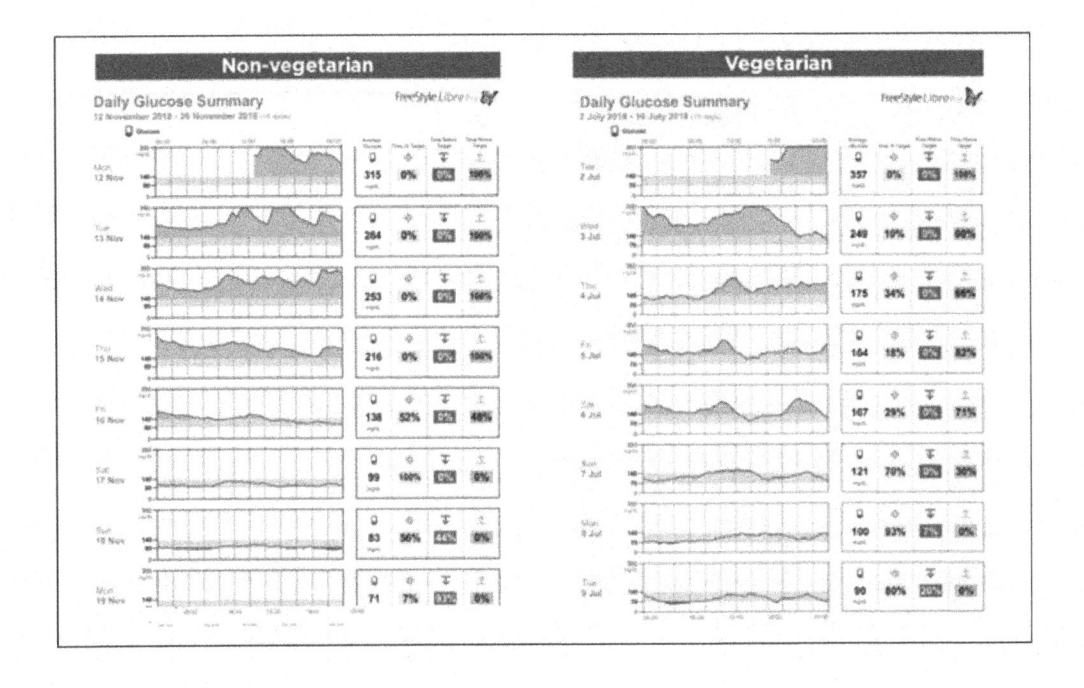

Freestyle Libre Pro Reader

- The reader stays in the clinic
- No need to worry about patients losing or damaging components.
- One reader device starts multiple patients
- Multiple patients per reader minimizes waiting time and scheduling issues.
- Lower costs for the clinic

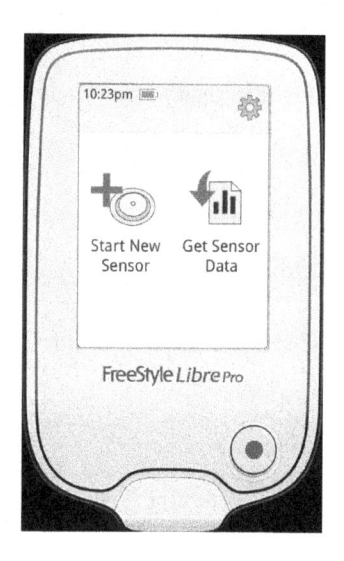

B. **Libra-Freestyle** (Clients)

The FreeStyle Libre Pro Flash Glucose Monitoring System is a professional continuous glucose monitoring (CGM) device indicated for detecting trends and tracking patterns and glucose level excursions above or below the desired range, facilitating therapy adjustments in persons (age 18 and older) with diabetes.

7. Heavy Metal Testing

Urine Toxic Metals

Urine Elements are traditionally used to evaluate exposure to potentially toxic elements and wasting of nutrient elements. Additionally, the comparison of urine element concentrations before and after administration of a chelator can be used to estimate not retention of potentially toxic elements. Subsequent urine element analysis, also following the administration of a chelator are useful for monitoring the efficacy of metal detoxification therapy. Results are expressed per 24 hours or creatinine corrected to account for urine dilution effects.

Metal

Aluminum	Mercury
Antimony	Nickel
Arsenic	Palladium
Barium	Platinum
Beryllium	Tellurium
Bismuth	Thallium
Cadmium	Thorium

Cesium: urine
Gadolinium: urine
Lead: urine
Tin: urine
Tungsten : urine
Uranium: urine

This Test is useful for

Toxic Element Exposure	Gastrointestinal Symptoms
Alopecia	Hypertension
Bone Density	Immune Function
Cardiovascular Disease	Impaired Glucose Tolerance
Depression	Inflammation
Dermatitis or Poor Wound Healing	Kidney Function
Detoxification Therapy	Nutritional Deficiencies
Fatigue	Parkinson's-like Symptoms

8. Omega-3 Testing

The Omega-3 Index is a measure of the fatty acids called EPA (eicosapentaenoic acid) and DHA (docosahexaenoic acid) in your red blood cell membranes, what they do is measure all of your fatty acids in a red blood cell membrane and then take the amount of EPA and DHA over all of the fatty acids and get a percentage. So your result could be 4% or 6% or 8% and so on. For example, if your result is 6%, then that means 6% of your fatty acids are represented by EPA and DHA.

Research has consistently shown that an Omega-3 Index level of 8-12% is linked to better health outcomes for general wellness, as well as for your heart, brain, eyes and joints. However, most people globally have an Omega-3 index below 8%. Let's understand why.

Not surprisingly, most people eating a low-fish Western diet (i.e., typical American diet) have a low Omega-3 index. In fact, according to OmegaQuant research, the average American has an Omega-3 index of around 5%. Younger people tend to have lower levels than older people and men tend to have lower levels than women.

People who eat more fish have higher Omega-3 index levels. Likewise, people who take an omega-3 supplement have higher Omega-3 index levels. In a paper published a year ago by OmegaQuant researchers William S. Harris, PhD, and Kristina

Harris Jackson, PhD, RD, they found that those who ate three fish meals per week and took an omega-3 supplement were the most likely to hit a target Omega-3 index of 8% or higher.

Individuals reporting no fish intake and taking no omega-3 supplements had an average Omega-3 index of about 4.1%, which reflects the average for most Americans and is considered "deficient."

People with a RBC Omega Score >6.8% (cf 4.2%) had:
- 39% lower risk for cardiovascular disease
- 34% lower risk of death from any cause
- 5 year increased life expectancy

Note: Only 1300mg of added EPA/DHA supplements can move your Omega Index from 4.2 to 6.8%.

9. Advanced Immunological Testing

Lymphocytes are the next most abundant white blood cells in the blood stream and can be divided into subsets that have specific functions and characteristic changes with age and disease states.

Many cells of the body are identified by molecule markers that produce out of ("are expressed on" in biology lingo) their cell membranes. These molecules enable the cell to communicate with other cells and receive instructions from signaling molecules, such as those that direct them to a site of infection. Lymphocytes can be subdivided by these "cluster designation" or "CD" markers into Natural Killer (NK) cells, B-cells, and T-cells etc.

T Cell Ratio. T Cell Ratio is calculated by dividing the number of CD4 (Helper T-cells) by the number of CD8 (Suppressor T-cells). It is important because a number of landmark studies of adults older than 60 have shown that when the ratio is less than 1 (more suppressor cells than helper cells) the mortality rate increases by 50% regardless of other medical conditions. This "inversion" of the T-cell ratio occurs because of a simultaneous decline in helper cells with age and an even greater increase in senescent suppressor cells, most often because of longstanding CMV infection. You may wonder why a ratio between 1.5 and 2.5 is optimal while a higher ratio is just healthy. This is the case because in CMV negative adults ratios above 2.5 occur because of a decrease in naïve suppressors –

which can fight off new infections and higher numbers are desirable and not an increase in senescent suppressor cells that occurs in CMV positive adults.

B-Cells. B-Cells are designated by expression of the CD19 marker and are derived from the bone marrow. They are the part of the adaptive immune system that produces antibodies that travel in the bloodstream looking for the antigens found on the surface of pathogens. Through a complex process of DNA rearrangement during maturation, each B-cell produces only one type of antibody. However, the large number of B-cells produced by a healthy young immune system enables it to recognize virtually any pathogen that may invade the body. When an antibody encounters its unique antigen, it initiates the process that results in the invader's destruction. Unfortunately, the number of B-cells decreases linearly with age, which may be one of the reasons older adults are more susceptible to bacterial infections and cancer.

NK Cells. NK Cells carry the CD56 and CD16 proteins on their surface. They are part of the innate immune system because they do not have a T cell-receptor and can kill virally infected and certain tumor cells. Recent research has demonstrated that they are deeply involved with the adaptive immune system. In healthy adults, the function of individual NK-cells decreases with age, but as for neutrophils, their number increases to compensate.

Helper T-Cells. Helper T-Cells Help to orchestrate the functions of other WBCs by releasing cytokines (attracting and stimulating molecules) or by binding to them. They don't actually kill infectious agents or tumor cells (they are not cytotoxic) by themselves but rather recruit other cells to do so. They do not significantly decrease in number with age.

Senescent Suppressor Cells. Senescent Suppressor Cells are suppressor cells that have undergone multiple rounds of cell division, often in response to chronic viral infections. They are no longer able to divide but do not die; far from being inert, they secrete inflammatory cytokines that can damage tissues. In older adults, they can comprise over 50% of the circulating suppressor cells. It is the increase in their number that is usually the cause of the decrease in the CD4/CD8 ratio which defines the major component of the immune risk profile.

Naïve Suppressor Cells. Naïve Suppressor Cells are designated by lack of expression of the CD95 molecule which is involved in apoptosis. They are known as "virgin T-cells" because they have not encountered the antigen for their TCR and can be thought of as the reservoir of cells able to fight off new infections and tumors. They reach a peak of up to 50% of suppressor cells in young adulthood, but gradually decline as the thymus involutes. By the ninth decade, they can circulate in the single digits.

CMV Antibodies (IGG). CMV Antibodies (IGG) is a ubiquitous virus from the herpes virus family that includes the common HSV1 (cold sores), and HSV4 (Epstein-Barr virus-mononucleosis). While it causes up to 15% of mononucleosis cases, most commonly the initial infection occurs without significant symptoms. In the United States, about 60% of the population has been infected with CMV, similar to HSV1 frequency. As with all the other herpes viruses, the infection is quickly controlled, but then remains latent in the walls of the arteries and monocytes. After the initial infection, IGG antibodies specific for the virus are produced and form the basis for the test to detect infection. If the antibody level is above 0.91, then one is considered to have been infected i.e., seropositive. In some studies, higher levels of the antibody titer have been associated with greater morbidity and mortality.

Most physicians still think infection with CMV is benign and only causes problems for neonates or immunosuppressed individuals, but recent studies have demonstrated conclusively that it often causes significant shortening of lymphocyte telomeres and accumulation of senescent T-cells. This results in weakening of the ability of the immune system to fight off infections and can result in earlier death from infection in older adults. The accumulation of senescent T-cells is also a source of increased inflammation in even middle-aged adults. There is currently no treatment for CMV infection, though work continues on a vaccine. It is transmitted sexually and through blood, but also can be acquired through casual contact with saliva if a person is actively shedding virus. We test for it because it is important to know CMV status to properly interpret telomere and lymphocyte subset tests. There is primarily evidence that treatment with a telomere activator can reduce the accumulation of senescent T-cells that occurs after initial infection.

Biomarker	Optimum Range
T Cell Ratio	1.5-2.5
B Cells	100-300
NK Cells	150-250
Helper T-Cells	>900
Senescent Suppressor Cells	<50
Naïve Suppressor Cells	>250

Adapted from PhysioAge

By Joseph Raffaele, MD

10. Vitamins and Minerals

What SpectraCell Measures?

We have measured the functional levels of 31 micronutrients, from vitamins and minerals to fatty acids and metabolites, as well as an overall measurement of antioxidant capacity and immune function to provide you with a powerful tool for optimum health, performance, and insight into any health condition. We provide your unique nutrient status in the following areas:

Vitamins and Minerals

Discover your body's unique vitamin and mineral requirements and the disparities that exist within your makeup.

Energy, Fat and Metabolism

Know how well your body is metabolizing micronutrients for energy production.

Amino Acids

Learn how well your amino acids, the building blocks of protein, are functioning within your cells.

Antioxidant Status & Immune Function

Understand your body's ability to manage oxidative stress and your immune response to infections and disease.

I like the Micronutrient Test Panel from SpectraCell if a more detailed evaluation is needed as correlating micronutrient deficiencies not only slows aging and degenerative disease progression, it can also prevent as well as repair cellular dysfunction, and by extension, disease.

11. Leaky-Gut Testing

Intro

Microbes are everywhere, they live in and on all animals and plants they fill our oceans. Right now, they are on your phone, your hands (even if you wash them), in your drinking water (about a million per one milliliter), in aerosols around you and present at any moment in time. In fact, the ecosystem of planet earth, which is composed of a multitude of habitats, contains different sets of microbes that are essential for proper ecosystem functioning. As the ecosystems of planet Earth have a series of habitats with specific organisms that are essential for a proper ecosystem functioning, so does the human body. On a smaller scale, the human body is also an ecosystem, with different body sites providing different habitats for microbial communities. The microbial communities living in and on our body are collectively called the microbiome and we have distinct microbiomes at each of our body sites.

What is the Gut Microbiome?

The gut microbiome is a collective name for the 40 trillion cells and up to 1000 microbial species that include bacteria, viruses, fungi, parasites, and archaea which reside in our gut. The number of gut bacterial cells is approximately equal to the total number of human cells in our body, so if we consider only cell counts, we are only about half human. In terms of gene counts, the microbiome contains about 200 times more genes than the human genome, making bacterial genes responsible for over 99% of our bodies' gene content of all the microbial communities in the human body, the gut microbiome is by far the most dense, diverse and physiologically important ecosystem to our overall health.

The importance of your Gut Microbiome

Our body lives in a symbolic relationship with the microbes within us, which are significant contributors to our health and overall wellness.

Health: In recent years science has discovered various associations between the microbiome and various health conditions including obesity, allergies, and autoimmune conditions, vascular diseases, gastrointestinal diseases and disorders (IBS, IBD, Crohn's, colitis) and even neurodegenerative disorders and mental conditions. Dietary composition and calorie intake appear to swiftly regulate intestinal microbial composition and function.

Energy: Bacterial breakdown of food provides approximately 10-20% of our energy supplies. The extent of energy extracted from foods depends on the microbiome, and it can differ dramatically between people.

Essential Nutrients: The human body cannot produce all the nutrients required for its proper functioning, so some nutrients must be either acquired from diet, or produced by the gut microbiome. For example, the gut microbiome is a key producer of essential vitamins, like vitamin K and many vitamin B derivatives. Additionally, while many food components are absorbed early in our digestive tract (i.e. the small intestines), some kinds of dietary fiber can only be broken down in the large intestines by specific members of the gut microbiome. Important products of this process include short chain fatty acids (SCFA) that are important for energizing colon cells, have anti-inflammatory properties and are even associated with hunger levels and the release of the hunger hormone, Leptin.

Immunity: There is a growing evidence that the microbiome is regulating our immune system. Our microbiome is important in developing our immune system, helps by making our body tolerate food molecules and harmless substances, helps in recognizing invaders and protects against pathogens by constantly communicating with the immune system in the intestines.

A. Day Two Lab Testing
Taxonomic Hierarchy

	Home Sapiens	*Bacteroides fragilis*
KINGDOM	Animalia	Bacteria
PHYLUM	Chordata	Bacteriodetes
CLASS	Mammalia	Bacteroidia
ORDER	Primates	Bacteroidales
FAMILY	Hominidae	Bacteroidaceae
GENIUS	Homo	Bacteroides
SPECIES	H. Sapiens	B. fragilis
STRAIN		gcf_000297735

Interpretation of your Results

The results in this report are based of identification and quantification of microbial DNA sequences from your stool sample. In some cases, your results are compared to microbiome positions of others in DayTwo's cohort. Therefore, some of the analyses provide relative scores with respect to the entire DayTwo cohort (for example, diversity score of 10 will be given to the individual with the most diverse microbiome in our cohort while a grade of 1 will be given to the individual with the least diverse microbiome in our cohort).

The report includes:

- Ecological analysis of your gut microbiome composition (Richness, Evenness, Diversity)

- Your Microbiome composition in the phylum and genus level

- Important bacterial ratios in the phylum and genus level

- Probiotic Bacteria abundance and composition

- Important Microbiome members abundance

- Unique bacteria from your gut microbiome

- Important nutritional functions by your microbiome (B-vitamins and Short Chain Fatty Acids)

- In cases where multiple stool samples are provided, comparative analyses of the changes are performed so you can track and see how your microbiome changes with time

B. KBMO Diagnostic Lab

Zonulin. Zonulin is a protein that is made in intestinal and liver cells. It is a key biomarker for intestinal permeability and is the only regulator of intestinal permeability that is reversible.

It is estimated that anywhere between 50-100% of food tolerance sufferers have increased intestinal permeability.

Increased permeability (leaky-gut) can be caused by faulty diet, lectins, stress, infections, low stomach acids, medications, artificial sweeteners among other causes.

Elevated Zonulin is found in many Autoimmune diseases like Hashimoto's, Multiple Sclerosis, Psoriasis, Rheumatoid Arthritis and other chronic diseases. In a leaky gut the villi are damaged, there is a poor absorption and the cell junctions are loose. This means that bacteria and other protein fragments can pass through the gut and caused an autoimmune disease through molecular mimicry.

Optimum Level = <40ng/ml

Zonulin IgG Antibody Screening Assay Featuring A Unique Recombinant Zonulin protein.

Measurement in ELISA Assays

1. Cross reactivity: Haptoglobin, Properdin, Complement fragments block Zonulin binding and results in love positivity rates

2. Sample timing: Concentration in serum varies widely during the day which results in difficulty getting an accurate measurement.

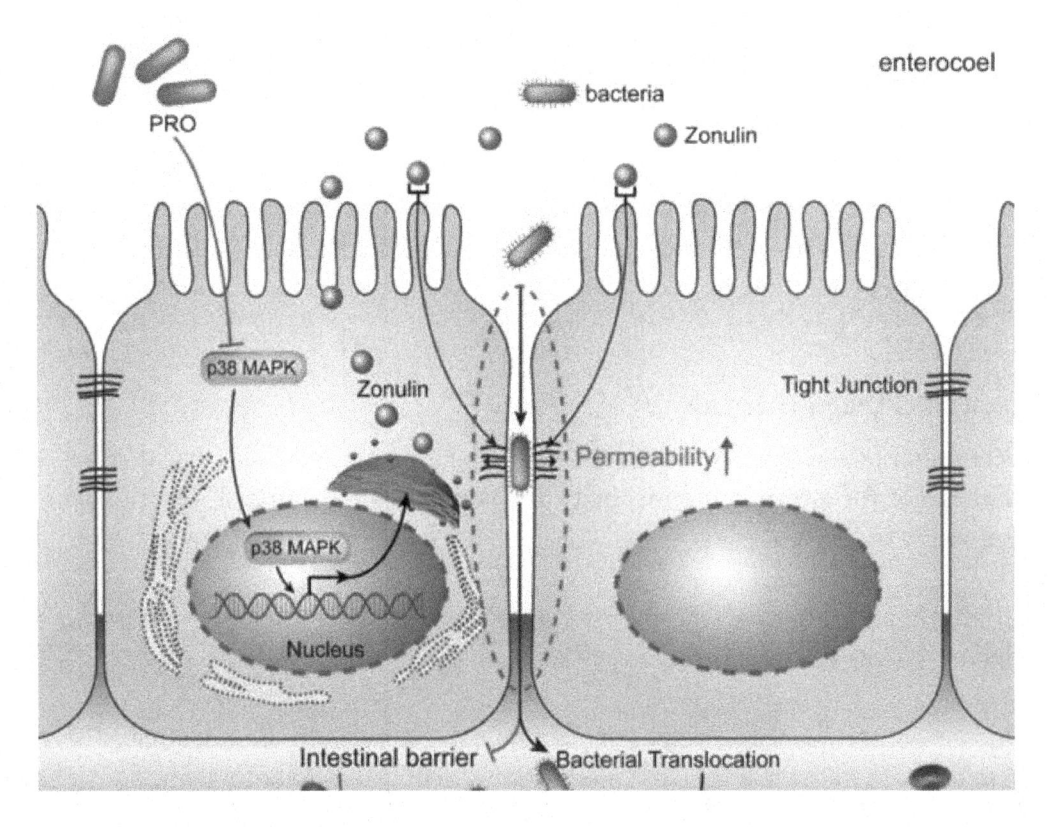

3. Sample type: Serum or fecal?

How KBMO Diagnostics Zonulin IgG Antibody Measurement Resolves Problems with Zonulin Protein ELISA

1. Eliminates Cross reactivity: Unique recombinant Zonulin protein eliminates Haptoglobin, Properdin, Complement fragment cross reactivity.

2. Positivity rate: KBMO assay matches similar positivity rate per Dr. Fasano's Lancet Letter

3. Sample timing: Serum IgG concentration is stable, which assures an accurate measurement.

4. Sample type: Serum or Blood Spot not Fecal

12. Food Sensitivity Testing

We measure up to 176 different foods, coloring and additives. It is the most sensitive food test available using patented technology.

The Food Inflammation Test (FIT Test) measures IGG and complement reaction to a 176 items that cause delayed sensitivity. Food sensitivities begin when food antigens cross the gut mucosa and evoke an immune response leading to the production of IgG antibody and the formation of immune complexes which activate complement. In most cases immune complexes are cleared from the circulation and do not cause any symptoms. However in some people, the immune complexes may lead to various symptoms that can affect almost any tissue or organ. Adverse symptoms include irritable bowel syndrome (IBS), joint pain, chronic headaches, migraines, fatigue, eczema and psoriasis to name a few.

These symptoms usually occur days after the food is ingested which makes the offending food hard to identify without proper testing.

13. Cancer Screening (Liquid Biopsy)

Liquid biopsy tests, which rely on NGS-based circulating tumor DNA (ctDNA) analysis, are a promising and growing area in clinical oncology. Liquid biopsy assays can accurately identify a single tumor variant in the presence of thousands of healthy cells. The most sought-after applications in the ctDNA field include early detection of disease, personalization of therapy, monitoring response to therapy, and monitoring for relapse of disease. Developing and standardizing these ultra-sensitive yet accurate ctDNA-based assays is paramount to ensure the resulting analysis from the test informs clinical decisions reliably. The Galleri Test detects more than 50 types of cancer.

14. Whole Genome Sequencing

Genes are areas of the DNA that carry instructions for the synthesis of proteins.

Every gene carries a specific combination of nucleotides marked with Letters A, T, C, and G where an individual combination determines a specific protein. Sometimes a mutation occurs in the process of DNA replication and the nucleotide sequence is not adequate resulting in incorrect functioning of the protein.

The type of mutation that occurs in the locus of the DNA is called the genotype. We inherit the DNA from our mother as well as our father and we therefore have every gene present in two copies. It is thus possible for a mutation to occur only in one copy of the genes or in both copies or not to occur at all.

The various genotypes are one of the most important factors which make people different. We have different eye color, different skin, talents, we are susceptible to different illness and have unique eating requirements. In genetic analysis where this information is known, heritability is shown.

It is a measure we use to determine how much our genes influence the formation of certain characteristics. The bigger the heritability is the greater influence our genes have and the lower the influence of our lifestyle and environment.

15. Braintap Brain Scan

How we experience our world is governed in large part by the structure and function of our brains and nervous systems. All change starts in our brain.

Neuroplasticity, also known as neural plasticity, or brain plasticity, is the ability of neural networks in the brain to change through growth and reorganization. These changes range from individual neuron pathways making new connections, to systemic adjustments like cortical remapping. We all have the power of neuroplasticity!

With brain wave entrainment, we are using the auditory (sound) and visual (light) senses, engaging the brains natural ability to sync to the environment.

Light – the flickering light works on the optic nerve causing it to follow the frequencies being presented, which positively guides the mind into a calmer and more relaxed state. The drowsy and comfortable feeling you get is actually a natural byproduct of the brain being gently guided into the Alpha and Theta frequencies.

Dr. Nogier light therapy is also delivered through the earphones via auriculotherapy.

To talk about binaural beats, we'll have to travel back in time again to 1839 where an associate professor at the University of Berlin named Dove discovered that if a person is made to hear different frequencies in each ear, he or she can actually hear a third frequency. This extra frequency had the ability to synchronize the brain of a listener into specific mindsets, like Alpha, to guide them into a state of awareness.

These are called binaural beats. They are produced when the brain combines the separate tones and makes a single tone. The single tone pulses according to the brain frequency you prefer, thus creating the perfect, relaxed state for you. Once the central nervous processor relaxes as it synchronizes with the frequency that generates a natural reaction from it, it causes your body to follow suit. Incidentally, this experience is exactly what you get when you use brainwave entrainment technology in combination with a Self-Mastery Technology audio session.

Let's say we want to create the Alpha brain wave state at 10Hz frequency. To do that we'd place 190Hz frequency in one ear and 200Hz in the other. The subject's brain will synchronize to produce the 10Hz, the difference between the two frequencies, and begin to function in the Alpha state. In this state you can visualize your desires and gain the confidence you need to realize your goals in real life.

This ideal state of mind is achievable with brainwave entrainment technology. Through modern science and this light and sound technology, everyone can experience the deep states of Theta that are necessary for weight loss, pain-free childbirth, stress reduction, sports enhancement, or kicking the smoking habit.

Hebb's Law- The basis of Neuroplasticity

One such scientific principal that has been part of biological and neuropsychological science for over 50 years is Hebb's Law named after Donald Hebb, which states that neurons that fire together wire together. This is a theory in neuroscience, which proposes an explanation for growth and change of neurons in the brain during the learning process. It describes how the brain's synapses have the ability to strengthen or weaken over time in response to activity or lack of activity. In other words, if you use it – it will get stronger! If you fail to exercise your brain's abilities, it can get weaker – such as in the aging process, while under stress, or when we fall into routines. Our brains are programmed to be able to strengthen, rewire and grow with practice and repetition of skills.

This theory is the basis of neuroplasticity. Neuroplasticity is the way in which our brain recognizes itself in response to our environment, experiences or injuries. For example, if someone has a stroke and part of the brain tissue is injured, very often the person can still recover the skills lost during the stroke with practice and repetition. Why? Not because the brain health itself in the particular damaged area, but because the brain can adapt to the new situation and create new neurological pathways. The functions previously performed in that region of the brain are simply shifted to other places on new paths.

This can occur when our brain is made to pay attention such as when learning new skills or practicing skills. When we are learning, we are wiring each experience into our brain's computer for future use. This is basically like exercise for the brain. It causes blood to flow to the prefrontal cortex, which allows hormone release, and hormones protect our brains as we age. Think about it – if you exercise your brain each day utilizing brainwave entrainment, you're not only creating new pathways and strengthening your brain each time, but you're also protecting your brain against the ravages of aging.

What is Self-Mastery Technology (SMT)?

We are devoted to helping people correct brain stress better, faster and more permanently. Most people are aware that they need to do something. The problem is they have no idea what that something is. They either don't have the tools or they set the bar too high with unrealistic expectations.

Stress is, unfortunately, a part of all our lives. In the 21st Century it has become a more prevalent problem than ever before in human history. What people need to realize is there is no magic potion to get rid of stress completely. Instead, we should be focusing on finding ways to control stress and cope with it more effectively. We need to accept that we will never be stress free, but we can neutralize it and allow ourselves to rebalance and heal more successfully.

The number one thing you need to know about Self-Mastery Technology is that it allows us to change our belief systems. We have to learn that it's not normal to feel lousy all the time. We have to learn to create a new normal; one in which we feel energized, powerful and able to live life to the fullest.

When individuals undergo SMT, they simple need to lie with their eyes closed and the BrainTap's precise frequencies of light and sound waves are fed into the brain using specially-designed phones and glasses.

Light and sound is used in SMT because it models the structure of the brain. The brain uses light and sound to create our space and place in the universe. When we walk into a room, our brain evaluates the light and sound and projects an image of the room. SMT helps us balance the two hemispheres of the brain using the light and sound waves being projected. When the brain begins to synchronize, the body begins to synchronize along with it. The brain is taken from Beta mode and is guided with a very specific algorithm to create a balanced, full spectrum of brain wave activity.

SMT Audio Processes

Dr. Porter and his team have created several hundred different audio series – each on is specifically designed to imprint positive suggestions into the mind of the user and integrate them so they become positive habits.

As he is fond of saying "You get what you rehearse in life, not necessarily what you intend." Conscious commitment leads to subconscious action. By learning this visualization process using the audio series you will learn to release the things you want and desire. Remember, the subconscious cannot tell the difference between real and imagined, so by using the visualization process to imagine what you want, your problem solving brain will find ways to make it so.

Three problems I have found BrainTap especially helpful for are: -

- Stress
- Sleep
- Weight Loss

Note: I spent more time on this diagnostic and therapy (Brain waves can be recorded before and after treatment to show the remarkable changes that can be made) and have used my friend Dr. Porter's original voice to explain his experiences over the past 30 years.

16. Advanced Lipid Testing

Standard lipid tests may not completely represent your cholesterol-related risk for heart attack and stroke. Do you have diabetes, insulin resistance, or cardiovascular disease? Those conditions may progress even when your low-density lipoprotein (LDL) is at its best level. You may want advanced lipid testing.

In addition to a standard lipid panel that measures total cholesterol, LDL, high-density lipoprotein (HDL) cholesterol and triglycerides, commonly-used advanced tests are apolipoprotein B (ApoB) and LDL particle number (LDL-P). Unlike standard lipid tests, apoB, LDL-P do not require fasting.

When the test might be helpful

When you don't seem to have risk factors to explain your cardiovascular disease and you are not responding to treatment, advanced lipid testing might help, especially if you also have a sibling or parent with cardiovascular disease. An advanced test may reveal that a person with a seemingly normal LDL has a large amount of small, dense LDL particles, which increase risk. A doctor might prescribe a statin like atorvastatin (Lipitor) or pravastatin (Pravachol), or increase the dose of a statin, to reduce all forms of LDL.

17. Biotoxin Testing

A Portable Immunoassay Platform for Multiplexed Detection of Biotoxins in Clinical and Environmental Samples

The proposed SpinDx platform meets the stringent sensitivity and diagnostic time window requirements for effective treatment of individuals exposed to biotoxins. Our system is designed for direct analysis of samples (blood, urine, white powder, etc.) with no additional sample prep required and diagnostic results in less than 15 min. Unique signal and enrichment background suppression elements inherent to the assay approach enable sensitivities unmatched by conventional approaches. But perhaps key to the assay's successful adoption by its anticipated end-users and market is its generic architecture and adaptability to many clinical tests with minimal assay development effort. By this characteristics the proposed diagnostic system not only meets an urgent unment need for biodefense, but also provides revolutionary instrumentation and capabilities for the public health community.

RSC Publishing Jan 2012, Cy Koh and Me Piccini

18. Periodontal Disease (PD) Testing

Oral microbiology is the study of the microorganisms (microbiota) of the oral cavity and their interactions between oral microorganisms or with the host. The environment present in the human mouth is suited to the growth of characteristic microorganisms found there. It provides a source of water and nutrients, as well as a moderate temperature. Resident microbes of the mouth adhere to the teeth and gums to resist mechanical flushing from the mouth to stomach where acid-sensitive are destroyed by hydrochloric acid.

Anaerobic Bacteria in the oral cavity include: - Actinomyces, Arachnia, Bacteroides, Bifidobacterium, Eubacterium, Fusobacterium, Lactobacillus, Leptotrichia, Peptococcus, Peptostreptococcus, Propionibacterium, Selenomonas, Treponema, and Veillonella.

Genera of fungi that are frequently found in the mouth include Candida, Cladosporium, Aspergillus, Fusarium, Glomus, Alternaria, Penicillium, and Cryptococcus, among others.

Bacteria accumulate on both the hard and soft oral tissues in biofilms. Bacterial adhesion is particularly important for oral bacteria. Oral bacteria have evolved mechanisms to sense their environment and evade or modify the host. Bacteria occupy the ecological niche provided by both the tooth surface and gingival epithelium. However, a highly efficient innate host defense system constantly monitors the bacterial colonization and prevents bacterial invasion of local tissues. A dynamic equilibrium exists between dental plaque bacteria and the innate host defense system. Of particular interest is the role of oral microorganisms in the two major dental diseases: dental caries and periodontal disease. Additionally, research has correlated poor oral health and the resulting ability of the oral microbiota to invade the body to affect cardiac health as well as cognitive function.

Look at both the oral microbiota and the entire gut microbiome with our partners. PD may contribute up to 40% of acute myocardial infarctions (MI) as well as neurocognitive disease, diabesity, arthritis and other systemic disease. Similar bacterial signatures are found in the mouth and thrombus of MI patients.

Tanja Pessi
Circulation 2013

MyPerioPath

Early Warning of Oral Pathogens

MyPerioPath is our most widely used test for the detection of oral pathogens that cause gum disease and threaten oral & systemic health. MyPerioPath provides early warning of oral pathogens to enable the personalization of periodontal treatment.

The pathogens tested for in MyPerioPath can help determine if a patient is at increased risk of Cardiovascular Disease, Diabetes, Stroke and birth complications. MyPerioPath test identifies the following type(s) of oral bacteria:

High Risk Pathogens

- Aggregatibacter actinomycetemcomitans
- Porphyromonas gingivalis
- Tannerella forsythis
- Treponema denticola

Moderate Risk Pathogens

- Eubacterium nodatum
- Fusobacterium nucleatum/periodonticum
- Prevobella intermedia
- Campylobacter rectus
- Peptostreptococcus (Micromonas) micros

Low Risk Pathogens

1. Eikenella corrodens
2. Capnocytophaga species (gingavalis, ochracea, sputigena)

Note: There must be much more collaboration between Doctors and Dentists so we can improve both the Healthspan and Lifespan of our clients.

Doctors and Dentists Need To Work Together

19. Carotid Intima Media Thickness (CIMT)

Atherosclerosis and Heart Disease

Heart disease remains the number one health problem in the world today, accounting for more deaths than the next five causes combined – including all cancers.

What we call heart disease is often found in the 60,000 miles of our body's arteries and blood vessels that supply nutrients to the body as much as in the heart itself.

What many think of as "heart disease" actually starts in the body's system of arteries and blood vessels, not the heart. Atherosclerosis, also referred to as arteriosclerosis, is a progressive disease characterized by a buildup of plaque within the arteries leading to what is called hardening of the arteries.

Plaque is formed from fatty substances, uric acid, cholesterol, cellular waste, calcium and fibrin, which build up in the vascular wall. This process is exacerbated by inflammation of the body caused by, among other things, high triglycerides and blood sugar levels.

As individuals grow older, it is normal to develop some thickening of the arteries. However, if the atherosclerosis is advanced, heart disease is likely. Plaque will eventually intrude into the artery and may partially or totally block blood's flow through an artery.

Cardiologists now recognize that plaque composition and stability are more important than size. The danger is with the intermediate stage "soft" plaques that are unstable and vulnerable to rupture, which can cause a heart attack or stroke even though they are not sufficiently large to block blood flow.

Cardiovascular imaging: seeing into your arteries

There is no substitute for looking at the actual state of your arteries with cardiovascular imaging. There are two major tests that look for plaque that are far more predictive of future heart disease and stroke than risk factors can be. There are
1. **Carotid intima media thickness (CIMT)** using ultrasound. CIMT is a measurement of the thickness of the innermost layers of the carotid artery wall by ultrasound imaging. This is where atherosclerosis begins. CIMT tests may also identify soft plaques that are vulnerable to rupture, causing heart attacks or stroke.

Atherosclerosis can be reversed, and because there is no radiation, CIMT can be safely used in all age group and as often as needed to monitor the progression or regression of disease.

20. Coronary Calcium Score (CAC)

This is one of my favorite tests as it is non-invasive, takes 15 minutes and is usually under 100$. Another simple test for seeing into your arteries. I often use this for those clients who have diabesity and men who have erectile dysfunction as ED is often the "canary in the coal mine" and may herald a future heart attack. (The arteries in the penis are the same size as the coronary arteries)

The heart scan uses a specialized x-ray technology called multidetector row or multislice computerized tomography (CT). The scan creates multiple images that can show any plaque deposits in the blood vessels. A heart scan provides an early look at levels of plaque. **CAC's** determines the coronary calcium score, proven the most powerful predictor of future heart attacks. It measures the actual build-up of the calcified plaque in the arteries of the heart. During one deep breath, 35-45 pictures taken of the heart allow you and your physician to understand whether you are at low, medium, or high risk for a heart attack. A zero score is very common and provides reassurance that the chances for a heart attack in the foreseeable future are extremely low.

Already in 2006, leading preventive cardiologists from the Screening of Heart Attack Prevention and Education (SHAPE) Task Force recommended that CIMT and calcium scoring be utilized as the preferred initial tests for determining risk in middle-aged adults. The degree of plaque burden measured by these techniques helps determine how aggressively one needs to address modifiable risk factors and is a window of opportunity to prevent heart disease and stroke from affecting you and your family.

Score	Mortality Risk
<10	Very Low
10-100	Low
101-400	High
>400	Very High

Using AI with CAC scoring (for example the company Cleerly) greatly enhances the images for diagnosis.

21. Sphygmocor and Arterial Stiffness

Why is arterial stiffness important?

Measurements of arterial stiffness in the larger arteries with devices like the Sphygmocor or AngioScan can predict the likelihood of a heart attack or stroke. As the arteries stiffen your heart needs to work harder. With each contraction of the heart a pulse wave travels through the circulatory system. The pressure and volume of this directly effects the wear and tear on organs like the arteries, brain and kidneys.

Measurements that help predict a problem

Aortic Pulse Pressure is the difference between the aortic systolic (ASBP) and the aortic diastolic pressure (ADBP). An optimum Aortic Pulse Pressure is <25.

Augmentation Pressure (AP) is the increment in the aortic pressure above its first systolic shoulder thought to be determined primarily by the pressure wave reflection. This changes with age are seen in the AP Table below.

Augmentation Pressure (mmHg)				
Age	Ideal	Low Range	Mid Range	High Range
20-30	< -3	-3	(-3) -2	>2
30-40	-3	(-3) -2	2-7	>7
40-50	<2	2-7	7-12	>12
50-60	<7	7-12	12-17	>17
60-70	<12	12-17	17-22	>22
>70	<17	17-22	22-27	>27
	No further action required	Manage other factors (eg. Cholesterol, exercise) and add nutritional supplementation to maintain arterial elasticity.	Requires 1 medication and monitoring. (yearly check-ups)	Requires intensive (2 or more) medications and monitoring. (6 monthly check-ups)

Augmentation Index (AI). The AI is an indirect measure of the arterial stiffness and increase with age shown in the table below and is calculated as augmentation pressure divided by pulse pressure x 100 to give a percentage. With increased stiffness there is a faster propagation of the pulse pressure as well as a more rapid effected wave.

Augmentation Index (%)				
Age	Ideal	Low Range	Mid Range	High Range
20-30	<0	0-5	5-10	>10
30-40	<5	5-10	10-15	>15
40-50	<10	10-15	15-20	>20
50-60	<15	15-20	20-25	>25
60-70	<20	20-25	25-30	>30
>70	<25	25-30	30-35	>35
	No further action required	Manage other factors (eg. Cholesterol, exercise) and add nutritional supplementation to maintain arterial elasticity.	Requires 1 medication and monitoring. (yearly check-ups)	Requires intensive (2 or more) medications and monitoring. (6 monthly check-ups)

How arterial stiffness (measured by Augmentation index) can be reduced

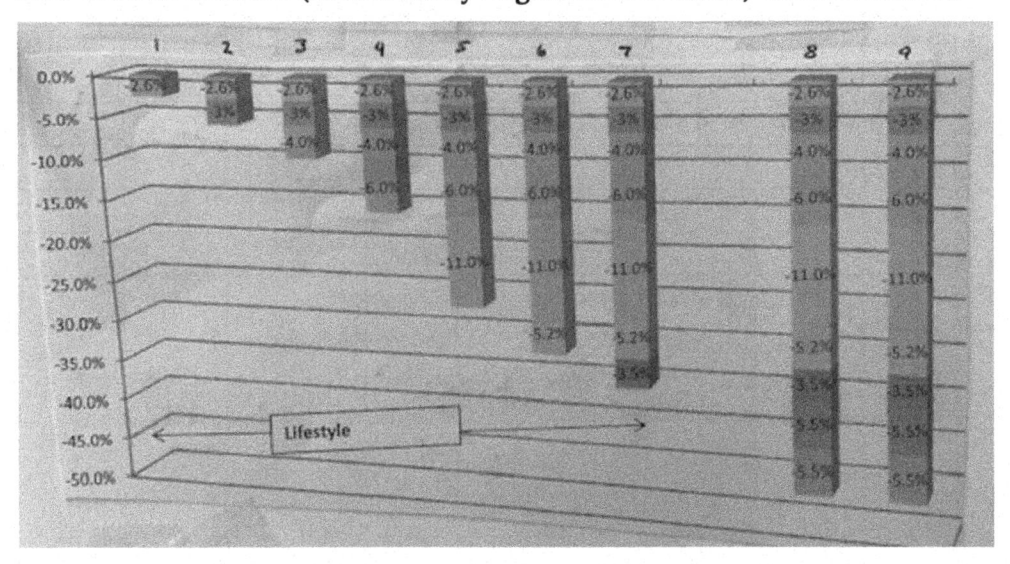

1. Exercise; 2. +Smoking cessation; 3. Reduce fruit juice; 4. + Reduce Stress; 5. + Reduce salt with low sodium diet; 6. +250ml beetroot juice; 7. + fish oil supplementation; 8. + one vasodilating medication; 9. +2nd vasodilating medication

Note: Lifestyle is the **major way** to reduce arterial stiffness and prevent cardiovascular disease.

Both the Sphygmocor and AngioScan together with the Endopat and Endothelix are important **functional tests** which often predate the structural changes we see in the CAC and IMT previously mentioned.

22. Endopat (Endothelial Dysfunction)

For more than a decade endothelial dysfunction has been recognized by the medical community as the critical junction between risk factors and clinical disease. It is the earliest detectable stage of cardiovascular disease. Furthermore, it is treatable, and unlike atherosclerotic plaque that it causes, it is even reversible.

The endothelium is the inner lining of all blood vessels, considered a "super organ" that regulates key natural biological processes that ensures homeostasis, amongst them inflammation, oxidative stress and autoimmune disease.

The endothelium is the thin layer or flat, smooth cells that line the inner walls of the 60,000 miles of blood vessels in the body.

As major negative lifestyle factors begin to increase, oxidative stress damages the endothelial tissue throughout the body by stiffening the veins and arteries, leading to a host of medical concerns, including erectile dysfunction, kidney disease, peripheral vascular disease, heart attack, and stroke.

Numerous studies positioned Endothelial Dysfunction as the "ultimate risk of risk factors" and is the earliest clinical detectable stage of cardiovascular disease.

23. Endothelix (Vendys) – Endothelial Dysfunction

Like the Endopat the Endothelix diagnostic machine, that is also FDA approved, again measures **functional changes** in the endothelium. Clearly we know functional changes occur long before structural changes that often take years to develop which is why I like functional diagnostics so we can intervene early.

Early Diagnosis (Functional Changes)	Late Diagnosis (Structural Changes)
Brachial Vasoreactivity	Coronary Calcium Score
Vascular Compliance (Radial Tonometry)	IMT
Endopat	MRI (measures aortic/ carotid plaque)
Endothelix	Ankle Brachial Index
Sphygmocor	

In simple terms, Vendys® measures vascular reactivity.

Vendys® uses an standard arm-cuff vascular activity procedure, which includes a temporary occlusion of blood flow in the arm. During the cuff occlusion, the lack of blood flow (ischemia) elicits a microvascular dilative response (opening small vessels). Upon releasing the cuff, blood flow rushes into the forearm and hand, not only restoring baseline flow but also resulting in an overshoot (reactive hyperemia). This overshoot causes shear stress in the larger (conduit) arteries, which stimulates these arteries (macrovessels) to dilate and accommodate the increased blood flow.

Vendys® monitors, records and analyzes fingertip temperature during the above cuff occlusion and release procedure. Temperature changes serve as a surrogate marker of blood flow changes that result from vascular reactivity.

24. Ultrasound

Medical ultrasound includes diagnostic techniques using ultrasound, as well as therapeutic applications of ultrasound. In diagnosis, it is used to create an image of internal body structures such as tendons, muscles, joints, blood vessels, and internal organs, to measure some characteristics or to generate an informative audible sound. Its aim is usually to find a source of disease or to exclude pathology.

25. Dexa Scan

A DEXA scan is **an imaging test that measures bone density (strength)**. DEXA scan results can provide helpful details about your risk for osteoporosis (bone loss) and fractures (bone breaks). This test can also measure your body composition, such as body fat and muscle mass.

26. CAT –Scan

CT or CAT-scans are special X-ray tests that produce cross-sectional images of the body using X-rays and a computer CT-Scans are also referred to as computerized axial tomography. CT was developed independently by a British engineer named Sir Godfrey Hounsfield and Dr. Alan Cormack. It has become a mainstay for diagnosing medical diseases. For their work, Hounsfield and Cormack were jointly awarded the Nobel Prize in 1979.

CT scanners first began to be installed in 1974. CT scanners have vastly improved patient comfort because a scan can be done quickly. Improvements have led to higher-resolution images, which assist the doctor in making a diagnosis. For example, the CT scan help the doctors to visualize small nodules or tumors, which they cannot see with a plain film x-ray.

CT Scan Facts

CT scan images allow the doctor to look at the inside of the body just as one would look at the inside of a loaf of bread by slicing it. This type of special X-ray, in a sense, takes 'pictures' of slices of the body so doctors can look right at the area of interest. CT scans are frequently used to evaluate the brain, neck, spine, chest, abdomen, pelvis and sinuses.

27. MRI

Whereas a CT scan uses X-ray a MRI scan uses strong magnetic fields and radio waves – Magnetic Resonance Imaging.

CT scans are more common and less expensive, but MRI scans produce more detailed images. Again, combining AI with, for example, a brainscan by Combinostics, greatly enhances the diagnosis of Alzheimers.

28. PET Scan

A Position Emission Tomography (PET) scan **is an imaging tests that allows a doctor to check for diseases in the body**. The scan uses a special dye containing radioactive tracers. These tracers are either swallowed, inhaled, or injected into a vein in your arm depending on what part of the body is being examined.

29. SPECT SCAN

SPECT (Single photon emission computed tomography) scan

What does a SPECT scan show?

A SPECT scan is primarily used to view how blood flows through arteries and veins in the brain. Tests have shown that it might be more sensitive to brain injury than either MRI or CT scanning because it can detect reduced blood flow to injured sites.

30. TruAge Diagnostic

What is Epigenetics?

If your DNA is your body's big book of recipes, and your genes are carefully describing each step in the many recipes... then epigenetics is your body's way of adding sticky notes to those recipes, to change how much of a step is read, or to skip a step entirely!

Epigenetics is how your body changes gene expression throughout your life. It actually changes how your cells read your own DNA by using little markers that are added or subtracted based on experiences you have and what you inherited from your parents.

Epigenetics is a major factor in Aging, so we use epigenetics to analyze it and create our TruAge Epigenetic Collections.

Discover your True Age. The epigenetic marker we analyze is called Methylation. It is currently the most useful and accurate way to measure the biological processes of aging.

Different areas of our body age at different rates due to differences in cell type and stressors. Since those different aging rates also impact health and lifespan in different ways, we realized there is no single, perfect measurement of aging. No single "Biological Age" number could express all the useful things we can tell you about aging, and how it impact your health!

So, we expanded TruAge into a collection of reports instead of just a single number.

By looking at different aspects of epigenetic aging, along with trait reports and other advanced metrics, we offer a larger and more complete picture of your ever-changing health and lifespan.

Why Measure Age?

Ever wonder why some people look and act 10 years younger than they are? A person's Epigenetic Age matters far more than the number of candles on birthday cake, when it comes to estimating their health and age-related disease risks.

Aging itself, from a biological perspective, is the gradual loss of function at a cellular and molecular level. Epigenetics play a big part in regulating and controlling those functions, so it also plays a big part in aging.

Accelerated Epigenetic Aging is actually the #1 risk factor of developing most age-related chronic disease. With TruAge, you can measure your epigenetic aging, and use our reports as a reference point to begin tracking how your lifestyle changes are affecting your aging at a molecular level.

We measure aging, so you can more effectively manage it.

It is important to remember that computers run on microchips - they are the brains of the machine. The first microchip contained 4,000 transistors that cost a dollar a piece. Today's state-of-the-art microchips feature more than six trillion transistors that cost an infinitesimal fraction of a penny. They're 6,500 times faster and 4.2 million times cheaper.

Since 2012 the computational power of computers has doubled every three and a half months. That is a 300,000 fold increase in the last 10 years. This is why we can masure over 850,000 CPG units on your DNA from 2 drops of blood and quiclky analyze key methylation data that will help reverse your biological age.

CHAPTER 5: HEALING THE TOXIC TRIAD

Diabesity due to "insulin resistance" affects half of the world's population and is responsible for 80% of all deaths and 80% of all healthcare costs. We "connect the dots" for health professionals and clients and show that all the major chronic disease – Obesity, Diabetes, Heart Disease, Strokes, Hypertension, Cancer, Alzheimer's, Kidney Disease, Liver Disease and even Aging itself is due to Metabolic Stress (Insulin Resistance) and Psychological Stress.

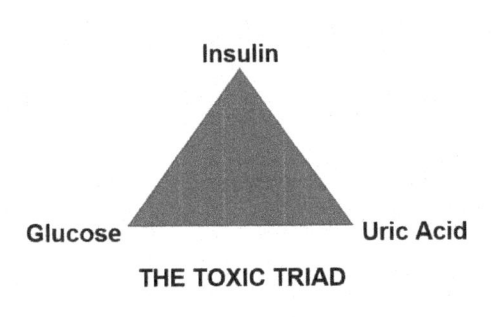

THE TOXIC TRIAD — Insulin, Glucose, Uric Acid

I have included a video from my earlier company, Eternity Medicine, from our work on Diabetes Reversal in the Middle East, Europe, and Asia: https://youtu.be/-HABYjssNEs

A. What Is Insulin Resistance?

The diagnosis of being "insulin resistance" is critical to understanding how we get fat and develop chronic disease.

Every time you eat sugar foods your insulin levels spike which results in a sharp drop in blood sugar. This triggers craving for more sugar which leads to another spike in insulin and so on. When this "up and down" cycle continues over time your cells lose their sensitivity to insulin and ever-increasing levels of insulin are needed to move glucose into cells. This is known as insulin resistance and is the primary cause of cardio-metabolic disease.

The problem is the body was never designed to burn sugar as its primary fuel. Sugar is the body's 'turbo charged' fuel that you need to 'fight or flee' in more urgent situations when we had predators in our close environment like saber tooth tigers. Unfortunately in our modern world, there is an overabundance of sugars and carbohydrates and we rarely get to burn the sugar as fuel hence the obesity and cardio-metabolic epidemic.

New research shows that half the world's population now has "insulin resistance."

Fat around the belly (increased waist size) is a good indication of insulin resistance (apple shape). Most people (80%) who are obese have increased body fat and have insulin resistance. However 40% of normal looking people have insulin resistance – these are the 'skinny fat' or TOFI's (Thin on the Outside but Fat on the Inside).

B. What Does Fructose and A High Uric Acid Tell Us?

1. 21% of the US population have hyperuricemia (high uric acid).

2. Asymptomatic hyperuricemia causes systemic inflammation and chronic disease.

3. Elevated uric acid correlates with diabetes, obesity, high blood pressure etc.

4. High uric acid is responsible for 16% of all-cause mortality.

5. High uric acid causes 39% of total cardiovascular disease.

6. High uric acid is closely correlated with insulin resistance.

7. **Fructose** is the primary cause for elevated uric acid.

8. High uric acid causes gout and kidney disease.

9. **Purines** are also an important contributor to high uric acid.

10. Elevated uric acid leads directly to increased fat storage.

11. **Alcohol** also increases uric acid.

12. Uric acid also important in cognitive decline (dementia).

13. Humans lost the uricase enzyme in evolution (↑ uric acid and turns on fat-swtich).

14. Even a slight increase in uric acid increases mortality in men and women.

15. High fructose (uric acid) silences hormone leptin (helps us stop eating).

16. High uric acid directly increases fat in the liver that leads to NAFLD.

17. High uric acid is correlated with increases in CRP.

18. High uric acid can amplify existing inflammation in the body.

19. Uric acid increases during sleep and reaches highest level at 5am (most heart attacks here).

20. Uric acid a key marker for metabolic syndrome (40% ↑ in all cause mortality).

21. High uric acid increases chance by 2.6 times in Covid-19 patients chance of being on ventilator.

22. Increased uric acid decreases Nitric Oxide (increases insulin).

23. Increased uric acid associated with erectile dysfunction (ED).

24. Increased uric acid decreases autophagy.

25. Increased uric acid diminishes the anti-inflammatory capacity of cell.

26. High uric acid damages our mitochondria.

27. Fructose only found in Nature as fruit and honey.

28. Fructose does not trigger insulin or leptin which leads to obesity.

29. High uric acid correlates with BMI and waist circumference.

30. High uric acid decreases AMPK (antiaging enzyme).

31. Uric acid alters gut health and permeability (↑ pro-inflammatory strains).

32. Uric acid is missing link between fructose consumption and illness.

33. High uric acid keeps fructokinase in activated state (↑ body fat).

34. High uric acid increases free radical formation.

Note: 7, 9 and 11 only sources of elevated uric acid.

Lower Uric Acid By Lifestyle Changes

1. Simple dietary changes (A WFKD is best – Avoid **all** fructose).

2. Decrease purines found in certain seafood, meat, multigrain bread, beer and some legumes and vegetables.

3. Get quality sleep.

4. Get adequate exercise.

5. Avoid drugs which increase uric acid (see below).

6. Nurture your microbiome.

7. Add cherries, coffee, broccoli etc.

8. Add supplements – Vit C, Quercetin, Luteolin, DHEA, Chlorella

9. Time restricted eating (intermittent fasting)

10. Manage stress

11. Drugs like allopurinol will lower uric acid

12. Avoid all sodas (including artificial sugars)

13. Decrease alcohol consumption (1 glass wine/night ok) – avoid drinks made from yeast

14. Psoriasis, Kidney Disease, Thyroid Disease, Lead and Tumor Lysis Syndrome all ↑ uric acid.

15. Metformin inhibits mTOR and decreases uric acid

Top 10 Dietary Rules To Lower Uric Acid Levels

1. Go gluten and GMO free

2. Eat mostly plant based diet

3. No refined carbs, added sugar or artificial sweeteners

4. No organ meats

5. Limit purines especially meat and fish, especially sardines and anchovies

6. Eat nuts and seeds

7. Eat organic eggs

8. Confine yourself to small amounts of dairy

9. Add plenty of olive oil

10. Add uric acid lowering foods, cherries, broccoli, sprouts and coffee

Food and Uric Acid
- Seafood: 31% increased risk
- Red meat: 29% increased risk
- Fructose: 114% increased risk
- Alcohol: 158% increased risk
- Dairy Products: 44% reduced risk
- Soy Products: 15% reduced risk
- Vegetables: 14% reduced risk
- Coffee: 24% reduced risk

Drugs That Increase Uric Acid
- Aspirin (in doses of 60-300 mg daily)
- Testosterone (in testosterone-replacement therapy for men)
- Topiramate (eg. Topamax, an anticonvulsive)
- Ticagrelor (eg. Brilinta, a blood thinner)
- Sildenafil (eg. Viagra)
- Omeprazole (eg. Prilosec, for acid reflux)
- Cyclosporine (an immunosuppressant)

- Niacin (vitamin B; eg. Niacor)
- Acitretin (eg. Soriatane, to treat psoriasis)
- Filgrastim (eg. Neupogen, to treat low white blood cell count)
- L-dopa, or levodopa (eg. Sinemet, to treat Parkinson's disease)
- Theophylline (eg. Theo-24, to treat lung disease such as asthma and chronic bronchitis)
- Diuretics (water pills)
- Beta-blockers (eg. propranolol and atenolol)

Our modern day health problems began just 10,000 years ago in our two million years history due to changes in the diet.

Our Early Ancestors Were Hunter-Gatherers
The Major Dietary Changes Throughout History

The Agricultural Revolution

When: About 10,000 years ago

The Defining Change: The planting and sowing of grains

Health Changes that Occurred As a Result: A reduction in stature; an increase in bone abnormalities and bone diseases; an increase in tooth decay and dental enamel effects; an increase in infectious diseases; an increase in iron-deficiency anemia; a shorter lifespan.

The Industrial Revolution

When: The late 1800's

The Defining Change: The refining of grains and sugar

Health Changes that Occurred As a Result: Nutrient deficiencies; development of degenerative diseases in the masses.

The Fast-food Revolution

When: The mid-1900's to the present

The Defining Change: The combining of refined grains with unhealthy fat, sugar, salt, and/or chemical additives to make convenience foods.

Health Changes that Occurred As a Result: Huge increase in obesity and Type 2 diabetes and chronic degenerative disease.

You Can Completely Reverse Type 2 Diabetes Today

According to the journal of American Medical Association (JAMA) 53% of adult Americans have diabetes or pre-diabetes. In fact, nearly half of the world are fat, diabetic and sick!

That's a sobering thought, but forget the wider statistics for a moment: what does this really mean for you? While genetics certainly plays a part in the likelihood of succumbing to this disease, by and large our Western diet is the main culprit.

And while medications will help you manage the symptoms, I'm here to tell you they are not your best weapon in the fight against diabetes. The easiest and most effective solution lies in your own hands, simply through what you eat.

Basically, you need to stick to a diet of pure, natural foods and ditch everything else. So what should you include and what should you avoid? Here are the 3 most important dietary changes to make: -

1. **Quit Sugar**

According to Dr. Robert Lustig, author of Fat Chance: The Hidden Truth about Sugar, sugar is pure poison. Every time you eat sugary food your insulin level spike, which results in a sharp drop of blood sugar. This triggers cravings for more sugar, leading to another spike in insulin and so on. Over time, your cells lose their sensitivity to insulin and your body becomes insulin resistant which can not only lead to type 2 diabetes but also a number of other problems – think obesity, cardiovascular disease, stroke, and hypertension.

If Lustig is right, our excessive consumption of sugar is the primary cause of increasing rates of diabetes and obesity (Diabesity). Not only has diabesity sky-rocketed in the past 30years but so has most cardio-metabolic disease like heart disease, stroke, cancer, kidney disease, hypertension, Alzheimer's, Autoimmune disease and more. I believe that sugar is far more important than alcohol and cigarettes combined as a cause of disease.

Refined sugar (sucrose) is made up of 1 molecule of glucose plus one molecule of fructose (50/50). Fructose is twice as sweet as glucose. The more fructose in a substance the sweeter it is for example high fructose corn syrup (HFCS) is 55% fructose and 45% glucose and is now known to be more toxic than other sources of sugar.

The fructose component of sugar and HFCS is metabolized primarily in the liver, while the glucose from sugar and starches is metabolized by every cell in the body. When fructose hits the liver in sufficient quantity and speed, the liver will convert most of it to fat. This induces the condition of "insulin resistance" the underlying cause of obesity and diabetes.

If all this sounds a little scary, there's more: high sugar and insunlin levels also cause inflammation of the endothelium, the single layer of cells that line the blood vessels – which kick starts the process that leads to chronic disease. I list over 100 negative effects of sugar in my book, "The Metabolic Miracle."

So what can you do? In addition to the obvious culprits such as sweets, chocolate and cakes, you need to cut out all sweeteners and 'liquid carbs' – fruit juices and sweet, carbonated drinks. And beware the 'hidden sugars' found in processed foods. They may be labeled differently – corn syrup, dextrose, fructose, glucose, lactose, maltose, sucrose, syrup – but they do all the same thing: increase insulin levels. And remember to be careful of fruit, as it's nature's candy.

2. **Go Grain Free (And Use Non-Starchy Vegetables)**

Since the Agricultural Revolution, grains have become a cheap staple of the Western diet. As I pointed out in Metabolic Miracle. "The first mistake in our nutrition occurred over 10,000 years ago (just 400 generations ago) in our 2.5 million history when we began growing grains."

Today, grains are, regrettably, a cheap stable of the Western diet. They can be found in foods you are probably feeding your family on a daily basis, including breads, pasta, cereals, rice, pastries and cakes. However, being high in carbohydrates they are a definite no – no if you want to avoid diabetes.

In basic terms, when you eat anything containing carbohydrates your body breaks the carbs down into simple sugars and releases them into the bloodstream, which again leads to insulin spikes. This causes underlying inflammation throughout the body and triggers a process that cannot only result in chronic disease but can actually accelerate ageing as well. People you hear about who have supposed "good genes" and look great into their 50s, 60s and beyond – you can bet a high percentage of them eat a low-carb diet, too. Want more reasons to avoid grains? They also contain phytic acid, which can prevent our bodies from absorbing important minerals such as calcium, magnesium and iron hurting our bones. And they can contribute to the onset of leaky gut syndrome. This is where gaps occur in the intestinal membrane, allowing undigested food and bacteria to leak from the gut into the bloodstream and react with different tissue to cause autoimmune disorders. Sounds nasty, doesn't it?

The first mistake in our nutrition occurred over 10,000 years ago (just 300 generations ago) in our 2.5 million year history when we began growing grains (the seeds of grass). Together with the domestication of animals (dairy) agriculture marked a dramatic shift in the diet of humans who were predominantly hunter-gatherers before this period.

Wheat and corn, the two most widely grown and consumed grains in the world, have been extensively changed over the past 50 years by agribusiness.

As William Davis MD writes, "Grain elimination is revolutionary appropriate for a member of the species Homo Sapiens; it is consistent with your physiology and metabolism." The elimination of all grains, wheat and others including "healthy whole grains" is essential if you want to optimize your health. (Recent research from Israel reveals we ate mostly meat for 2 million years and only began eating plants 80 million years ago).

Humans about 10,000 years ago found ways to eat the only edible part of the einkorn plant which are the seeds (the outer husk had to be removed once the seed is crushed) and then heated over a fire. Similar processes occurred with maize (corn) in the Americas and rice in Asia.

Dental decay affected less than one percent of teeth before we began consuming the seeds of grass. Modern wheat now accounts for 20% of all calories consumed by humans and these grains are very different from those of the 20th Century.

Paul Dudley White, MD., President Dwight D. Eisenhowers personal physician during his two heart attacks, explained that when he graduated from medical school in 1911, he had never heard of coronary thrombosis (heart attack). But, by 1943, is was responsible for more than 50% of all deaths.

It's worth noting that even after agriculture developed in other parts of the world, the majority of humanity didn't eat gluten-containing grains. In Asia, rice was the cultivated staple, while in Africa sorghum and millet were, and in the Americas, corn.

The main refined grain in the diet today is white flour used to make bread, pasta, pizzas, bagels etc, many snack foods and desserts. Other refined products from the grain/grass family and fructose and sugar are often combined with white flour.

This "complex carbohydrate" of grain is highly digestible and yields some of the highest sugars of any foods and is why the GI of grains are very high even higher than sugar. Thus a lifestyle of "whole healthy grains" will cause repeated highs in blood sugar followed by an increased likelihood of pre-diabetes and diabetes. White flour and whole grains both lead to colon-cancer, heart disease, weight gain and diabetes!

Remember a single slice of pumpernickel bread or a handful of pretzels can cause inflammation for weeks or months before it subsides.

Corn (Maize), oats, triticale, bulgur, teff, sorghum and rice are like wheat, the seeds of grasses. Humans eat more than 200lbs of grains each year (300 loaves of bread). Some of the highest blood sugars you will ever see follow consumption of grains, even if "whole", organic, stoneground, sprouted or sourdough fermented are eaten.

Note: Rice can contain less than 1% protein and thus exerts less potential damage by proteins such as GI toxicity, allergy and autoimmune disease but it does not mean it is harmless as rice raises the blood sugar to the highest of all grains. (Rice has the ability to concentrate inorganic arsenic from the soil). One serving of basmati rice contains 10 teaspoons of sugar.

The agribusiness multinationals of our time control the flow of commodity crops (wheat, corn, and rice) with a lot of say so in government circles. Political contributions are another way agribusiness influences policy, read "Eat More Healthy Grains." Agribusiness is up there with Big Pharma and Big Food!

Research is probing what Hippocrates (the father of Western Medicine) stated thousands of years ago – "All disease begins in the Gut" which was also echoed more recently by the prophet Mohammed. The bacteria that live in our gut (100 trillion compared to our 50 trillion human cells) have co-evolved with all life on earth and have mutually beneficial effects on our gut.

Eating refined carbohydrates alters our gut by encouraging abnormal growth of bacteria in the mouth and small intestine (SIBO) while also causing the growth of pathogenic harmful bacteria in the large intestine. (Remember eating indigestible fiber can result in fatty acids like butyrate that can nourish intestinal cells).

Furthermore, these changes in our gut allow for increased levels of lipopolysaccharides (LPS) to make its way into our circulation causing low grade inflammation throughout our body. Studies on non-Western populations show little inflammation and disease provided the carbohydrates consumed are non-processed and come mostly from fruits, vegetables and tubers.

Eating refined grains thus not only promotes pathological bugs in our gut but also the immunogenic properties of some foods (depending also on a person's genetics) can damage the lining of the gut causing it to become "leaky" which sets the stage for autoimmune disease. Most is due to "molecular mimicry" where certain peptides can cross react with select organs in the body for example:

Gut →	Crohn's Disease
Myelin Sheath →	Multiple Sclerosis
Pancreas →	Diabetes
Joints →	Rheumatoid Arthritis
Thyroid →	Hashimoto's or Graves
Skin →	Psoriasis

For those of you concerned about autoimmune disease an excellent resource is "The Paleo Approach" by Sarah Ballantyne PhD who was herself a victim of autoimmune disease. Another good resource is the "The Wahl's Protocol" by Terry Wahl MD who cured herself of debilitating Multiple Sclerosis.

Common Grains

Grain	Gluten	Lectin
1. Barley	+	+
2. Quinoa	-	+
3. Amaranth	-	+
4. Buckwheat	-	+
5. Teff	+	+
6. Oats	-	+
7. Farro	+	+
8. Bulgar wheat	+	+
9. Rice	+	+
10. Millet	-	-
11. Sorghum	-	-
12. Rye	+	+
13. Spelt	+	+
14. Kamut	+	+
15. Wheat	+	+
16. Corn	-	+

Of all the grains, wheat is the most problematic and is largely due to the fact it has the most gluten. The longer people go undiagnosed with celiac disease the greater the chance of developing autoimmune disease. Luigi Greco, MD listed over 200 symptoms in a paper he presented in the fall of 2000.

Starchy VS Non-Starchy Vegetables

Vegetables can be classified into two main types based on their starch content. Starchy vegetables include potato, corn, peas, and lentils, while non-starchy varieties include broccoli, tomatoes, cauliflower and mushrooms.

Starch is the main type of carbohydrate in your diet. It is made up of a string of glucose molecules that are joined together (it is often referred to as complex carbs).

3. Beware Adulterated Plant Oils While Cooking

The chemical structure of saturated fat has each carbon molecule linked or 'saturated' with hydrogen so when the fat is heated the molecules remain stable. This means they won't become oxidized or rancid with heat. So, saturated fats are the best for cooking at temperatures over 180°C.

Use:
- Butter
- Ghee
- Lard
- Coconut oil
- Avocado oil
- Tallow

Note: High quality virgin 'olive oil' used cold is ideal for salad dressings.

A low carb high fat (LCHF) eating plan (AKA Keto diet) follows the habits of our hunter-gatherer ancestors who stuck to a diet full of natural foods. This eating regime is based on fresh meats, salads, vegetables, nuts, seeds, and eggs.

These types of foods are all easily available in their natural form and can be used to create healthy and tasty meals that contain none of those added chemicals, preservatives and sugars.

The Keto diet has been shown in more than 60 research articles to quickly reverse type 2 diabetes often in just weeks. A Well Formulated Keto Diet (WFKD) is a high fat (70 percent), moderate protein (20 percent), low carb (10 percent) diet. In a recent Virta Study, 262 type 2 diabetics, 60 percent saw their diabetes reverse after completing one year on the program. They came off all medications or took only metformin.

Finally, I believe Intermittent Fasting is also a key to reversing diabetes. This simply means eating dinner early (6pm) and breakfast late (12pm). You can have a bulletproof coffee (coffee with butter/ghee and MCT oil) or tea for breakfast. Here you eat in an eight-hour window while your body switches from its usual sugar burning mode to burning your fat. My preference for the most effective way to restore metabolic flexibility (insulin sensitivity) is a WFKD and time restricted eating of 20/4 hours – usually a meal around 5pm once a day until you heal the toxic triad.

Summary Era I: Recovering Metabolic Flexibility

The first part of your LB100 program is to **Prevent The Preventable** – this is done by healing the **Toxic Triad™.** You must get these 3 biomarkers to **<5**!

- **HbA1c – less than 5**

- **Fasting Insulin – less than 5**

- **Uric Acid – less than 5**

This is primarily done with a HFLC diet and Time Restricted Eating. With this we are able to restore insulin sensitivity in a few weeks. By reversing insulin resistance you are able to increase your Healthspan. Remember by reversing your Biological Age by just 7 years you cut your risk of chronic disease in half.

Those with "insulin resistance" (diabetes or prediabetes) will be given a Continuous Glucose Monitor (CGM) or Keto-Mojo device to help restore insulin sensitivity more rapidly. You will be provided with a personalized nutritional program with select nutraceuticals and pharmaceuticals together with regular support from the physicians and coaches.

Our health professionals are experts in implementing a Well Formulated Keto Diet (WFKD) or other Low Carb diet so that you can regain your metabolic flexibility.

Once you have regained insulin sensitivity we move to Part Two of the LB100 Program – **Delay The Inevitable.** By implementing the latest science in Anti-Aging we target the 10 Hallmarks of aging. Each year we measure your Biological Age and Pace of Aging (PoA) our goal is to help you reverse your Biological Age 20 years!

ERA II Medicine (local)

Reduce Mind-Body Stress (LB100)

Simple can be harder than complex. You have to work hard to get your thinking clear enough to make it simple. But it is worthwhile in the end, because once you get there you can move mountains.

Steve Jobs

Hallmarks of Aging

What follows in chapter 6 to Chapter 15 are the 10 Hallmarks of Aging – 9 described by Carlos Lopez-Otin in June 2013 in a landmark paper. Most researchers believe these hallmarks all play a role in causing aging.

I have added a 10th that was not appreciated in 2013 and that is Microbiome Dysfunction covered in Chapter 7.

I have tried to pull these and other research together with my own experience over the last 40 years, to present a unified theory not unlike the Harvard Researcher David Sinclair.

As space is limited, I briefly cover each hallmark and provide some examples of therapeutic interventions at the end of each chapter.

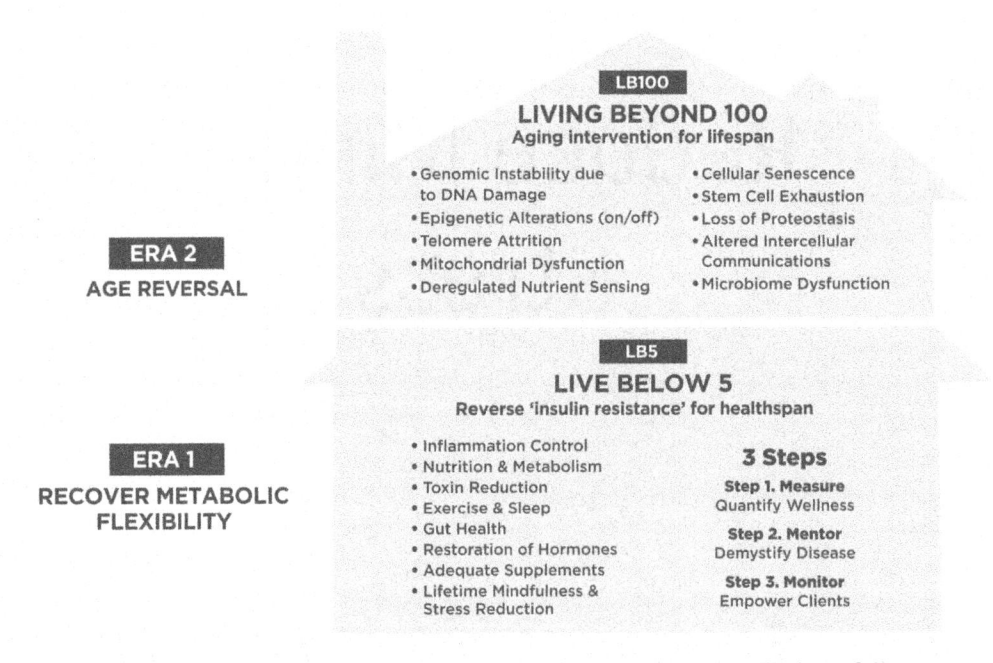

LB100
LIVING BEYOND 100
Aging intervention for lifespan

- Genomic Instability due to DNA Damage
- Epigenetic Alterations (on/off)
- Telomere Attrition
- Mitochondrial Dysfunction
- Deregulated Nutrient Sensing
- Cellular Senescence
- Stem Cell Exhaustion
- Loss of Proteostasis
- Altered Intercellular Communications
- Microbiome Dysfunction

ERA 2
AGE REVERSAL

LB5
LIVE BELOW 5
Reverse 'insulin resistance' for healthspan

- Inflammation Control
- Nutrition & Metabolism
- Toxin Reduction
- Exercise & Sleep
- Gut Health
- Restoration of Hormones
- Adequate Supplements
- Lifetime Mindfulness & Stress Reduction

3 Steps
Step 1. Measure
Quantify Wellness

Step 2. Mentor
Demystify Disease

Step 3. Monitor
Empower Clients

ERA 1
RECOVER METABOLIC FLEXIBILITY

If you don't optimise Level 1, then progressing to Level 2 is likely to fail.

OUR PROGRAMS ARE BUILT ON THE HOUSE OF LONGEVITY

It is useful to remember when medicine first began to become "scientific".

This happened just around the time of the American Civil War in the 1860's.

Prior to that time almost everything physicians did to patients – leaching, bleeding, purging, for example was either ineffective or actually harmful. If we begin at this historical moment and come forward to the present, we can see three distinct historical eras that embody fundamentally different approaches to the nature of illness and healing.

Over 30 years ago my friend Larry Dossey and I independently came up with this 3 Eras of Medicine that we had both taken from John Wheeler and his 3 Eras of Physics. Larry describes these 3 Eras best when he writes as follows:

- **Era I:** the era of physicalistic medicine that dominated medicine from the 1860s to about 1950, and which is still influential.

- **Era II:** the era of mind-body medicine that arose in the 1950s and which is still developing

- **Era III:** our era of nonlocal science and medicine, which is just being recognized

I used Diabesity reversal (Chapter 1-5) as an example of Era I medicine - mostly a physicalistic medicine describable by classical concepts of space and time and happens within the individual(local).

The Hallmarks of Aging and the Chapter on Blue Zones are examples of Era II Medicine – the era of Mind – Body Medicine where the mind is the major factor in healing the individual(local).

Era III Medicine, unlike Era I and II Medicine, is Non-Local and is covered in more detail in Chapter 20.

Before we get to the Hallmarks of Aging it is worth noting the role of local mind on healing. One of the first real accounts of the placebo effect was discovered by an anesthesiologist named D. Henry Beecher, who had run out of morphine in the middle of a German bombardment. Desperate to ease the soldier's pain, Beecher's nurse injected a syringe of salt water but told the wounded man he was getting the powerful painkiller. To Beecher's astonishment, the saline soothed the soldier's agony and kept him from going into shock. After the war Beecher returned to Harvard Medical School to pioneer many "controlled" clinical studies to show that the mind contains the power to heal the body. Traditional medical science still cannot explain what happens here.

Another classic example of how the therapeutic relationship can be manipulated for good or ill was reported by Dr. Bruno Klopfer, who was treating a man for advanced lymphoma in the 1950s. The man was terminally ill, with large tumors throughout his body and fluid in his chest. All medical therapy except oxygen had been stopped, and Klopfer believed the man would die within 2 weeks. However, in a last ditch effort he injected Krebiozen, an experimental drug that was later said to be ineffective. Klopfer describes the amazing results:

"What a surprise was in store for me! I had left him febrile, gasping for air, completely bedridden. Now here he was, walking around the ward, chatting happily with the nurses, and spreading his message of good cheer to anyone who would listen…The tumor masses had melted like snow balls on a hot stove, and in only these few days they were half their original size! This is, of coarse, far more rapid regression than most radiosensitive tumor could display under heavy x-ray given every day… And he had no other treatment outside of the single useless "shot."

Within 10 days the man was practically free of disease. He began to fly his private airplane again. His improvement lasted for 2 months, until reports cropped up denouncing Krebiozen. When he read them, the man appeared cursed, and his attitude and medical condition quickly returned to a terminal state. At this point, Klopfer urged the man to ignore the negative news reports because a "new" super-refined, double-strength product" was now available – a complete fabrication – and injected him with sterile water. The man's response this time was even more dramatic than initially, and he resumed his normal activities for another 2 months. But his improvement ended when the American Medical Association released a report stating that nationwide tests had proved Krebiozen worthless in the treatment of cancer. A few days after reading this statement, he was admitted to the hospital, and 2 days following admission he died.

THE HALLMARKS OF AGING

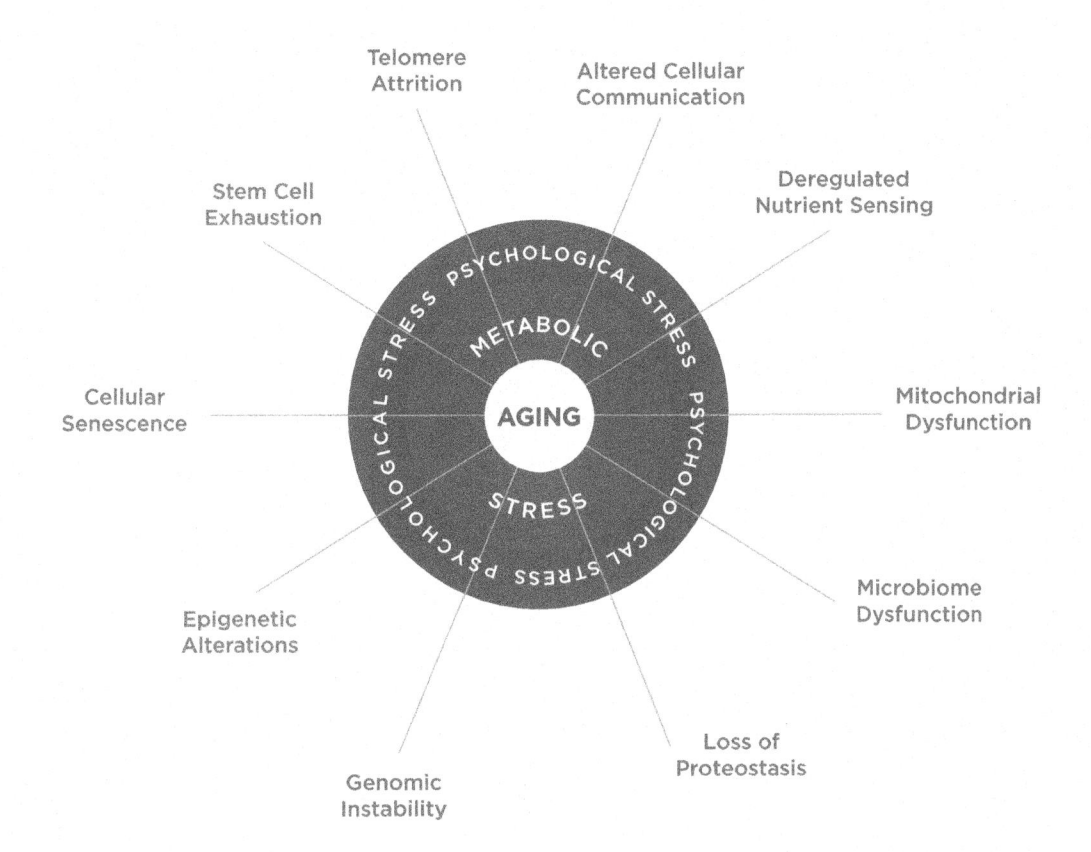

- Telomere Attrition
- Altered Cellular Communication
- Deregulated Nutrient Sensing
- Mitochondrial Dysfunction
- Microbiome Dysfunction
- Loss of Proteostasis
- Genomic Instability
- Epigenetic Alterations
- Cellular Senescence
- Stem Cell Exhaustion

Center: AGING — METABOLIC STRESS / PSYCHOLOGICAL STRESS

WHAT IF ALL HALLMARKS OF AGING ARE DUE TO METABOLIC AND PSYCHOLOGICAL STRESS?

CHAPTER 6: DEREGULATED NUTRIENT SENSING

When nutrients are abundant, cells and tissues respond by storing energy and growing, while nutrient scarcity activates homeostasis and repair mechanisms. In diabetes and obesity, cells are exposed constantly to abundant nutrients, causing the cellular mechanisms that sense nutrients to become desensitized. Deregulation of the nutrient sensing pathway also occurs during aging, and as a result, cells fail to respond properly to the cues that normally regulate energy production, cell growth, and other crucial cell functions.

The 5 most important proteins that regulate metabolism are: -

1. IgF1
2. AMPK
3. mTOR
4. Sirtuins
5. P13 Kinase

We call these proteins "nutrient sensing" because nutrient levels influence their activity.

1. IGF-1 and IIS pathway

Insulin-like growth factor (IGF-1) inhibits the secretion of growth hormone by binding to a special receptor on the surface of a cell. Like insulin, IGF-1 takes part in glucose sensing. Both it and insulin are part of the aptly named "insulin and insulin-like growth factor" (IIS) pathway.

Attenuation of the IGF-1/GH pathway appears to improve lifespan in several model organisms. For example, P13k mice, which have a weakened IIS pathway, live longer. Additionally, FOXO, a transcription factor (a protein that affects the production of RNA), lengthens lifespans in worms and fruit flies by attenuating IIS signaling. In other studies, IGF-1 improves healthspan even when it does not lengthen lifespan.

There's also evidence of harm when IGF-1 activity is high. Higher levels of IGF-1 are associated with increased risk of some types of cancer. This increased cancer risk might be due to IGF's ability to promote pathways that result in increased cell production.

IGF-1 expression and the IIS pathway are a bit of a paradox. Since it looks like turning down the IIS pathway promotes longevity, you might expect the IIS pathway to be very active in old organisms. It looks like high IIS ages us, after all. However, that's not the case. In both accelerated and normal aging models, we see that the IIS pathway decreases.

One explanation for this weirdness is that it's a last-ditch measure of the organism to increase its own lifespan. Yet, this short-term decrease in IIS activity can be harmful. In fact, it is so harmful that IGF-1 supplementation is beneficial. What this seems to point to is a dichotomy concerning the expression of IIS. Overall it looks like turning down the IIS pathway is good over the long term of longevity. This might be because it causes the reduction of metabolism and cell growth, which lessens wear and tear. However, the body's attempt to do the same in later life goes too far and too late to be truly beneficial.

How IGF-1 affects human lifespan is still fuzzy as well. On one hand, there is evidence that reduced IGF-1 activity promotes longevity in people with Laron syndrome (who don't have functional growth hormone receptors), female nanogenarians, and extremely long-lived people. Yet, the epidemiological data is not clear enough to be conclusive on IGF-1's effects on humans. This is partially due to the difficulty of structuring epidemiological studies on IGF-1, as many external factors, such as nutrition, can confound results.

2. **AMP-Kinase**

AMP-kinase is the cells fuel gauge. It knows the difference between full and empty. Anything that increases AMP-kinase like exercise, metformin, berberine will keep the mitochondria functioning optimally and improve insulin sensitivity. Anything that impairs AMP-kinase will drive fat synthesis and worsen insulin resistance. And what food impairs AMP-kinase most? Sugar!

AMP-activated kinase (AMPK) senses AMP (adenosine monophosphate) and ADP (adenosine diphosphate). These molecules are present in higher quantities when nutrients are scarce. Therefore, it is easiest to remember AMPK as a sensor of fasted or calorie-restricted states and catabolism. Molecularly, AMPK acts by adding phosphates to serine and threonine. By doing so, AMPK helps metabolism.

Like sirtuins, higher activity of AMPK has longevity-promoting effects. Metformin, a diabetes drug that appears to have a life extension effect, activates AMPK in mice, worms and humans. Calorie restriction, which is known to increase lifespan in short-lived animals and humans, can also increase the activity of AMPK. Conversely, less AMPK sensitivity due to cellular stress results in oxidative stress, reduced autophagy, metabolic syndrome, more fat disposition, and inflammation.

3. **Rapamycin M-TOR**

M-TOR determines a cells commitment to growth, quiescence or death. M-TOR is the holy grail of cell fats, and the target of many longevity drugs. M-TOR is highly sensitive to diet. A high protein diet will activate M-TOR promoting cell division and growth including insulin sensitivity and the development of lean body mass and cardiovascular health. Activating AMP-K or lowering calories will inhibit M-TOR. M-TOR is thus also dependent on the cells AMPK status.

Mechanistic target of rapamycin (mTOR) is composed of the mTORC1 and mTORC2 protein complexes. It senses amino acids and is associated with nutrient abundance. It is a kinase, which means it adds phosphates to molecules. mTOR is a champion regulator of anabolic metabolism, the process of building new proteins and tissues. In this way, how it functions is similar to the IIS pathway. At any given moment, the metabolism is either breaking down old parts (catabolism) or building new ones (anabolism). Both mTOR and the IIS are part of the anabolic side of metabolism.

Lower activity of mTOR lengthens lifespan in model organisms, such as mice, yeast, worms, and flies. Along those lines, mTOR activity increases in the hypothalami of aged mice, which promotes late-life obesity. With rapamycin, an inhibitor of mTOR, these effects are ameliorated. As is the case with, IIS, lowered expression on mTOR is not always beneficial. Low expression of mTOR can harm healing and insulin sensitivity and can cause cataracts and testicular generation in mouse models.

4. **Sirtuins**

Sirtuins are a family of proteins that acts as NAD(+) dependent histone deacetylases. Histones are the proteins that DNA wraps around. They serve as a way to compact the DNA (which is very long) in the nucleus, especially during cell division. Histones also help control the expression of genes by spatially making some genes more or less available for proteins like RNA polymerase to attach to. On histones, there are lysines, a type of amino acid. It is on these lysines that histone deacetylases remove acetyl groups, which are small molecules. In some, adding or removing acetyl groups helps control the expression of genes, and this is how sirtuins help control gene expression.

Sirtuins detect when energy levels are low by sensing the coinciding increase of NAD+. They also help control catabolic metabolism. Upregulating some sirtuins produces anti-aging or health-promoting effects. However, some sirtuins have only weak effects in some species, which makes summarizing their effects difficult. For example, in worms, higher expression of SIR2 yields only slight gains in longevity. Overexpression of SIR2's most similar counterpart in mice, SIRT1, appears to improve healthspan but not lifespan.

Another mouse sirtuin, SIRT6, seems to promote longevity more robustly. Mice deficient in it experience accelerated aging. Conversely, turning it up results in increased longevity. There is also SIRT3, which has been shown to help the regeneration ability of old hematopoietic (blood and immune cell producing) cells when overexpressed.

In summary sirtuins by stabilizing human DNA will prevent cellular senescence!

5. P13-kinase

Cancer cells import more than 200x the amount of glucose than normal cells do. Cancer cells have very high levels of P13-kinase that opens the glucose floodgates of the cell. Insulin drives cancer cells growth because its how the glucose gets into the cell in the first place – it's the key to the door and P13-kinase determines how wide the door swings open. Insulin & P13-kinase work together to flood the cell with glucose.

You can see how 3 of the 5 nutrient sensors, IgF1, mTOR and P13-kinase are all involved in anabolic metabolism (building tissue) and increase in states of nutritional abundance.

AMPK and sirtuins work to produce catabolic metabolism (breaking down tissues) and increase with nutrient scarcity. Both of these nutrient sensors help longevity.

The Hyperfunction Theory of Aging

In 2006 this new theory of aging had no name. Unlike the classical theory of aging which believes that functional decline is due to the increased accumulation of molecular damage over time, the Hyperfunction Theory of Aging believes instead that it results from the continuation of growth, driven in part, by hyperfunctional signaling pathways such as MTOR.

In 2013 David Gems named it Hyperfunction Theory. Mikhail Blagosklonny is a strong proponent of this theory. Although he doesn't deny that molecular damage can ultimately kill you he feels that increased levels of MTOR is the real culprit of aging and will usually kill you much earlier by causing organ damage.

MTOR is essential for growth earlier in life but its expression in adulthood is a prime example of hyperfunction. By down regulating MTOR earlier in life we can slow down aging later in life.

Rapamycin inhibits cell proliferation, yet preserves (re)-proliferative potential (RPP). RPP is a "potential" of quiescent cells that is lost in senescent cells. MTOR drives conversion from quiescence to senescence (geroconversion). MTOR driven geroconversion is associated with cellular hyperfunction, which in turn leads to organismal aging manifested by age-related diseases. Thus cellular hyperfunction is the essence of cellular aging.

Rapamycin maintains the potential to proliferate enabling these quiescent cells to restart proliferation when needed. To become senescent, an arrested cell must undergo geroconversion with MTOR. MTOR driven geroconverscion is associated with cellular hypertrophy and hyperfunction such as hypersecretion (or SASP), ROS production and lysosomal activation. These hyperfunctions inturn provoke compensatory reactions such as growth factor and insulin resisstance, further lysosomal hyperactivation and loss of RPP. Because most cells within organisms are quiescent, senescence consists of slow geroconversion.

MTOR driven geroconversion is associated with tissue specific hyperfunction which drives age related diseases. For example vascular smooth muscle contraction, hypertrophy and hyperplasic all contribute to hypertension and atherosclerosis and together with thrombosis,clue to platelet hypersecretion, can culminate in stroke or myocordial infarction and loss of organ function. Thus, initial hyperfunction eventually leads to dysfunction and functional decline (aging).

It has been known since 2006 that Rapamycin delays most age related diseases by slowing cell growth and geroconversion in arrested (quiescent) cells.

Many of these hyperfunctions for example hyperglycemia, obesity, diabetes, hyperlipidemia, insulin resistance, hyperuricemia, hypercortisol can be measured by routine medical tests. Such systemic manifestation of hyperfunction also constitutes loss of homeostasis.

Koschei The Immortal and Anti Aging Drugs

In Slavic folkore, Koschei The Immortal was the bonny, thin and lean. I believe that diabesity and hyperinsulinemia are the primary factors driving the Hyperfunction Theory of Aging. We know that if you are obese and insulin resistant you will not be a centenarian! A well formulated Ketodiet and intermittent fasting will decrease MTOR. Exercise is another powerful way to decrease MTOR and improve longevity.

We now employ several AntiAging Drugs that will lower MTOR including Metformin, Berberine and Rapamycin that all decrese obesity and insulin resistance. Rapamycin is best given in low doses and infrequently usually once a week. Rememeber MTOR drives growth early in life and aging later in life. Rapamycin slows down geroconversion: conversion from quiescence to irreversible senescence.

Aspirin, an antiinflamitory agent, decreases proinflammation, a marker of senescence as well as hyperfuncion of blood platelets and endothelial cells.

Since Angiotensin II activates MTOR partially and is involved in aging, Angiotensin Receptor Blocker (ARB's like Losartan) and Angiotensin Converting Enzyme Inhibitors (ACE inhibitor like Lisinopril) - these drugs prolong life by lowering blood pressure and also lower the risk of cancer.

Therapy For Deregulated Nutrient Sensing

1. A Low Carb High Fat Diet (LCHF)

A WFKD and Intermittent Fasting will improve nutrient sensing.

2. AMPK Activation

There is upregulation of NLRP 3 inflamma-some in patients with diabesity. Metformin and Berberine, by activating AMPK and inhibiting the MTOR pathway, will improve autophagy and decrease NLRP3.

3. Sirtuins

A number of the sirtuins appear to improve deregulated nutrient sensing and improve longevity.

4. Rapamycin

Activating AMPK or limiting calories and a high protein diet will lower m-TOR. Recent research indicates the judicious use of Rapamycin once a week in the older client may enhance longevity.

5. Excercise

6. Magnificent 7

Clinical Applications

- Reverses diabetes
- Weight loss
- Lowers HOMA-IR by 50%
- Supports Mitochondrial function
- Lowers risk of heart disease
- Lowers risk of cancer
- Improves memory
- Anti-aging effects
- Protection against Covid-19

Introduction

Relying on lowering blood sugar with medications or insulin will not improve one's health nor will it counteract the effects of diabetes.

In one large study, the Accord study, published in the NEJM in 2008, the 10,000 patients treated with blood sugar lowering drugs or insulin were monitored for the risk of heart attacks, strokes and death. The National Institute of Health (NIH) ended the study early because the medical intervention was leading to MORE deaths, heart attacks and strokes.

Many conventional hypoglycemia drugs actually increase insulin levels—Hyperinsulinemia and not hyperglycemia is what increases the endothelial dysfunction and death.

Turning off the Fat-Switch

The first enzyme in fructose metabolism, fructokinase, consumes ATP while it metabolizes fructose. The process not only generates AMP, but also activates AMPD and intracellular uric acid accumulates damaging the mitochondria. Uric acid is a powerful biological signaling molecule and is recognized as a biomarker of metabolic syndrome.

During summer squirrels accumulate fat in preparation to winter AMPD activity is high.

During winter squirrels switch to burning the fat, and AMPK activity is high.

Unfortunately, unlike animals in the wild and our hunter-gatherer forefathers we are exposed to sugar, grains and processed foods 24/7 365 days a year and never turn off our fat switch. When this happens, the individual loses control of their appetite, develops the Metabolic Syndrome characterized by insulin resistance and increased fat stores, and in addition to hunger has fatigue due to the loss of energy from reduced ATP production in the mitochondria. Eventually, the mitochondria decrease in number and we become "locked in" to our new weight. Our approach to break this deadlock is twofold first to turn off the fat switch by increasing AMPK and secondly to repair mitochondrial biogenesis—to restore energy production.

Our Magnificent 7 product has 4 natural substances that increase AMPK and 3 that increase mitochondrial biogenesis. When this is taken together with a Keto diet and Intermittent Fasting, we can often reverse diabetes in a few weeks and also restore "insulin sensitivity" that will help you finally lose weight and reverse diabesity and metabolic syndrome.

Ingredients that increase AMPK

1. **Berberine** a natural plant alkaloid, has many health benefits and has been used in Indian and Chinese Medicine for more than 2,500 years.

Diabetes Reversal – An excellent therapy to help reverse diabetes including diabetic neuropathy, kidney disease and cardiomyopathy:

- Berberine increases the major nutrient sensor AMPK
- Berberine lowers blood sugar
- Berberine decreases HbA1c
- Berberine decreases post-prandial glucose
- Berberine decreases glucose production in the liver
- Berberine slows the digestion of carbohydrates
- Berberine increases glycolysis –the breakdown of glucose inside cells
- Berberine improves HOMA-IR by 50%
- Berberine increases insulin sensitivity

Note: Berberine is as effective as Metformin which also showed that it significantly lowered the chances of dying from Covid-19.

Weight Loss – Adults taking 500mg of berberine 3 times daily for 12 weeks easily lost on average 5 pounds.

- Berberine inhibits fat storage and lowers visceral fat.
- Berberine reduces the size of fat cells and reduces their number.
- Berberine increases adiponectin and helps normalize metabolic function.
- Berberine enhances "brown fat" that burns energy instead of storing it.
- Berberine increases the number of beneficial bacteria in the gut.

Cardiovascular Health

- Berberine lowers LDL-cholesterol
- Berberine lowers triglycerides (TG)
- Berberine lowers blood pressure
- Berberine lowers inflammation
- Berberine lowers HbA1c

- Berberine lowers oxidative stress in the mitochondria

Cancer Inhibition
- Research shows Berberine leads to cell cycle arrest and apoptosis
- Berberine reduces inflammation
- Berberine helps regulate microRNA's
- Berberine inhibits NF-KB (including P52)
- Berberine enhances chemotherapy

Enhanced Memory and Cognitive Function
- Berberine improves both memory and learning
- Berberine has been found to improve a number of neurodegenerative disorders

Anti-Aging Effects
- Like Metformin, Berberine improves heart health, hypertension, immune functions, low bone density, cognition, diabesity and provides cancer prevention as we age.

2. **Quercetin** is the most abundant flavonoid. It is found in many plant-based foods and is concentrated in the peel. Like Berberine it increase AMPK and reverses insulin resistance.

- lowers blood sugar
- lowers inflammation
- lowers blood pressure
- powerful antioxidant
- lowers risk of cancer
- reduces fatty live disease
- lowers risk of degenerative brain disease
- acts as a senolytic and slows aging
- helps lower the risk of Covid-19

3. Gynostemma pentaphyllum is from the cucumber or gourd family and is widely used in Asia. Extracts of saponins from this plant increase AMPK and a wide range of health benefits.

- lowers blood sugar
- anti-obesity effect and lowers visceral fat and fatty liver
- lowers BMI and weight—lowers ht/waist ratio
- lowers triglycerides and cholesterol
- lowers anxiety
- improves microbiome
- neuroprotective function
- increases longevity (upregulates sirtuins)

4. Epicatechin is a flavonoid from chocolate. A study in the American Journal of Clinical Nutrition found "ingesting 100 grams of dark chocolate resulted in a decrease in blood pressure and improves insulin sensitivity in healthy people." Epicatechin also works by increasing AMPK.

- lowers blood sugar
- stimulates fat burning
- decreases appetite
- lowers inflammation
- lowers blood pressure
- increase blood flow by increasing NO
- inhibits angiogenesis and fat gain
- protects against cancer
- improves bone density
- helps muscle growth
- improves athletic endurance
- reduces aging of the skin
- helps build immunity
- helps neurodegenerative disease
- also increases mitochondrial biogenesis
- increases longevity

Note: The other 3 ingredients of Magnificent 7 increase Mitochondrial Biogenesis (Chapter 8).

CHAPTER 7: MICROBIOME DYSFUNCTION

The human gastrointestinal track hosts more than 100 trillion bacteria and archaea, which together make up the microbiota. The amount of bacteria in the human gut outnumbers human cells by a factor of 10, but some finely tuned mechanisms allows these microorganisms to colonize and survive within the host in a mutual relationship. In it's entirety, the microbiome is estimated to contain 150-fold more genes than our own host genome. The human gut microbiota co-evolved with humans to achieve a symbiotic relationship leading to physiological homeostasis. The microbiota provides crucial functions that human cannot exert themselves while the human hosts provides a nutrient-rich environment. Chaotic in the early stages of life, the assembly of the human gut microbiota remains globally stable over time in healthy conditions and absence of perturbation. Following perturbation, such as antibiotic treatment, bacteria will recolonize the niches with a composition and diversity similar to the basal level since the ecosystem is highly resilient. Yet, recurrent perturbations lead to a decrease in resilience capacity of the gut microbiome. Shifts in the bacterial composition and diversity of the human gut microbiota have been associated with intestinal dysfunctions such as inflammatory bowel disease and obesity. More than specific bacteria, a general destructuration of the ecosystem seems to be involved in these pathologies. Application of metagenomics to this environment may help in deciphering key functions and correlation networks specifically involved in health maintenance. Fecal transplant and synthetic microbiome transplant might be promising therapies for dysbiosis-associated disease.

Metabolic Disease

The prevalence of obesity and related disorders such as metabolic syndrome has vastly increased throughout the world. Recent insights have generated an entirely new perspective suggesting that our microbiota might be involved in the development of these disorders. Studies have demonstrated that obesity and metabolic syndrome may be associated with profound microbiotal changes, and the induction of a metabolic syndrome phenotype through fecal transplants corroborates the important role of the microbiota in this disease. Dietary composition and caloric intake appear to swiftly regulate intestinal microbial composition and function.

The human gut microbiome with its collection of bacteria, protozoa, fungi, and viruses that coexist in our bodies are essential in protective, metabolic, and physiologic functions of human health.

Today, we recognize that the gut microbial balance (dysbiosis) may lead to dysfunction of the host machineries, thereby contributing to pathogenesis and/or progression toward a broad spectrum of diseases. Some of the most notable diseases namely *Clostridium difficile* infection (infectious disease), inflammatory bowel disease (intestinal immune-medicated disease), celiac disease (multisystemic autoimmune disease), obesity (metabolic disease), colorectal cancer, and autism spectrum disorder (neuropsychiatric disorder).

Diabesity

William Davis, M.D. shows how our modern wheat is very different from 80 years ago. Norman Borlaug genetically modified the wheat which produced semi-dwarf high yield wheat which helped avert a global famine. Borlaug received a Nobel Prize for this. However, since this time autoimmune disease has increased by a factor of 4 over the past two decades due to unintended consequences.

We now realize that the new paradigm for autoimmunity is made up of 3 ingredients:

1. you must be genetically predisposed.
2. an environmental factor that triggers the immune response.
3. a breach of the barrier so 1+2 can interact.

Some of us, when we eat wheat and don't have a genetic predisposition, the tight junction (TJ) opens for a short time only as compared with a celiac client where the TJ stays open much longer and much more material comes through from the environment and interacts with the immune system.

Opiate activity of semi-digested peptide fragments from the gliadin protein stimulates the appetite centers of the brain, causing constant hunger resulting in increased calorie intake (to the tune of an extra 440 cals/day). Little wonder why half the world is fat, diabetic and sick. Amylopectin found in wheat also causes hyperglycemia and insulin resistance which makes matters even worse.

In summary:
- Wheat protein fragments (peptides) act as opiates and increase appetite.

- Wheat amylopectin raises blood sugar higher than most foods.
- Wheat germ agglutin (a lectin) is directly toxic to the GI tract.
- Most wheat today is sprayed with glyphosate which is also extremely toxic to the GI tract.

Modern wheat is inherently unhealthy and should be eliminated from the diet. This applies to most people, not just to celiac clients and those who are gluten sensitive.

A number of years ago, I went to Amsterdam and visited with Prof. Max Niewdorp who was one of the first to use Fecal Microbiome Transplants (FMT) that showed he could transplant fecal microbes from young healthy donors that would increase insulin sensitivity in overweight individuals with Metabolic Syndrome and type 2 diabetes. Many of those treated with FMT were able to lose weight and reverse their diabetes.

Another important observation is when lipopolysaccharide (LPS), the primary component of the outer membrane of gram negative bacteria, leak from the gut into the blood they cause a low grade inflammation that can contribute to insulin resistance and diabesity.

The ratio of certain bacteria in the gut are also important for who gets obesity and diabetes. Fermicutes/Bacteroidetes is one such ratio. Increased obesity is seen when there is a larger number of Fermicutes and relatively less Bacteroidetes.

Clearly the gut microbiome can increase 'insulin resistance' which will increase most cardio-metabolic disease like heart disease, cancer and Alzheimer's. Colorectal cancer, for example, is the third most common cancer worldwide and research shows that the gut microbiome and inflammation gradually form a microenvironment that is associated with the development of colorectal cancer.

Gut bacteria (C. elegans) studied by Meng Wang and other researchers believe that the genetic composition of our microbiome is also important for longevity. Stay tuned to this exciting topic.

Autoimmune Disease

The human microbiome has emerged as the crucial moderator in the interactions between food and our body more than any other environmental factor. It is now recognized that the gut microbiome can change our mind and our body or switch on a wide range of diseases including cardio-metabolic disease, diabesity, cancer, autoimmune disease and allergies.

We tend to think more about our dogs and cats than we do about our real pets—our microbiome.

1. Wheat Gluten and Autoimmune Disease

William Davis, M.D. and Alessio Fasano, M.D. are two well-known doctors who have proved conclusively the connection between wheat, leaky-gut and autoimmune disease. For more than a century we have believed that the GI tract was a closed tube representing a sealed barrier that keeps 'bad things' like bacteria and larger macromolecules out of our body.

It is a major shift in the last decade to recognize the concept of a "leaky gut" and autoimmune disease (over 140 at last count). 1 in 4 people today are thought to have autoimmune disease like thyroid disease, psoriasis, multiple sclerosis, diabetes, rheumatoid arthritis, etc.

Electron microscopy from Japan first showed that the Tight Junction (TJ) between GI mucosal epithelial cells open and close in response to Zonulin.

Thanks to Alessio Fasano who discovered the Zonulin molecule, we now understand how leaky-gut comes about.

In genetically susceptible individuals, possessing the HLADQ gene, an excessive amount of Zonulin is released upon ingestion of gliadin, a protein found in wheat products. The excess Zonulin then opens the TJ between the GI epithelial cells allowing large macromolecules and bacteria to leak through together with food particles, proteins and peptide fragments which enter the blood stream.

These particles are recognized as foreign by our immune system which produces an inflammatory infiltrate in the wall of the GI tract and antibodies against certain tissues in the body through "molecular mimicry" and produces different autoimmune diseases.

For example, Grave's Disease, a thyroid condition, is thought to result from cross reactivity to the Yersinia organism that crosses over and enters the blood.

Autoimmune disease was thought by doctors not to be curable and was often managed by immunosuppressive drugs, which are often toxic to us. The simple fact is that most autoimmune disease can be cured by elimination of wheat from the gut.

I would like to end this with a quote from Alessio Fasano, MD, which gives an idea of the critical role the microbiome plays in health and longevity.

"The primary functions of the gastrointestinal tract have traditionally been perceived to be limited to the digestion and absorption of nutrients and to electrolytes and water homeostasis. A more attentive analysis of the anatomic and functional arrangement of the gastrointestinal tract, however, suggests that another extremely important function of this organ is its ability to regulate the trafficking of macromolecules between the environment and the host through a barrier mechanism. Together with the gut-associated lymphoid tissue and the neuroendocrine network, the intestinal epithelial barrier, with its intercellular tight junctions, controls the equilibrium between tolerance and immunity to non-self-antigens. Zonulin is the only physiological modulator of intercellular tight junctions described so far that is involved in trafficking of macromolecules and, therefore, in tolerance/immune response balance. When the finely tuned zonulin pathway is deregulated in genetically susceptible individuals, both intestinal and extraintestinal autoimmune, inflammatory, and neoplastic disorders can occur. This new paradigm subverts traditional theories underlying the development of these diseases and suggests that these processes can be arrested if the interplay between genes and environmental triggers is prevented by reestablishing the zonulin-dependent intestinal barrier function. This review is timely given the increased interest in the role of a 'leaky gut' in the pathogenesis of several pathological conditions targeting both the intestine and extraintestinal organs. Zonulin has been observed to be involved in the intestinal innate immunity and to be upregulated in several autoimmune diseases, including celiac disease and diabetes in which TJ dysfunction seems to be the primary defect."

As part of the LB5/LB100 program we use Dr. Fasano's test to determine if clients have a leaky-gut!

2. Other Changes In Our Diet and Auto-immune Disease

"I've discovered a significant part of the answer to the mystery of why our collective health has declined and our collective weight has risen so dramatically in just a few decades—and it starts with plant proteins called lectins."

The Plant Paradox, Steven Gundry, M.D.

The first mistake in our nutrition occurred over 10,000 years ago (just 400 generations ago) in our 2.5 million year history when we began growing grains (the seeds of grass). Together with the domestications of animals (dairy), agriculture marked a dramatic shift in the diet of humans who were predominantly hunter-gatherers before this period.

Long before humans (450 million years ago), plants protected themselves from predators by producing toxins, including lectins, in the plant and its seeds.

Lectins are found in almost all plants and other foods in our diet including meat, poultry and fish. Lectins bind sugars (especially polysaccharides) when we consume grains (and other foods)—these 'sticky proteins' because of this binding process can interrupt messaging between cells or cause toxic inflammatory reactions.

As Gundry notes, the reason wheat became the grain of choice in northern climates was due to a small lectin known as wheat germ agglutinin (WGA) which is responsible for wheat's weight-gaining propensity (WGA resembles insulin). WGA is also found in barley, rye and rice and is also very toxic to our gut (WGA can cause celiac disease).

Wheat, rye and other grains are also high in fructans—the gut bacteria can convert the fructans to fructose in the gut which can turn on the fat switch and also increase weight.

When cows and other animals eat grains (or soy) these proteins end up in the animal's meat or milk. The same happens in chicken and farm-raised sea foods. Knowing how the food you eat was grown and raised also directly affects your health.

We have five primary defenses against lectins:
1. mucus (nose and mouth)
2. stomach acid
3. microbiome
4. mucus (intestine)
5. cooking

Again, Gundry points out in The Plant Paradox that four other major changes in the eating patterns of humans have upset the delicate balance between humans and plants which had allowed us to co-exist and thrive for millennia and it's only very recently that we have recognized the role that lectins play:

1. Agricultural Revolution

Fish, lean meats, nuts, fruits and vegetables are part of a menu that's in harmony with our genetic makeup, which has not changed substantially for millennia. Our ancestors only ate from two food groups, "meat and fish" and "vegetables and fruits." Grains only appeared about 10,000 years ago in the Nile Valley and animal husbandry started more even recently, about 7,000 years ago.

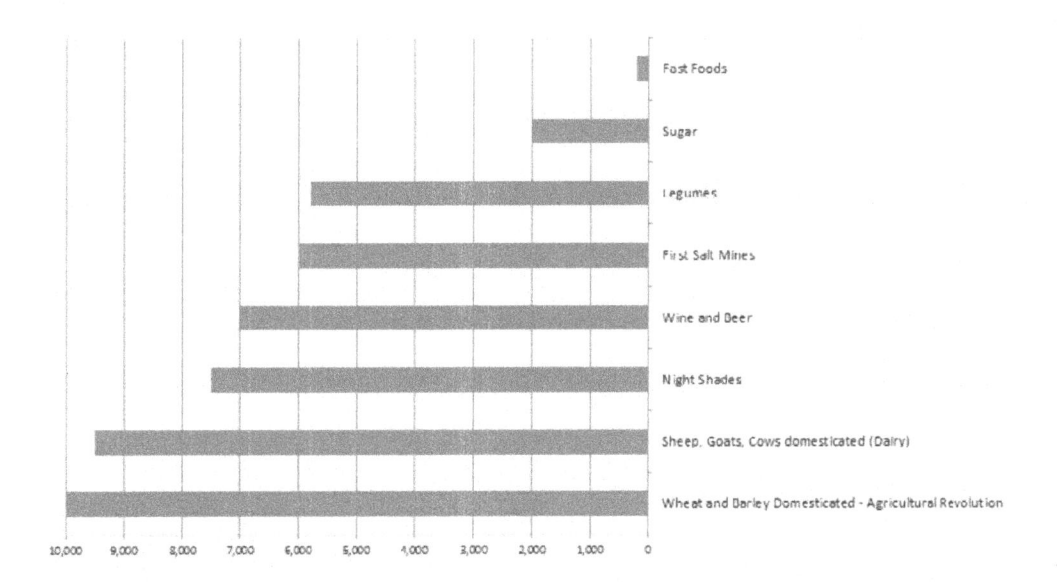

Years ago	Event
~500	Fast Foods
~2,500	Sugar
~6,000	Legumes
~6,000	First Salt Mines
~7,000	Wine and Beer
~7,500	Night Shades
~9,000	Sheep, Goats, Cows domesticated (Dairy)
~10,000	Wheat and Barley Domesticated - Agricultural Revolution

2. A Mutation in Cows

About 2,000 years ago, a mutation occurred in Northern Europian cows that caused them to make the protein casein A1 in their milk instead of the normal casein A2 that the Southern European cows make.

3. Plants from the New World

Christopher Columbus exposed the world to a whole new army of lectins not only from grains and pseudo-grains like amaranth and quinoa but also deadly nightshades, legumes, squash family, chia seeds etc. Half of the foods Europeans, Asians and Africans, who have been told to eat these foods for good health, have never been exposed to these New World plants—our microbiome and immune system are ill prepared to tolerate them.

4. Contemporary Innovations

Over the last few decades, a large amount of lectins in processed foods and recent GMO foods, together with antibiotics and other drugs and an avalanche of herbicides, pesticides and insecticides have devastated our microbiome. This chemical load has compromised our ability to deal with grains and legumes and other lectin breeding plants. Wheat and corn, the two most widely grown and consumed grains in the world, have also been extensively changed over the past 50 years by agribusiness.

10 Signs you have a Leaky Gut

1. Digestive issues such as gas, bloating, diarrhea or irritable bowel syndrome (IBS).
2. Seasonal allergies or asthma.
3. Hormonal imbalances.
4. Diagnosis of an autoimmune disease such as rheumatoid arthritis, Hashimoto's thyroiditis, lupus, psoriasis, or celiac disease.
5. Diagnosis of chronic fatigue or fibromyalgia.
6. Mood and mind issues such as depression, anxiety, ADD or ADHD.
7. Skin issues such as acne, rosacea, or eczema.
8. Diagnosis of candida overgrowth.
9. Food allergies or intolerances.
10. You are overweight and probably have insulin resistance.

Tight junctions are also opened by other dietary proteins, alcohol, elevated cortisol levels, some medications, some infections, microorganisms, and perhaps as yet unidentified substances.

Steven Gundry, M.D. lists seven deadly disruptors to our gut:

1. Broad Spectrum Antibiotics
2. Non-steroidal Anti-inflammatory Drugs (NSAIDs)
3. Proton Pump Inhibitors (PPIs)
4. Artificial Sweeteners
5. Endocrine Disruptors
6. GMOs and Roundup (glyphosate)

7. Constant Blue Light

3. Thyroid Disease, Dysbiosis and Autoimmune Disease

There are trillions of bacteria in your gut that play a vital role in thyroid health, yet the microbiome is so often overlooked in the treatment of hypothyroidism.

Thyroid disease and the microbiome are intricately intertwined and imbalances can set off a cyclical reaction. Low thyroid function can lead to inflammation and poor gut health while disturbances in the microbiome can suppress thyroid function and lead to an autoimmune condition called Hashimoto's Thyroiditis.

In practice, the emphasis is always on healing the gut (intestines) and balancing the colonies of bacteria that live there called the microbiome. Trillions of bacteria live on us and in us with the largest concentration located in the intestine where 70% of our immune system also lives.

In practical terms, when the bacteria that make up our microbiome are healthy and thriving, so are we. Dysbiosis or imbalances or overgrowth of unfriendly strains of bacteria can throw things off contributing to disease and immune issues.

Likewise our actions impact the bacteria as mentioned. Over-medicating with antibiotics and antacids destroys microbial populations. Environmental toxins, pesticides, heavy metal exposure, and chemicals in beauty and cleaning supplies also take a toll. Poor diets of sugary foods, refined carbs, GMO's, gluten, and chemical additives cause pathogenic strains to bloom. In the end the one who suffers is you.

How does the microbiome affect the thyroid?

Negative shifts in microbial populations can affect thyroid function, even triggering autoimmune disease.

The majority of hormone produced by the thyroid is actually inactive T4, which needs to be converted to T3 before being used by cells. 20% of the hormone gets converted or activated in the intestine with the help of gut bacteria. Negative shifts in microbial populations will impact the amount of usable hormone that's available, leading to a low thyroid state.

A major role of friendly gut bacteria is to strengthen the intestine wall, fortifying it against pathogens and preventing leaky gut. Without that barrier, foreign matter and large particles of food leak out of the intestine into the body setting off an immune response. Prolonged heightened immune response can trigger antibody production against healthy tissue creating autoimmune conditions like Hashimoto's thyroiditis – the number one cause of low thyroid in America today.

When the microbiome is unbalanced, long-term inflammation and damage may ensure causing the adrenal glands to produce the stress hormone cortisol. Over time, too much cortisol can also suppress thyroid function, lowering the amount of hormone produced while also inhibiting the conversion of T4 to T3.

H. Pylori is a pathogenic bacterium that colonizes areas of the stomach creating a wide range of digestive disorders including ulcers. Studies are now linking this bacterial infection to autoimmune conditions like Hashimoto's.

How does the thyroid affect the microbiome?

If thyroid function is sluggish, all systems can slow down.

1. The main communication highway linking the brain and the intestine is called the vagus nerve. Commonly patients suffering with low thyroid also have a down-regulation in vagus nerve activity reducing the speed at which the intestines are working and processing food. When gut movement slows, constipation takes hold and food lingers in the small intestine. This creates the ideal setting for pathogenic bacteria and candida to thrive and colonize. Patients often test positive for a condition called SIBO or small intestine bacterial overgrowth as a direct result of low thyroid. Symptoms are varied but may present as abdominal bloating and pain after meals, flatulence, constipation or diarrhea, heartburn, nausea, food sensitivities, headaches, fatigue, skin issues, and malabsorption.

2. Another consequence of low thyroid function is low stomach acid. While hydrochloric acid is our first line of protein breakdown, it also kills off bacteria hitching a ride on food. Without adequate HCL, proteins breakdown slower, nutrients aren't absorbed as well and bacteria and yeast often make it into the intestine where they can take hold. A lack of HCL has also been linked to increases in intestinal permeability and inflammation.

3. Since thyroid function affects the health of the intestine, the immune system is also affected. Dysbiosis will impact the way the immune system works mak-

ing us more susceptible to infections, viruses, and parasites. Parasites steal our nutrients, create inflammation, damage tissues, and further upset the balance of the body.

4. Thyroid hormone also strengthens the joints or tight junctions between cells that make up the intestine wall. If the thyroid is underactive, tight junctions may become loose and leaky compromising intestinal health.

Note: Above is adapted from Raphael Kellman, MD.

Dysbiosis and Brain Function

Alterations in the microbiota influences stress-related behaviors. New studies show that bacteria, including commensal, probiotic and pathogenic bacteria, in the gastrointestinal (GI) tract can activate neural pathways and central nervous system (CNS) signaling systems. Ongoing and future animal and clinical studies aimed at understanding the microbiota-gut-brain axis may provide novel approaches for prevention and treatment of mental illness, including anxiety and depression.

Dysbiosis and Aging

Gut dysbiosis has traditionally been linked to increased risk of infection, but imbalances within the intestinal microbial community structure that correlate with untoward inflammatory responses are increasingly recognized as being involved in diseases processes that affect many organ systems in the body.

Furthermore, it is becoming more apparent that the connection between gut dysbiosis and age-related diseases may lie in how the gut microbiome communicates with both the intestinal mucosa and the systemic immune system, given that these networks have a common interconnection to frailty.

When Hallmarks of Aging was initially published by Carlos Lopez-Otin in 2013 Microbiome Dysfunction had not been recognized for its important role in chronic disease and aging.

Interest toward the human microbiome, particularly the gut microbiome has flourished in recent decades owing to the rapidly advancing sequence-based screening and humanized gnotobiotic model in interrogating the dynamic operations of commensal microbiota.

Therapy for Microbiome Dysfunction

1. The 4R Program (Adapted from Dr. Kellman)

Healing the gut and microbial communities will improve the overall health of the patient as well as boost the immune system. Typically, start by **removing** pathogens like fungus, parasites, yeast, and especially SIBO. Potent herbal compounds can break through biofilms making it easier to eradicate overgrowth. Berberine, wormwood, garlic, oregano oil, grapeseed and olive leaf extracts, and caprylic acid are very helpful. Use a clay/charcoal compound to assist with clearing toxins from die off. Correcting the diet to support a healthy bacterial balance is also very important. Additionally discontinuing unnecessary medications like PPI's and avoid overuse of antibiotics that will protect our bacterial friends.

Replace stomach acid and pancreatic enzymes to ensure foods are broken down and assimilated as well as kill unfriendly bacteria on foods.

Next, **re-inoculate** with probiotics and good flora. After eradicating the harmful strains, replenishing the good is very important. Targeted strains like S.Boulardii have an immune modulating effect either boosting or calming the immune system.

In this phase, always concentrate on prebiotics food as well. The fibers found in superfoods like onion, garlic, apples, asparagus, Jerusalem artichokes, leeks, radish, and carrots feed the beneficial bacteria and ensure they thrive. Fermented foods really pack a punch when it comes to replenishing the microbiome with large quantities of healthy bacteria while also including prebiotics.

Finally, **repair** any damage in the intestinal wall, reducing inflammation and leaky gut. Use compounds like butyrate, quercetin, and curcumin to lower inflammation while glutamine, aloe, DGL, zinc carnosine, and Vitamin D can all help heal damage.

Sealing the deal by improving thyroid function.

Mainstream doctors only check levels of TSH and possibly T4 but that is just not enough to make an accurate thyroid diagnosis. At a minimum levels of TSH, Free and Total T3, Free and Total T4, Reverse T3, and antibodies to thyroid tissue TPO and TBG should be checked. Antibody levels are almost always omitted by routine testing yet necessary to understand if there is an autoimmune process going on in the thyroid.

When patients require thyroid treatment, work with a compounding pharmacy to mix the proportion of both T4 and T3 for the need of each individual person. The hormone used is pure without any filters or dyes that patients often react to.

Incorporating adaptogenic herbs to either soothe overworked adrenal glands or boost them after years of overuse can further protect the thyroid. Panax ginseng, rhodiola, ashwaganda, cordyceps, and IV's of high dose Vitamin C, vitamins, and minerals all help reboot and balance.

Additionally, supplements for gut health include Betaine HCL, digestive enzymes, probiotics, glutamine, and aloe.

2. Gut Health and Short-Chain Fatty Acids (SCFA)

Short-Chain Fatty Acids, or SCFAs, are the main source of energy for the cells lining the colon. They play an important role in colon health and are also involved in the metabolism of important nutrients like carbs and fat.

When boosting gut health, consider increasing SCFAs as it can help treat diseases of the gut such as inflammatory bowel diseases, or IBD. Moreover, these fatty acids have antagonistic effects on cancer and are involved in the body's immune response to pathogens.

How Short-Chain Fatty Acids are made and where to get them?

Short-Chain Fatty Acids are produced by the good gut bacteria by fermenting fiber in the colon. When prebiotic fiber reaches the body, the gut bacteria feed on it and this results in the postbiotic SCFA. There are three main types of SCFA in the body: **butyrate, acetate, and propionate**. Propionate is primarily involved in glucose production in the liver while acetate and butyrate are incorporated into other fatty acids and cholesterol.

The number of microorganisms present in the body affects the amount of SCFA's in the colon. The food source and the time it takes for the food to travel through the digestive system also determine SCFA number. It is therefore important to eat the right kinds of food that will nourish good gut bacteria.

Best of all is fiber. Research showed that **eating more fiber boost butyrate production** while decreasing your fiber intake reduces production.

Foods such as **artichokes, garlic, leeks, onions, rye and asparagus are rich in the fiber inulin. Meanwhile, apples, apricots, carrots and oranges are good sources of the fiber pectin.**

The Benefits of SCFAs

- SCFAs Anti-inflammatory effects in the gut help inflammatory bowel disease
- SCFAs can correct leaky gut and heal the wall of the colon
- SCFAs have strong immune enhancing effects and are anti-cancer
- SCFAs help T-cell production and function
- SCFAs regulate gene expression through histone deacetylases

Bottom line – The good bacteria ferment fiber in the gut so ensure you eat at least 35gm fiber per day.

3. Fasting

Breakfast, lunch and dinner are a relatively new thing. Snacking in between each of these meals only was introduced in the mid-60s. They are a product of civilization, work schedules and big business.

The idea of fasting aka "skipping a meal or two" really fits with our ancestry. I am firmly convinced after 40 years treating clients that most of us would benefit from eating once a day between 5-6pm i.e. a 20/4 hour window I believe is best.

4. An Ancestral Diet

Our modern diet with excess sugar, grains and adulterated plant oils is the single biggest factor for a shorter healthspan and lifespan as I have mentioned. A Paleo or Keto diet should be what we embrace if we wish to live long.

There is good evidence that a WFKD and Nutritional Ketosis is beneficial to our microbiome.

5. Add plenty of fermented food to your diet.

6. Microbiome Transplants For Reversing Hallmarks Of Aging

Changes in gut composition increase with age and adversely affect biological factors such as metabolism and immunity. This has been linked to age-related disorders, including inflammatory bowel diseases, cardiovascular disease, autoimmune and neurodegenerative disorders. Previous studies have proven the relationship between alterations in microbiota composition and infammaging, declines in tissue function, and increased subceptibility to age-related chronic disease.

Results of a 2022 study in Microbiome revealed that microbiota composition profiles could be successfully transferred via fecal microbiome transplant – which can modulate metabolic pathway profiles into young mice induced inflammation in the brain and elevated proteins responsible for retinal degeneration.

Microbiome Modulation For Longivity?

These findings implicate that gut microbiota regulates age-related degeneration, driving detrimental changes in the gut-brain and gut-retina axes. They also open up the possibility of developing gut microbe-based therapies aimed at combatting inflammation related tissue decline in later life and potentially reversing hallmarks of aging in the eye and brain. If these results can be replicated in humans, such therapies could greatly impact longevity science and the future of gastroenterological care.

Head of the Gut Microbes Health Research Program at the Quadram Institute, Professor Simon Carding, concluded: "This ground-breaking study provides tantalizing evidence for the direct involvement of gut microbes in aging and the functional decline of brain function and vision, and offers a potential solution in the form of gut microbe replacement therapy"

Summary of How to Optimize Your Gut Microbes

1. Boost intake of soluble and insoluble fiber
2. Eat plenty of fermented food
3. Avoid all antibiotics as much as possible
4. Avoid all artificial sweeteners (including stevia)
5. Take a probiotic
6. Get your hands dirty in the garden
7. Avoid chlorinated/fluoridated water
8. Avoid all processed foods
9. Wash your dishes by hand—not the dishwasher
10. Opening your windows helps change the microbiome at home
11. Avoid agricultural chemicals like glyphosate (RoundUp)
12. Avoid antimicrobial soaps
13. Avoid the Seven Deadly Gut Disruptors mentioned earlier
14. Get good sleep
15. Manage your stress
16. Try a Keto diet and Intermittent Fasting
17. Use L-glutamine, zinc, curcumin, magnesium, Vit D3/K2
18. Use only top-rated organic brands of yogurt:
19. Beware foods containing lectins
20. Opt for Vaginal rather than C-section delivery

CHAPTER 8: MITOCHONDRIAL DYSFUNCTION

Free radicals, or reactive oxygen species (ROS), form a natural byproduct of energy production in the mitochondria. Although they have a role in cellular signaling, **in high doses free radicals can be damaging to the cell.** The free radical theory of aging proposes that over time, increasing ROS production triggers mitochondrial dysfunction, which causes further increases in ROS production and cellular deterioration. Mitochondrial dysfunction may also affect other important cellular signaling pathways and processes. Eventually the cell becomes less efficient at producing energy, and at the same time, levels of oxidative stress increase, causing damage to other cellular components. As a result, mitochondrial dysfunction contributes to various age-related conditions such as myopathies and neuropathies.

Mitochondria are the tiny energy factories located in the body's 60 trillion cells. This is where we get our energy from. When mitochondrial dysfunction occurs, our cells are not able to function properly. Fructose is very toxic to the mitochondria.

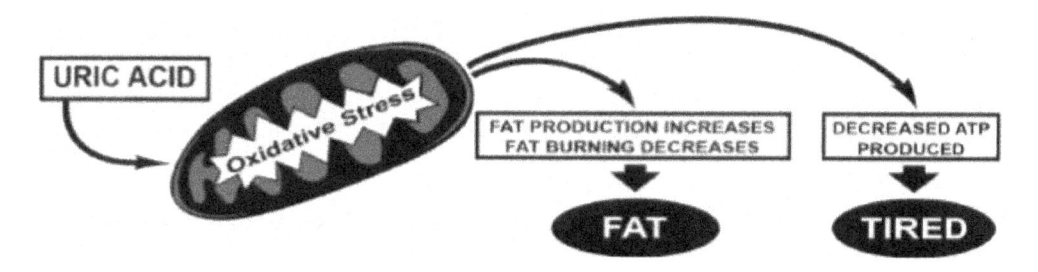

Uric acid affects mitochondria, causing oxidative stress. This results in stimulating fat synthesis, blocking fatty acid oxidation, and reducing ATP production. The net effect is to preferentially shunt the energy from food into fat stores.

The Connection Between Mitochondria and a Ketogenic Diet

What follows is adapted from Dr. Gabriela Seguras excellent article. She is a Consultant Cardiologist and recognizes the essential role of mitochondria for good cardiac function and general health.

Ketosis is an often misunderstood subject. Its presence is thought to be equal to starvation or a warning sign of something going wrong in your metabolism. But nothing could be further from the truth, except if you are an ill-treated type 1 diabetic person. Ketones - contrary to popular belief and myth - are a much needed and essential healing energy source in our cells that come from the normal metabolism of fat.

The entire body uses ketones in a more safe and effective way than the energy source coming from carbohydrates - sugar AKA glucose. Our bodies will produce ketones if we eat a diet devoid of carbs or a low carb diet (less than 60 grams of carbs per day). By eating a very low carb diet or no carbs at all (like a caveman) we become keto-adapted.

Our body organs and tissues work much better when they use ketones as a source of fuel, including the brain, heart and the core of our kidneys. If you ever had a chance to see a heart working in real time, you might have noticed the thick fatty tissue that surrounds it. In fact, heart surgeons get to see this every day. A happy beating heart is one that is surrounded by layers of healthy fat. Both the heart and the brain run at least 25% more efficiently on ketones than on blood sugar.

Ketones are the ideal fuel for our bodies unlike glucose - which is damaging, less stable, more excitatory and in fact shortens your life span. Ketones are non-glycating, which is to say, they don't have a caramelizing ageing effect on your body. A healthy ketosis also helps starve cancer cells as they are unable to use ketones for fuel, relying on glucose alone for their growth. The energy producing factories of our cells - the mitochondria - work much better on a ketogenic diet as they are able to increase energy levels in a stable, long-burning, efficient, and steady way. Not only that, a ketogenic diet induces epigenetic changes which increases the energetic output of our mitochondria, reduces the production of damaging free radicals, and favours the production of GABA - a major inhibitory brain chemical. GABA has an essential relaxing influence and its favored production by ketones also reduces the toxic effects of excitatory pathways in our brains. Furthermore, recent data suggests that ketosis alleviates pain in addition to having an overall anti-inflammatory effect.

Mitochondrial Dysfunction

Mitochondria are best known as the powerhouse of our cells since they produce the cell's energy. But they also lead the genetic orchestra which regulates how every cell ages, divides, and dies. They help dictate which genes are switched on or off in every single cell of our organism. They also provide the fuel needed to make new brain connections, repair and regenerate our bodies.

Whether we are housewives, sportsmen or labourers, energy is a topic that concerns us all, every day and in every way. Our wellbeing, behavior and ability to perform the tasks put in front of us is all to do with our individual levels of energy. But how do we derive energy from the foods that we eat?

There are many man-made myths surrounding energy production in the body and which foods supply energy. Mainstream science says that carbohydrates are what mitochondria use as fuel for energy production. This process is called oxidative metabolism because oxygen is consumed in the process. The energy produced by mitochondria is stored in a chemical "battery", a unique molecule called adenosine triphosphate (ATP). Energy-packed ATP can then be transported throughout the cell, releasing energy on demand of specific enzymes. In addition to the fuel they produce, mitochondria also create a by-product related to oxygen called reactive oxygen species (ROS), commonly known as free radicals. But what we are not told is that mitochondria were specifically designed to use fat for energy, not carbohydrate.

Mitochondria regulate cellular suicide, AKA apoptosis, so that old and dysfunctional cells which need to die will do so, leaving space for new ones to come into the scene. But when mitochondria function becomes impaired and sends signals that tell normal cells to die, things go wrong. For instance, the destruction of brain cells leads to every single neurodegenerative condition known including Alzheimer's disease, Parkinson's disease and so forth. Mitochondrial dysfunction has wide-ranging implications, as the health of the mitochondria intimately affects every single cell, tissue and organ within your body.

The catalysts for this destruction is usually uncontrolled free radical production which causes oxidative damage to tissues, fat, proteins, DNA, causing them to rust. This damage, called oxidative stress, is at the basis of oxidized cholesterol, stiff arteries (rusty pipes) and brain damage. Oxidative stress is a key player in dementia as well as autism.

We produce our own anti-oxidants to keep a check on free radical production, but these systems are easily overwhelmed by a toxic environment and a high carb diet, in other words, by today's lifestyle and diet.

Mitochondria have also interesting characteristics which differentiate them from all other structural parts of our cells. For instance, they have their own DNA (referred as mtDNA) which is separate from the widely known DNA in the nucleus (referred as n-DNA). Mitochondrial DNA comes for the most part from the mother line, which is why mitochondria are also considered as your feminine life force. This mtDNA is arranged in a ring configuration and it lacks a protective protein surrounding, leaving its genetic code vulnerable to free radical damage. If you don't eat enough animal fats, you can't build a functional mitochondrial membrane which will keep it healthy and prevent them from dying.

If you have any kind of inflammation from anywhere in your body, you damage your mitochondria. The loss of function or death of mitochondria is present in pretty much every disease. Dietary and environmental factors lead to oxidative stress and thus to mitochondrial injury as the final common pathway of diseases or illnesses.

Whereas the nDNA provides the information your cells need to code for proteins that control metabolism, repair, and structural integrity of your body, it is the mtDNA which directs the production and utilization of your life energy. A cell can still commit suicide (apoptosis) even when it has no nucleus nor nDNA.

Because of their energetic role, the cells of tissues and organs which require more energy to function are richer in mitochondrial numbers. Cells in our brains, muscles, heart, kidney and liver contain thousands of mitochondria, comprising up to 40% of the cell's mass. According to Prof. Enzo Nisoli, a human adult possesses more than ten million billion mitochondria, making up a full 10% of the total body weight. Each cell contains hundreds of mitochondria and thousands of mtDNA.

Since mtDNA is less protected then nDNA because it has no "protein" coating (histones), it is exquisitely vulnerable to injury by destabilizing molecules such as neurotoxic pesticides, herbicides, excitotoxins, heavy metals and volatile chemicals among others. This increases free radical production to the extreme which then leads to oxidative stress damaging our mitochondria and its DNA. As a result we got overexcitation of cells and inflammation which is at the root of Parkinson's disease and other diseases, but also mood problems and behavior problems.

Enough energy means a happy and healthy life. It also reflects in our brains with focused and sharp thinking. Lack of energy means mood problems, dementia, and slowed mental function among others. Mitochondria are intricately linked to the ability of the prefrontal cortex – our brains captain – to come fully online. Brain cells are located in mitochondria that produce the necessary energy to learn and memorize, and fire neurons harmoniously.

The sirtuin family of genes works by protecting and improving the health and function of your mitochondria. They are positively influenced by a diet that is non-glycating i.e. a low carb diet as opposed to high carb diet which induces mitochondrial dysfunction and formation of reactive oxygen species.

Therapy for Mitochondrial Dysfunction

1. **The Ketogenic Diet**

Ketone bodies production through intermittent fasting and the ketogenic diet is the most promising treatment for mitochondrial dysfunction. The longevity benefits seen by caloric restriction research is due to the fact that our bodies shift to a fat burning metabolism within our mitochondria. With a ketogenic diet, we go into a fat burning metabolism without restricting our calorie intake.

Ketosis deals effectively with all the problems of a diet rich in carbs – the one recommended by mainstream science. Namely a ketogenic diet deals with anxiety, food cravings, irritability, tremors, and mood problems among others. It is a crime to discourage the consumption of a high fat diet considering that a ketogenic diet shrinks tumors in human and animal models, and enhances our brain's resilience against stress and toxicity.

In addition to increasing the production of our body's natural valium – GABA – the increased production of acetyl-CoA generated from the ketone bodies also drives the Krebs cycle to increase mitochondrial NADH (reduced nicotinamide adenine nucleotide) which our body uses in over 450 biochemical reactions – including the cells signaling and assisting of the ongoing DNA repair. Because the ketone body beta-hydroxybutyrate is more energy rich than pyruvate, it produces more ATP. Ketosis also enhances the production of important anti-oxidants that deal with toxic elements from our environments, including glutathione.

Mitochondria from the hippocampus of ketogenic diet-fed animals are also resistant to mtDNA damage and are much less likely to commit cell suicide – apoptosis – at inappropriate times. As hominins slowly began to evolve larger brains after having acquired a more secure and abundant food supply, further brain expansion would have depended on significant fat stores and having reliable and rapid access to the fuel on those fat stores. Fat stores were necessary but were still not sufficient without a coincident increase in the capacity for ketogenesis. This unique combination of outstanding fuel store in body fat as well as rapid and abundant availability of ketones as a brain fuel that could seamlessly replace glucose was the key fuel reserve for expanding the hominin brain, a reserve that was apparently not available to other land – based mammals, including nonhuman primates.

It is indisputable that a ketogenic diet has protective effects in our brains. With all the evidence of its efficacy in mitochondrial dysfunction, it can be applied for all of us living in a highly stressful and toxic environment. Ketone bodies are healing bodies that helped us evolved and nowadays our mitochondria are always busted in some way or another since the odds in this toxic world are against us. Obviously, there are going to be people with such damaged mtDNA or with mutations they were born with, who can't modify their systems (i.e. defects in L-carnitine metabolism), but even in some of those cases, they can halt or slow down further damage. Our healthy ancestors never had to deal with the levels of toxicity that we live nowadays and nevertheless, they ate optimally. Considering our current time and environment, the least we can do is eat optimally for our physiology.

The way to have healing ketone bodies circulating in our blood stream is to do a high fat, restricted carb and moderate protein diet. Coupled with intermittent fasting which will enhance the production of ketone bodies, and resistance training which will create mitochondria with healthier mtDNA, we can beat the odds against us.

What is considered nowadays a "normal diet" is actually an aberration based on the corruption of science which benefits Big Agra and Big Pharma. If we would go back in time to the days before the modern diet became normalized by corporative and agricultural interests, we will find that ketosis was the normal metabolic state. Today's human metabolic state is aberrant. It is time to change that.

2. Intermittent Fasting

There is evidence to suggest that the circadian rhythm fasting approach, where meals are restricted to an eight to 10-hour period of the daytime, is effective.

But why does simply changing the timing of our meals to allow for fasting make a difference in our body? An **in depth review of the science of IF** recently published in *New England Journal of Medicine* sheds some light. Fasting is evolutionarily embedded within our physiology, triggering several essential cellular functions. Flipping the switch from a fed to fasting state does more than help us burn calories and lose weight. The researches combed through dozens of animal and human studies to explain how simple fasting improves metabolism, lowers blood sugar levels; lessens inflammation, which improves a range of health issues from arthritic pain to asthma; and even helps clear out toxins and damaged cells, which lowers risk for cancer and enhances brain function.

1. **Avoid sugars and refined grains.** Instead, eat fruits, vegetables, beans, lentils, whole grains, lean proteins, and healthy fats (a sensible, plant-based, Mediterranean-style diet).

2. **Let your body burn fat between meals.** Don't snack. Be active throughout your day. Build muscle tone.

3. **Consider a simple form of intermittent fasting.** Limit the hours of the day when you eat, and for best effect, make it between 10am to 6pm (but definitely not in the evening before bed).

4. **Avoid snacking or eating at nighttime,** all the time.

Note: I believe the single best approach is to eat **one meal a day** around 5-6pm. Coffee, tea, and other healthy beverages can be consumed anytime. This will reverse your Biological Age.

3. Magnificent 7 (Final 3 ingredients)

Vitamin C (ascorbic acid) can lower uric acid and blocks mitochondrial oxidative stress and tames the 'fat switch.' Vitamin C can block the effects of fructose to cause metabolic syndrome.

- lowers blood sugar throughout the day (and minimizes spikes in sugar)
- lowers blood pressure
- good antioxidant and is vital for body's healing process
- supports synthesis of proteins for blood vessels
- helps absorb and stores iron
- stimulated white blood cells and helps immunity
- lowers the risk for cardiovascular disease
- may have role in common cold and cancer prevention.

Alpha-lipoic acid (ALA) is an antioxidant found in many foods. It is important for mitochondrial health—acts as heavy metal chelator and is important cofactor for mitochondrial enzymes like AMPK. It is both fat and water soluble.

- lowers blood sugar and improves insulin resistance
- powerful antioxidant and recycles CoQ10, Glutathione, Vit C and E
- lowers NF-Kappa B and inflammation
- increases mitochondrial biogenesis
- helps detoxify the liver
- ALA inhibits AMPK in the hypothalamus and decreases appetite
- lowers risk of cardiovascular disease
- slows brain aging and wrinkling and improves immunity

Resveratrol a natural product found in grapes, mulberries, wine and peanuts. Induces mitochondrial biogenesis in endothelial cells throughout the body.

- enhances insulin sensitivity (can be seen from a single glass wine)
- improves mitochondrial biogenesis
- enhances effects of metformin
- lowers blood pressure
- lowers body weight
- improves neurodegeneration in brain
- cardiovascular protection (French Paradox)
- promotes longevity by activating on sirtuins 1–7

4. Beware Heavy Metals

Heavy metals are especially toxic to the mitochondria as are several other toxins.

We encourage most of our clients to do a challenge test and collect their urine to test for heavy metals that might be increasing mitochondrial dysfunction. Several remedies are available to remove heavy metals from the body.

5. MitoQ

Coenzyme Q10, also known as ubiquinone or CoQ10, is a vitamin-like substance found in the bodies of almost all life forms. CoQ10 is found primarily within **mitochondria,** the power plants of the cell, where it is a vital part of the energy production process and also acts as a free radical neutralizing antioxidant.

Natural production of CoQ10 can decrease with age, illness and lifestyle factors like diet and smoking. When CoQ10 levels diminish, we tend to see poorly functioning mitochondria and increased **free radical** damage which is now known to contribute to a whole host of health issues.

Since we know that CoQ10 levels can decline in aging and with poor health, why don't we try and increase them?

Actually people have been trying, it just hasn't worked particularly well. CoQ10 supplements have been widely available for many years, however, the research has shown us that supplementing with standard CoQ10 just isn't as effective as hoped. Although some benefits have been noted in scientific studies, the overwhelming body of evidence is just particularly strong for many of the conditions it is claimed to help. This is mainly down to one important factor.

CoQ10 is poorly absorbed

CoQ10 is a fairly large fat-soluble molecule which needs to be taken with foods containing oil or fat. Only a very small amount of CoQ10 actually makes it inside our mitochondria due to their impermeable membranes. That includes the active form of CoQ10 ubiquinol which is quickly oxidized back into ubiquinone (inactive form of CoQ10) inside the body. Yet the mitochondria is the very place you need CoQ10 to target in order for levels to be supported.

CoQ10 Breakthrough

The real breakthrough was discovered in New Zealand by two biochemists in the late 1990s. They realized that mitochondria have a significant negative charge compared to the rest of the cell, attaching the right positively charged molecule to CoQ10 should finally solve the absorption problem. After years of experimenting with different molecules, they found the optimal formulation and "MitoQ" was born.

Enter MitoQ

This mitochondria-targeting of CoQ10 worked amazingly well, with high levels of the MitoQ molecules finding their way into the mitochondria. It is also effective that the dose can be reduced to ten times less than the normal CoQ10 dose yet still provide a significantly high amount of this advanced form of CoQ10 directly into the mitochondria. Additionally, once it neutralizes a free radical, MitoQ is recycled back to its active form allowing it to perform this task over and over again.

Here are some of the benefits you may see by investing in your mitochondrial health with MitoQ:

- Sustains your body's optimal energy production

- **Supports normal blood pressure,** blood sugar and cholesterol levels

- Sustains healthy energy production in muscles, joints and other connective tissues, helping you stay strong and fit for longer and recover from physical exercise faster, and potentially reducing the risk of injury

- **Maintain healthy liver** and kidney function leading to normal metabolic function

- Healthy brain and nervous system function are supported, helping to sustain mental clarity and alertness as you age

- Supports balanced immune and allergic-pathways which can help to normalize the potentially damaging effects of the body's natural responses to both harmful and normal aggressors

- Helps with the reduction of **oxidative stress** from both internal and environmental sources, which can lead to healthier aging of skin

MitoQ has shown significant promise in over 50 different health conditions including seven of the top ten most costly to human lives. **Over 500+ peer reviews research papers have now been published.**

6. Melatonin

The majority of melatonin is made inside your mitochondria in response to near-infrared radiation from the sun. (Only 5% of your melatonin is produced in your pineal gland at night). These rays penetrate deep inside your body and activate cytochrome oxidase which stimulates the production of Melatonin in your mitochondria.

As discussed the energy currency of your body is ATP produced by your mitochondria. A by-product of ATP is reactive oxygen species (ROS) that can damage your mitochondria causing chronic inflammation and chronic disease like obesity, diabetes and thrombosis and even aging itself.

Melatonin mops up the ROS that damages your mitochondria. Good sleep and plenty of sun exposure during the day will ensure plenty of Melatonin which will reduce oxidative stress.

Not too long ago humans received 10 hours a day (70 hours/week) living and working outside. Today most of us spend less than 30 minutes a day (3 hours/week) in daylight according to Dr. Daniel Kripke (UCSD).

Another problem today is that linoleic acid (LA) makes up 60-80% of the omega-6 fat you consume and is a primary driver of most chronic disease. LA acts as a metabolic poison and impedes your body's ability to generate ATP.

Over the past 150 years LA has increased from 3 grams/day to 30 grams/day. Primary sources are seed oils and processed foods and conventional raised chicken and pork due to the LA rich grains they are fed.

Are Vegetables and Seed Oils Bad for Your Health?

As I pointed out sugar, grains and most adulterated vegetable oils are the primary cause of "insulin resistance" and chronic disease.

Their health benefits (or not) depend on what fatty acids they contain, what plants they are extracted from and how they are processed.

Refined vegetable oils were not available until the 20th century, when the technology to extract them became available. They are extracted from plants using a chemical solvent or oil mill. You should look for oils that are made by crushing or pressing plants or seeds rather than those produced using chemicals which can be chemically altered.

In the past century the consumption of vegetable oils has increased at the expense of other fats like butter and lard. The reason that polyunsaturated oils were in preference to butter/lard they were mistakenly thought to be 'heart healthy' compared to saturated fat which is false.

This is especially true of omega-6 fats. Both omega-6 and omega-3 fatty acids are essential, meaning you need some of them in your diet because your body can't produce them. Whereas in the past the ratio was 1:1, this ratio has shifted to as high as 20 (omega-6s):1 (omega-3s). The problem with polyunsaturated fats is that all their double bonds make them susceptible to oxidation and can damage your cell membranes throughout your body.

Coconut oil and olive oil are excellent choices but you should try to avoid the following plant oils due to their high omega-6 contents:

- Soybean oil
- Corn oil
- Cottonseed oil
- Sunflower oil
- Peanut oil
- Sesame oil
- Rice bran oil

Melatonin and Cancer

"Melatonin in Mitochondria: Mitigating Clear and Present Dangers," by Dr. Roger Seheult, further explains important additional benefits of melatonin.

Again, melatonin is important for fighting cancer, and mitochondrial dysfunction and plays a central role in most all chronic disease, including cancer, Parkinson's, Alzheimer's disease, Heart disease and Type 2 diabetes, just to name a few. The paper also describes in far greater detail the mechanism for how melatonin is created within the mitochondria:

"In normal cells, mitochondria account for energy (ATP) production, which results from glucose metabolism (glycolysis) and cellular respiration (oxidative phosphorylation or OXPHOS) in the inner mitochondrial membrane.

Glycolysis, which occurs in the cytosol, generates pyruvate, which is actively transported into the mitochondrial matrix. Here, pyruvate is converted to acetyl-CoA, the latter linking glycolysis with the citric acid cycle in the mitochondrial matrix and thus coupling it to ATP production.

Acetyl-CoA is also an essential co-factor for N-acetyltransferase (AANAT), which converts serotonin to N-acetylserotonin, the precursor of melatonin; AANAT activity rate limits melatonin synthesis.

In contrast to normal cells, many solid tumor cells allow the metabolism of glucose to pyruvate in the cytosol but restricts the transfer of pyruvate into the mitochondria; this is known as the Warburg effect... The Warburg effect allows cancer cells to rapidly proliferate, avoid apoptosis, and enhance the invasiveness and metastatic processes characteristic of tumors."

CHAPTER 9: LOSS OF PROTEOSTASIS

In our cells, proteins are constantly being synthesized and degraded in a process known as protein homeostasis, or proteostasis. Proteins are like tools which must be assembled in the correct way to perform their many crucial cellular functions, and an important part of assembly is folding proteins into the proper shapes. Various mechanisms have evolved to better stabilize or restore correctly folded proteins, and to remove and degrade improperly shaped proteins which could otherwise accumulate and damage the cell. When these mechanisms become less efficient over time, damaged and aggregated protein components cause dysfunction or even cell toxicity, as seen in diseases like Alzheimer's.

Wikipedia describes "proteostasis" as the dynamic regulation of a balanced functional proteome. The "proteostasis" network includes competing and integrated biological pathways within cells that control the biogenesis, folding, trafficking and degradation of proteins present within and outside the cell.

Proteostasis ensures that proteins are produced and folded appropriately before they are trafficked to precise locations. It also acts to ensure that abnormal or excess proteins are degraded to prevent the accumulation of unwanted products.

The proteostasis network within human cells contains over 1,400 proteins. Proteostasis regulates the functional properties of the proteome to minimize the damage of misfolded and aggregated proteins through this network.

With age, the ability of many cells and organs to preserve proteostasis under resting and stress conditions is gradually compromised.

With age, negative processes increase. Oxidative stress accumulates randomly in the cells proteins, healthy synthesis and degradation slow down and like-overfilled garbage cans – the activity of keeping proteins properly folded is exceeded. The tipping point to cell death happens when the negative overwhelms the positive.

Loss or dysfunction of proteostasis is at the root of many well studied human neurological diseases, such as Alzheimer's and recently has been implicated in the aging process as reports show that the long live animals have improved proteostasis.

At Stanford University School of Medicine, researchers noted that by measuring certain proteins in the blood they could predict the age of patients – they developed an Age clock initially from over 373 proteins that they were able to refine it to 9.

As we age protein damage occurs from exposure to various chemicals, UV radiation, diet and environmental toxins. Reduced mitochondrial function as we age means less ATP and thus this inhibits proteostasis leading to an increase in incorrect folding. Proteasomal degradation is also dramatically reduced in older cells.

Studies have shown that the process of proteostasis can be maintained by restricting calorie intake. (This has been shown to increase the lifespan of rats by 50%). This appears to be due to hormesis of the endoplasmic reticulum.

The first component of this network is the ribosome that synthesis polypeptide claims via the translation of RNA. Once this happens the proteostasis network can aid protein folding.

The Proteostasis capacity to sustain brain healthspan

Sustaining neuronal proteostasis during the course of our life is a central aspect required for brain function. The dynamic nature of synaptic composition and abundance is a requisite to drive cognitive and motor processes involving a tight control of many aspects of protein biosynthesis and degradation. Through the concerted action of specialized stress sensors, the proteostasis network monitors and limits the accumulation of damaged, misfolded, or aggregated proteins. These stress pathways signal to the cytosol and nucleus to reprogram gene expression, enabling adaptive programs to recover cell function. During aging, the activity of the proteostasis network declines, which may increase the risk of accumulating abnormal protein aggregates, a hallmark of most neurodegenerative diseases. Pharmacological and gene therapy strategies to intervene and boost proteostasis are expected to extend brain healthspan and ameliorate disease state.

Studies of some of the longest lived people – in what researchers called "The Blue Zones" – had nine important lifestyle factors that help them avoid diabetes, heart disease, cancer and dementia. 5 out of 9 of these lifestyle factors depended on a healthy brain.

Any therapy directed at improving brain function is critical to improving our healthspan and lifespan.

Conclusion:

Aging is the main risk factor for a variety of neurodegenerative disease, such as AD and PD Recent studies indicate that there is a dramatic age-associated collapse of proteostasis responses, leaving the cells vulnerable to physiological and environmental stressors, and more susceptible to disease. In the case of diseases associated with protein misfolding, the proteostasis machinery takes initial care of the abnormal protein aggregates. However, as the clearance ability gets compromised, the accumulated aggregates cause cellular toxicity, tissue dysfunction, and disease. Therefore, boosting up the proteostasis machinery by the use of natural compounds emerges as a potent pharmacological tool with promising effects to treat and protect against neurodegenerative disorders. In this study we compile a list of natural modulators of the proteostasis network. Not surprisingly, majority of them are of plant-origin. However, it is remarkable to note that we report some compounds of marine-animal-origin as well. It is indeed necessary to explore more alternative sources of natural compounds. In addition, further studies are required to understand the precise mechanism of action of the natural proteostasis activators, their off-target effects and their in vivo bioavailability. We foresee that the development of innovative, natural and safe therapeutic strategies to tackle the accumulation of misfolded protein aggregates through the modulation of the proteostasis machinery, will have exceptional effects to prevent and treat disorders related to age-dependent protein aggregation.

Therapy for Improving Proteostasis

1. Calorie Restriction

Several studies show that calorie restriction is one sure way to boost proteostasis.

2. Fasting and Keto Diet

Recent evidence also has shown that fasting and periods of Nutritional Ketosis will improve the proteostasis network.

3. Improve Mitochondrial Function

The Magnificent 7 product mentioned in Chapter 8 will improve mitochondrial biogenesis.

4. Stress Reduction

MTORC1 is suppressed by psychological stress and is implicated in regulating both protein folding and proteasomal degredation.

5. Improve Sleep

Evidence shows that if sleep is chronically poor the proteostasis regulatory mechanisms are less efficient and the cell is inundated with misfolded proteins and suffer a collapse in homeostasis.

6. Nutritional Compounds as Modulators of Proteostasis

Proteostasis failure has been reported in the context of aging and neurodegeneration such as Alzheimer's and Parkinson's disease. A variety of natural products are known to be neuroprotective for protein homeostasis interaction.

Recent hypothesis suggest that a progressive reduction in the repair capacity of the proteostasis network may generate a "pathological aging" that results in protein aggregation and a higher incidence of neurodegenerative disease. Functional studies indicate that altered proteostasis at the level of the endoplasmic reticulum is one of the major contributors to aging. In addition, neurodegenerative diseases have in common autophagy failure. The inhibition of autophagy response is known to exacerbate protein toxicity and accelerate disease progression.

Chaperones are highly conserved proteins that exist and mediate the proper 3-D conformation of proteins. Chaperones play important roles during stress response, hence they are known as heat shock proteins (Hsp).

To date several natural products have been identified as Hsp modulators. These include: -

- Curcumin
- Proanthocyanide (present in cranberry extract)
- Celastrol (extracted from the thunder god vine)
- Paconiflorin (from plant ferns)
- Glycyrrhizin (from licorice root)
- Geldanamycin
- Herbamycin A
- Radicicol

Several studies have pinpointed a down regulation of important components of the **autophagy** pathway during aging and neuro degenerative disease. Several products have been seen to induce autophagy and reduce the accumulation of misfolded protein. In this regard polyphenolic compounds are known potent activators of the autophagy response. They include: -

- Quercetin (red wine)
- Kaempferol (grapes/tomatoes)
- Caffeine (coffee)
- Resveratrol (grapes)
- Olive oil
- Spermidine (mushrooms/cheese)
- Ginseng
- Berberine
- Corynoxine B
- Marine organisms

Unfolded Protein Response (UPR)

Three branches of a conserved signaling pathway collectively termed as the unfolded protein response (UPR) are triggered in response to ER stress (ATF6, PERK, IRE). When ER stress is chronically activated, proteostasis cannot be restored with devastating consequences to the brain, leading to synaptic impairment and neurodegeneration. Recent studies indicate the relation of ER stress with chemical chaperones alleviate synapse and memory loss.

Only a few naturally occurring compounds have been explored to modulate the UPR in the context of neurodegeneration.

They include the following:
1. Bajijiasu (Chinese medical herb)
2. Kaempferol (phytoestrogen from G. biloba)
3. Gingko Biloba extract
4. Honokiol (Magnolia trees)

7. CRISPR Gene Editing Treatment

A study using a simple CRISPR editing technique more than doubled the lifespan of progeroid mice in January 2021.

On the same day another study found that CRISPR edit of just one senescent-accelating gene (KAT7) increased the lifespan of mice by 25%. These mice also had improvements in overall appearance and grip strength.

A study by Dr. George Church in mice showed that a single dose of combination treatment gave impressive results:

1. 55% increased function after heart failure
2. 38% reduction in vascular disease markers
3. 75% reduction in kidney atrophy
4. Complete reversal of obesity and diabetes

The **Ubiquitin Preteasome System** (UPS) is the main system responsible for degrading intracellular damage proteins. Several products enhance proteasome activity including: -

- Resveratrol
- Quercetin
- Corydalis bungeana

Boosting up the proteastasis machinery by the use of these natural compounds emerge as a potent tool to increase longevity. Although the majority of these compounds come from plants several come from marine-animal origin as well.

8. Peptides

Peptides are short chains of amino acids linked by peptides bond. Chains of fewer than twenty amino acids are called oligopeptides, and include dipeptides, tripeptides, and tetrapeptides. A polypeptide is a longer, continuous, unbranched peptide chain.

Protein-protein interactions (PPIs) execute many fundamental cellular functions and the peptides smaller size and flexibility have made them promising candidates for targeting challenging binding interfaces with satisfactory binding affinity and specificity. These peptide-protein recognition mechanisms together with peptides safety record promise great results for the Anti Aging physician in the decades ahead.

Already more than 90 peptides have been approved and administrated globally in clinics. Since the isolation and commercialization of insulin, a 51 amino acid, done in the 1920's, peptide drugs have and will greatly shape medicine and longevity in the years ahead. Peptides also have favorable tissue penetration and have high affinity interactions with endogenous receptors.

Six of my favorite peptides include:

1. Semaglutide – weight loss and glucose management

2. Sermorelin – stimulates and balances growth hormone

3. PT 141 - sexual arousal in both men and women

4. MK 677 – optimizes growth hormone and ghrelin

5. BPC 157 - activates growth factors and tissue healing

6. VIP – good for water damaged buildings (WDB) and the treatment of chronic inflammatory response syndrome (CIRS) – often dosed nasally.

CHAPTER 10: GENOMIC INSTABILITY

Genome instability refers to a high frequency of mutations within the genome of a cellular lineage. These mutations can include changes in nucleic acid sequences, chromosomal rearrangements or aneuploidy. Genome instability does occur in bacteria. In multicellular organisms genome instability is central to carcinogenesis, and in humans it is also a factor in some neurodegenerative diseases such as amyotrophic lateral sclerosis or the neuromuscular disease myotonic dystrophy.

Exposure to smoke, chemicals or other exogenous agents over time can damage our genome, as can factors like simple DNA replication errors or oxidative stress. Although we have evolved a complex network of DNA repair mechanisms, DNA damage accumulates over the course of our lives, causing mutations in cells that can in the worst cases lead to cancer formation.

A host of factors contribute to "silent inflammation" which impacts all the Hallmarks of Aging ultimately causing genomic instability.

Inflammation is essential in protecting us against foreign pathogens. However, when left unchecked, it becomes chronic inflammation, a potential precursor to carcinogenesis. While inflammatory signalling provides pro-survival stimuli, it also causes genomic instability and allows mutant cells to escape cell cycle arrest and apoptosis. This occurs through the release of reactive oxygen/nitrogen species (ROS/RNS), the increased expression of activation-induced cytidine deaminase (AID), inhibition of p53 function and the reactivation of TERT expression. Because chronic inflammation can ultimately lead to genomic instability, there is a need to target chronic inflammation, through the suppression of effector pathways with biologics.

My good friend Giuseppe Mucci is the CEO of Bioscience Institute and developed one of the first 'liquid biopsy' tests to detect risk of cancer with a simple tube of blood. I have quoted from a white paper from his lab which focused on the role of inflammation and genomic instability.

Inflammation And Aging

According to the research field that studies the molecular link between aging and chronic diseases related to age (the so-called "geroscience") inflammation is one of the mechanisms shared by age-related diseases. In particular chronic, low-grade inflammation occurring in the absence of infection that takes place during aging is called "inflammaging".

Inflammaging is primarily driven by endogenous signals, including the presence of cell debris, misplaced cell molecules and misfolded or oxidized proteins. Macromolecular damage, metabolism, epigenetics, stress, proteostasis and, stem cell regeneration are all interconnected factors influencing this low-grade inflammation state, which is characterized by a chronic activation of the innate immune system which can become damaging.

There are several cellular and molecular mechanism involved: cellular senescence: the dysfunction of mitochondria, defective mechanisms of autophagy and mitochondria degradation; the activation of the intracellular multiprotein complex that detects biological and non-biological stressor (the inflammasome: the dysregulation of the system controlling protein degradation, the activation of the response to DNA damage; changes in the composition of the microbiota (dysbiosis); and nutrient excess and overnutrition, which can generate a specific type of chronic inflammation called "metaflammation" associated with metabolic diseases such as obesity and type 2 diabetes. All these stimuli converge on a small number of sensors which trigger that innate immune response causing inflammation and an adaptive metabolic response. This response is critical for survival until middle age, but with aging the inflammatory response usually increases, becoming detrimental – and eventually leading to inflammation – in post-reproductive age. The increase of senescent cells and their accumulation and the hyperactivation of the immune response play an important role in this phenomenon, moreover, according to the garbaging theory, the age-related progressive impairment of cell debris elimination systems largely sustains inflammaging.

The inflammatory tone can increase progressively during several years or decades, depending on genetics, anatomical features, immunological history, and lifelong lifestyle habits. Nutrient excess and overnutrition fuel inflammaging; metaflammation contributes to the onset of insulin resistance, activating inflammatory responses that affect organs such as brain, muscle, pancreas and liver, and adipose tissue.

Lipids play a central role in metaflammation, increasing oxidative stress and cytokines such as IL-6. After a high-fat meal blood levels of lipopolysaccharide (LPS, the endotoxin associated with sepsis) increase too; this generates a state called metabolic endotoxemia associated with low-grade inflammation with the development and the progression of cardiometabolic diseases. Finally, high-fat diets can alter gut microbiota, further increasing LPS production; dysregulation in meal timing contributes to this metabolic and inflammatory dysregulation, whereas nutrient-dense diets induce the increase of adipocytes size, until they reach a structurally critical condition that contribute to metaflammation.

Endothelial Dysfunction

The endothelium lines our 60,000 miles of blood vessels. Metabolic stress like diabesity can negatively effect this lining with widespread effects in every organ system.

Recent studies have revealed the functional link between immune and metabolic systems, which are two central pillars of the survival pathways which evolved from common ancestors. The human complement system is a global mediator of our innate immune system. It is recently understood that the complement system not only contributes substantially to homeostasis by eliminating infectious microbes, and cellular debris, complementing immunological and inflammatory processes and immune surveillance, but also contributes to various immune, inflammatory-related diseases.

David Sinclair's Information Theory of Aging

I am going to quote extensively from Lifespan written by David Sinclair PhD in 2019. One of his most important insights occurred in October 28, 1996 over 25 years ago.

"Broken DNA causes genomic instability which distracts SIR2 protein, which changes the epigenome, causing the cells to lose their identity and become sterile while they fixed the damage." This was the foundation for understanding the survival circuit and its role in aging.

Epigenetic noise, driven in large part by highly disruptive insults to the cell (often due to certain lifestyles) and this according to Sinclair's Information Theory of Aging, is why we age – "It's why each one of the hallmarks of aging occurs, from stem cell exhaustion and cellular senescence to mitochondrial dysfunction and rapid telomere shortening."

These results were first recognized in old yeast cells that lost their fertility.

The rDNA was in a state of chaos. The genome, it seemed, was fragmenting. DNA was recombining and amplifying, showing up on the Southern blot as dark spots and wispy circles, depending on how coiled up and twisted they were. We called those loops extrachromosomal ribosomal DNA circles, or ERCs, and they were accumulating as the mutant yeast cells aged.

Sinclair published their work in December 1997 in the scientific journal *Cell*, and the news broke around the world: "Scientists figured out a cause of aging." Sinclair continues to explain his origins of the Information Theory of Aging: -

It was there and then that Matt Kaeberlein, a PhD student at the time, arrived at the lab. His first experiment was to insert an extra copy of SIR2 into the genome of yeast cells to see if it would stabilize the yeast genome and delay aging. When the extra SIR2 was added, ERCs were prevented, and he saw a 30 percent increase in the yeast cells' lifespan, as we'd been hoping. Our hypothesis seemed to be standing up to scrutiny: the fundamental, upstream cause of sterility and aging in yeast was the inherent instability of the genome.

What emerged from those initial results in yeast, and another decade of pondering and probing mammalian cells, was a completely new way to understand aging, an information theory that would reconcile seemingly disparate factors of aging into one universal model of life and death. It looked like this:

Youth → broken DNA → genome instability → disruption of DNA

packaging and gene regulation (the epigenome) → loss of cell identity

→ cellular senescence → disease → death

It took another twenty years to learn if those findings in yeast were relevant to organisms more complex than yeast. We mammals have seven sirtuin genes that have evolved a variety of functions beyond what simple *SIR2* can do. Three of them, SIRT1, SIRT6, SIRT7, are critical to the control of the epigenome and DNA repair. The others, SIRT3, SIRT4, and SIRT5, reside in mitochondria, where they control energy metabolism, while SIRT2 buzzes around the cytoplasm, where it controls cell division and healthy egg production.

But the true extent to which the survival circuit is conserved between yeast and humans wasn't fully known until 2017, when Eva Bober's team at the Max Planck Institute for Heart and Lung Research in Bad Nauheim, Germany, reported that sirtuins stabilize human *t*DNA. Then, in 2018, Katrin Chua at Stanford University found that, by stabilizing human *t*DNA, sirtuins prevent cellular senescence – essentially the same antiaging function as we had found for sirtuins in yeast twenty years earlier.

That was an astonishing revelation: over a billion years of separation between yeast and us, and, in essence, the circuit hadn't changed.

Sinclair noticed that yeast cells fed with lower amounts of sugar were not just living longer, but their rDNA was exceptionally compact – significantly delaying the inevitable ERC accumulation, catastrophic numbers of DNA breaks, nucleolar explosion, sterility, and death.

Our DNA is constantly under attack. On average, each of our forty-six chromosomes is broken in some way every time a cell copies its DNA, amounting to more than 2 trillion breaks in our bodies per day. And that's just the breaks that occur during replication. Others are caused by natural radiation, chemicals in our environment, and the X-rays and CT scans that we're subjected to.

If we didn't have a way to repair our DNA, we wouldn't last long. That's why, way back in primordium, the ancestors of every living thing on this planet today evolved to sense DNA damage, slow cellular growth, and divert energy to DNA repair until was fixed – what I call the **survival circuit**.

Can long-lived species teach us how to live healthier and for longer?

In terms of their looks and habitats, pine trees, jellyfish, and whales are certainly very different from humans. But in other ways, we're very similar. Consider the bowheads. Like us, they are complex, social, communicative, and conscious mammals. We share 12,787 known genes, including some interesting variants in a gene known as FOXO3. Also known as DAF-16, this gene was first identified as a longevity gene in roundworms by University of California at San Francisco researcher Cynthia Kenyon. She found it to be essential for defects in the insulin hormone pathway to double worm lifespan. Playing an integral role in the survival circuit, DAF-16 encodes a small transcription factor protein that latches onto the DNA sequence TTGTTTAC and works with sirtuins to increase cellular survival when times are tough.

In mammals, there are four DAF-16 genes, called. FOXO1, FOXO3, FOXO4, and FOXO6. If you suspect that we scientists sometimes intentionally complicate matters, you'd be right, but not in this case. Genes in the same "gene family" have ended up with different names because they were named before DNA sequences were easily deciphered. It's similar to the not uncommon situation in which people have their genome analyzed and learn they have a sibling on the other side of town. DAF-16 is an acronym for *dauer* larvae formation. In German "dauer" means "long lasting", and this is actually relevant to this story. Turns out, worms become *dauer* when they are starved or crowded, hunkering down until times improve. Mutations that activate DAF-16 extend lifespan by turning on the worm defense program even when times are good.

I first encountered FOXO/DAF-16 in yeast, where it is known as MSN2, which stands for "multicopy suppressor of SNF1 (AMPK) epigenetic regulator." Like DAF-16, MSN2's job in yeast is to turn on genes that push cells away from cell death and toward stress resistance. We discovered that when calories are restricted MSN2 extends yeast lifespan by turning up genes that recycle NAD, thereby giving the sirtuins a boost.

Hidden within the sometimes byzantine way scientists talk about science are several repeating themes: low energy sensors (SNF1/AMPK), transcription factors (MSN2/DAF-16/FOXO), NAD and sirtuins, stress resistance, and longevity. This is no coincidence – these are all key parts of the ancient survival circuit.

But what about FOXO genes in humans? Certain variants called FOXO3 have been found in human communities in which people are known to enjoy both longer lifespans and healthspans, such as people of China's Red River Basin. These FOXO3 variants likely turn on the body's defenses against diseases and aging, not just when times are tough but throughout life. If you've had your genome analyzed, you can check if you have any of the known variations of FOXO3 that are associated with a long life. For example, having a C instead of a T variant at position n2764264 is associated with longer life.

It's worth pausing to consider how remarkable it is that we find essentially the same longevity genes in every organism on the planet: trees, yeast, worms, whales, and humans. All living creatures come from the same place in the primordium that we do. When we look through a microscope, we're all made of the same stuff. We all share the survival circuit, a protective cellular network that helps us when times are tough. This same network is our downfall. Severe types of damage, such as broken strands of DNA, cannot be avoided. They overwork the survival circuit and change cellular identity. We're all subject to epigenetic noise that should, under the Information Theory of Aging, cause aging."

Yet different organisms age at very different rates. And sometimes, it appears, they do not age at all. What allows a whale to keep the survival circuit on without disrupting the epigenetic symphony?

In animal studies, the key to engaging the sirtuin program appears to be keeping things on the razor's edge through calorie restriction – just enough food to function in healthy ways and no more. This makes sense. It engages the survival circuit, telling longevity genes to do what they have been doing since primordial times: boost cellular defenses, keep organisms alive during times of adversity, ward off diseases and deterioration, minimize epigenetic change, and slow down aging.

Today, human studies are confirming that periodic "intermittent fasting" can have tremendous health benefits.

Why would exercising delay the erosion of telomeres?

Dr. Sinclair Continues: "If you think about how our longevity genes work – employing those ancient survival circuits – this all makes sense. Limiting food intake and reducing the heavy load of amino acids in most diets aren't the only ways to activate longevity genes that order our cells to shift into survival mode. Exercise, by definition, is the application of stress to our bodies. It raises NAD levels, which in turn activates the survival network, which turns up energy production and forces muscles to grow extra oxygen-carrying capillaries. The longevity regulators AMPK, mTOR, and sirtuins are all modulated in the right direction by exercise, irrespective of calorie intake, building new blood vessels, improving heart and lung health, making people stronger, and, yes, extending telomeres. SIRT1 and SIRT6, for example, help extend telomeres, then package them up so they are protected from degradation. Because it's not the absence of food or any particular nutrient that puts these genes into action; instead it is the hormesis program governed by the survival circuit, the mild kind of adversity that wakes up and mobilizes cellular defenses without causing too much havoc.

There's really no way around this. We all need to be pushing ourselves, especially as we get older, yet only 10 percent of people over the age of 65 do. The good news is that we don't have to exercise for hours on end. One recent study found that those who run four to five miles a week – for most people, that's an amount of exercise that can be done in less than 15 minutes per day – reduce their chance of death from heart attack by 40 percent and all-cause mortality by 45 percent. That's a massive effect."

What is unique in David Sinclair's thinking is that he believes that there is a single cause of aging upstream of all the Hallmarks of Aging.

Aging for him, quite simply, is a **loss of information**. As he points out there are two types of biological information. The first is **digital**, the nucleotides A, T, C, G of DNA.

The other type of information in the body is **analog** – this is the **epigenome** – meaning traits that are heritable that are not transmitted by genetic means.

As he writes - "Epigenetic information is what orchestrates the assembly of a human newborn made up of 26 billion cells from a single fertilized egg and what allows the genetically identical cells in our bodies to assume thousands of different modalities.

If the genome were a computer, the epigenome would be the software. That's why a neuron doesn't one day behave like a skin cell and a dividing kidney cell doesn't give to rise to two liver cells. Without epigenetic information, cells would quickly lose their identity and new cells would lose their identity, too. If they did, tissues and organs would eventually become less and less functional until they failed.

In the warm ponds of the primordial Earth, a digital chemical system was the best way to store long-term genetic data. But information storage was also needed to record and respond to environmental conditions, and this was best stored in analog format. Analog data are superior for this job because they can be changed back and forth with relative ease whenever the environment within or outside the cell demands it, and they can store an almost unlimited number of possible values, even in response to conditions that have never been encountered before.

The unlimited number of possible values is why many audiophiles still prefer the rich sounds of analog storage systems. But even though analog devices have their advantages, they have a major disadvantage. In fact, it's the reason we've moved from analog to digital. Unlike digital, analog information degrades over time – falling victim to the conspiring forces of magnetic fields, gravity, cosmic rays, and oxygen. Worse still, information is lost as it's copied.

Epigenetic noise causes the same kind of chaos. It is driven in large part by highly disruptive insults to the cell, such as broken DNA, as it was in the original survival circuit of M. Superstes and in the yeast cells that lost their fertility. And this, according to the Information Theory of Aging, is why we age. It's why our hair grays. It's why our skin wrinkles. It's why our joints begin to ache. Moreover, it's why each one of the hallmarks of aging occurs, from stem cell exhaustion and cellular senescence to mitochondrial dysfunction and rapid telomere shortening."

Overtime the "survival circuit" has evolved and researchers have now found more than two dozen of these systems within our genome – referred to as "longevity genes" for example sirtuins, AMPK and mTOR. These defense systems are all activated in response to biological stress.

Hormesis is generally good for organisms for example certain types of exercise, intermittent fasting, low carb, medium protein diets, and exposure to hot and cold temperature.

This is what people have been doing for centuries without even knowing it in the Blue Zones – activating their longevity genes.

"WE ARE ANALOG, THEREFORE WE AGE. According to the Information Theory of Aging, we become old and susceptible to disease because our cells lose youthful information. DNA stores information digitally, a robust format, whereas the epigenome stores it in analog format, and is therefore prone to the introduction of epigenetic "noise." An apt metaphor is a DVD player from the 1990s. The information is digital, the reader that moves around is analog. Aging is similar to the accumulation of scratches on the disc so the information can no longer be read correctly. Where's the polish?"

The "polish" is the survival circuit and longevity genes. These nutrient sensors and sirtuins together with the 4 Yamanaka factors is the **DVD polish** we have been looking for that can help cells that have lost their identity during aging and how they can be led back to their true selves.

What I suggest is that metabolic and psychological stress are the factors most responsible for the scratches on that DVD disc and that the key to longevity is to deal with insulin resistance and mental wellbeing.

Therapy for Genomic Instability

1. Frontiers in Anti-inflammatory Treatment: Removing Cytokines from the Blood

The demand for scientific tools to eliminate or at least significantly reduce residual cancer risk factors such as inflammation has been increasing day by day by healthy people (even if not included in classic risk groups). Among the newest tools for solid cancer prevention is CYTOBALANCE. Bioscience Institute instrument to find out and correct an increase of pro-inflammatory cytokines in the blood.

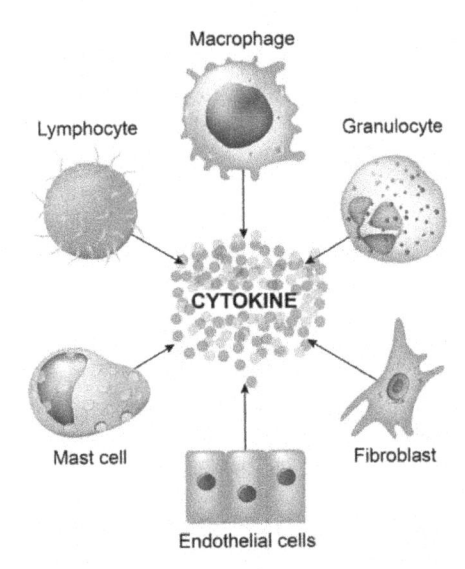

The procedure is aimed at controlling disease development predisposing or concurring conditions in healthy individuals, that is without diagnosed pathologies nor symptoms or genetic alterations making possible to hypothesize a pathway of genetic instability prodromic of cancer development, but in which it could be possible to identify or prevent physiologic or pre-pathologic conditions predisposing to the development of such alterations. Through a periodic monitoring of cytokine blood levels. CYTOBALANCE allows the detection of the increase of one or more inflammation mediators.

2. Cellphone use can damage DNA

As Lori Alton writes over 90% of American adults own one or more cellphones. While cellphones certainly make it easier to keep in touch with friends and family, to look up the nearest 4-star restaurant, and to navigate your way to new destinations, this seemingly benign technology isn't quite as benign as you might think.

The general public has NOT been properly informed about cellphone dangers. While most people don't think twice about using devices that expose their bodies to radiation in the form of radiofrequency waves or RFR, a spate of recent studies suggest that the widespread use of wireless technology presents a range of severe health risks. From increased incidents of malignant brain tumors to nervous system damage, DNA toxicity to compromised immune function – more than 1,800 studies indicate that wireless technology poses many threats to users, leading the Bioinitiative Working Group to describe wireless as "an unregulated experiment...on health and learning."

Here's what every consumer needs to know about the hidden dangers of wireless technology.

Wireless technology sends messages through RFR or a band of radiation ranging from 3kHz to 300,000 MHz. While people have regularly been exposed to RFR for more than a century, in the past decade, the amount of exposure has grown exponentially – thanks to the proliferation of cellphones, cell towers, and a variety of wireless devices.

Anytime someone uses a cellphone, laptop, tablet, or another device that utilizes Wi-Fi, they're exposed to RFR. But it's not just the users that are exposed; with about 5 million cell towers worldwide and growing, according to Scientific American, and smart-grids, Wi-Fi, Wi-Max and a vast array of commercial uses across sectors – it's almost impossible to avoid exposure to the electromagnetic fields created by these devices.

What are the health effects of wireless exposure?

As exposure levels reach new highs and continue to increase, health organizations and researchers worldwide are paying attention. For example, a meta-report from the Bioinitiative Working Group, a group of 29 independent scientists, reviewed the content and implication of about 1,800 scientific studies on the health effects of RFR exposure.

The results were sobering. Overall, the report found that:

- 68% of RFR studies indicate nervous system effects, an increase of 5% from just two years ago.
- 90% of extremely low-frequency radiation (ELFR) studies – generated by electronic equipment – show nervous system effects.
- 65% of RFR studies show DNA damage.
- 83% of ELFR studies show DNA damage.

In addition, specific studies evaluated by the report linked RFR and ELFR exposure to an increased risk of:

- Leukemia
- Brain tumors
- Neurodegenerative disease such as Alzheimer's
- Genotoxic effects
- Leakage between the blood-brain barrier
- Decreased immune function
- Increased inflammatory response
- Miscarriage
- Low sperm count and motility
- Poor cognition and memory
- Hyperactivity in children
- Insomnia
- Altered brainwave activity

What can you do to protect yourself?

The race of wireless coverage may provide convenience, but detrimental effects are too high of a cost. Seeking out wired alternatives, limiting phone call length, keeping devices off the lap, limiting wireless tech device use – especially amongst children – and using speaker options rather than holding phones up to the head offer some protection.

In addition, the World Health Organization recommends keeping wireless devices at least 30 to 40cm away from the body at all times during use to minimize RFR and ELFR exposure. If you have a cordless phone, at home, replace it with a corded telephone – it's much better.

3. **Novel exciting therapies to reduce Genomic Instability**

Very Small Embryonic-like Stem Cells (VSELS)

These cells are only 40nm and can easily go through the lung capillaries so after an IV injection of them they spread intact to all parts of the body. These cells are in everyone. They don't disappear with age. They can be extracted from your blood similar to PRP. They are like mesenchymal stem cells. They are pluripotential or tolipotential! – the ultimate stem cell. With these VSELS they are then activated by a laser so they can be activated and can respond to any environment they are placed into. Methylation data show multi year age reversal with these stem cells. The research on VSELS is continuing and is not accepted by several scientists.

Plasma Exchange

Often with one treatment methylation data we can see multiple years reduced. If you can get your Biological Age 7 years younger you can experience a 50% reduction of all chronic diseases. Remember aging is the number one risk factor for all chronic disease and death. Albumin helps bind certain proteins.

If there is one thing we all need to do is not age! This is why to have today an accurate biological age clock is essential.

Senolytics

There are several senolytics which I will cover in Chapter 13 that can also help the genome stability.

4. Endocrine Disrupting Chemicals (EDCs) or Environmental Endocrine Disruptors (EEDs)

This section is inspired by Dr. Shanna Swan's 2017 publication of her meta-analysis publication on sperm (and testosterone) decline in Western countries and her recent book *Count Down: How Our Modern World is Threatening Sperm Counts, Altering Male and Female Reproductive Development, and Imperiling the Future of the Human Race*—mostly driven by EDCs like phthalates.

Sperm and testosterone levels have fallen more than 50% in the last forty years. A massive sexual slump is underway due to people's sex drives and interest in sexual activity. Men, including younger guys I see each day, are also experiencing greater rates of erectile dysfunction.

The major cause of this crisis is the pollution we humans are doing to the planet, not just with fossil fuels, but the amount of trash we are dumping. For example, the "Great Pacific Garbage Patch," a convergence of more than 100,000 tons of floating debris including plastics, chemical sludge, and other litter. This has grown to twice the size of Texas.

A more serious problem, that directly effects our health, is the millions of pounds of chemicals found in herbicides, pesticides, and fungicides. This, together with plastic and other contaminants in our food and water supply, is creating untold hormone imbalance in our bodies. These endocrine disrupting chemicals (EDCs), that I have mentioned before, are playing havoc with the building blocks of our sexual health and reproductive development—and all living creatures that inhabit the Earth!

10 Common EDC's

1	**PHYTOESTROGENS**	Soy Flax Lavender Cannabis
2	**MYCOESTROGENS**	Fungal Contamination of Grains
3	**HERBICIDE-ESTROGENS**	Atrazine
4	**SOAP-ESTROGENS**	Triclosan and APE's
5	**SUN-SCREEN ESTROGENS**	BP and 4-MBC
6	**FOOD – COLORING ESTROGENS**	Red Numbers 3 and 40
7	**FRAGRANCE ESTROGENS**	Parabens
8	**PLASTIC ESTROGENS**	Phthalates and Parabens
9	**PLASTIC ESTROGENS**	BPA and BPS
10	**BIRTH-CONTROL ESTROGENS**	EE2 (17α-Ethynylestradiol)

These chemicals are found everywhere. Some common EDCs are seen in the table above. As Robert Hedaya, M.D., a clinical professor from Georgetown University School of Medicine writes, another problem is "Gender Fluidity." "It is nothing short of astounding that after hundreds of thousands of years of human history, the fundamental facts of human gender are becoming blurry. There are many reasons for this, but one, which I have not seen discussed as a likely cause, is the influence of endocrine disrupting chemicals (EDCs)." (One scientific theory suggests that in utero exposure to EDCs, particularly phthalates, which can lower a fetus' exposure to testosterone, may play a key role.)

Gender and sex are not the same. A person's sex is determined by biology (chromosomes, hormones, reproductive organs at birth), whereas gender depends on someone's fundamental inner sense of self, as well as the feelings, behaviors, and attitudes that go along with it.

Some members of the LGBTQ (lesbian, gay, bisexual, transgender, and questioning or queer) communities reject the born-this-way description because it doesn't necessarily apply to people whose sexuality and gender are fluid—a population that continues to grow. Research has found an association between high prenatal exposures to pesticides or phthalates and a higher risk of external genital malformations, smaller penis size, and a shorter anogenital distance (AGD) and less completely descended testes.

Reproductive Problems in Males

1. Erectile dysfunction
2. Low sperm count and quality
3. Low testosterone levels
4. Small penis and scrotum
5. Low libido
6. Infertility
7. Hormonal abnormalities e.g., thyroid/neurotransmitters
8. Ambiguous genitalia
9. Diabesity e.g., insulin
10. Prostate/testicular cancer
11. Undescended testes
12. Assisted Reproductive Technology (ART) failure

A recent publication lists the associations between phthalate exposure and a multitude of problems, both reproductive and non-reproductive:

"shorter gestational age, shorter anogenital distance, shorter penis, incomplete testicular descent, sex hormone alteration, precocious puberty, pubertal gynecomastia, premature thelarche (breast development), rhinitis, eczema, asthma, low birth weight, attention deficit hyperactivity disorder, low intelligence quotient, thyroid hormone alteration, and hypospadias in infants and children. Furthermore, many studies have suggested associations between phthalate exposure and increased sperm DNA damage, decreased proportion of sperm with normal morphology, decreased sperm concentration, decreased sperm morphology, sex hormone alteration, decreased pulmonary function, endometriosis, uterine leiomyomas, breast cancer, obesity, hyperprolactinemia, and thyroid hormone alteration in adults."

Remember, there are two main factors driving this health pandemic:

1. Chemical culprits

Phthalates, bisphenols, flame retardants, pesticides, per fluorinated chemicals, "legacy chemicals" found everywhere in plastic drinking bottles, cleaning supplies, house dust, home furniture, electronics, building materials, fragrances, food, food packaging, thermal cash register receipts, drinking water, personal care products.

2. Lifestyle factors

Poor nutrition, lack of exercise, smoking, alcohol, drugs, stress, diabesity. Many of these lifestyle factors are covered in the chapters included in this book.

How to Protect Yourself from EDCs

The following plan is taken from Estrogeneration by Dr. Anthony Jay:

Your Plan is to:
- Avoid ingredients that include "benz-" or "phen-"
- Eliminate dietary grains, including all corn products
- Eliminate dietary peanuts, cheap coffee, and cheap chocolate
- Eliminate liquid dairy products unless grass-fed and in glass
- Eliminate butter unless grass-fed
- Eliminate all dietary liquids stored in plastics, especially oils
- Eliminate fragrances in all personal care products
- Eliminate fragrances in laundry detergent and dryer sheets
- Travel and sleep with a pillow case washed without fragrance
- Eliminate processed foods
- Eliminate plastic shower curtains

- Eliminate vinyl flooring/tiling, wallpaper, and plastic countertops
- Avoid standard industrial bathroom hand-soaps
- Avoid cannabis
- Avoid candies except beeswax
- Avoid plastics in your environment, including plastic toys
- Eliminate carpets or use "Green-Label Plus" certified carpets
- Avoid foods canned in metal
- Only eat wild seafood from pristine waters
- Only eat grass-fed organic meats, preferably in wax paper
- Only eat grass-fed organic animal fats, with no plastic contacts
- Only eat free-range chicken eggs
- Use charcoal-filtered water for all drinking and cooking
- Use charcoal-filtered water for showering
- Use all glass and/or stainless steel coffee makers
- Use "Estrogenic-Free" cleaning products
- Use "Estrogenic-Free" kid's toys, especially chewable items
- Use "Estrogenic-Free" zinc sunscreen
- Avoid moldy environments
- Eliminate soy and soy byproducts
- Eliminate flax
- Eliminate lavender products
- Eliminate oral contraception
- Eliminate plastic cups, sippies, or plastic lined mugs
- Eliminate artificial red food dyes, including finger paints
- Eliminate microwaving food in plastics

How Can You Detoxify To Prevent Genomic Instability?

1. **Confirm You are Toxic**

Review your history and the Total-Body Toxic Load Test. An examination and select laboratory tests will confirm your toxicity level. Develop a plan to detoxify. (Doctors Data and other specialized labs can measure what you may be toxic to).

2. Identify Toxins in Your Environment

Do a room-by-room evaluation of your home and office, paying special attention to the kitchen, bathroom, and bedroom. Don't use toxic cleaners, especially in the bedroom, as you will lie all night inhaling toxic chemicals and awaken with a fatigued detox system. Get rid of EMF appliances in the bedroom, particularly those close to your head. Select all future products with awareness and phase out your unhealthy products.

3. Clean Up Your Air

Use plants such as spider plants, ferns, and philodendrons to filter toxins from your air. Avoid air fresheners and other chemicals that will make your air toxic. Use an air purifier in the bedroom. More than 90 percent of particulates can be handled by a HEPA (high-efficiency particle absorption) filter. Regularly open the windows and allow some good cross-ventilation. Don't jog or exercise near highways. Clean and monitor your heating system. Air out your dry cleaning.

4. Clean Up Your Water

Either buy a total household water filter or install one on each faucet. Reverse osmosis filters lower the pH of water. Consider installing a Water system. Ask your water utility for a copy of their annual water quality report. For further options, contact the NSF Consumer Affairs Office at 877-867-3435.

5. Clean Up Your Diet

Follow the Paleolithic or Keto diets. Eat organic whenever possible and avoid all processed and fast foods. Go easy on coffee and alcohol, but drink plenty of clean water and green tea. Choose foods that will help you detoxify. Remember to use nontoxic kitchen utensils—no aluminum pots. Fiji water is my favorite.

6. Get Down to Your Ideal Weight

The greater your percent of body fat, the greater the amount of toxins will be released and the more inflammation that will be generated. This inflammation causes more weight gain and a vicious cycle begins. You must break this cycle. Remember, the key is to reduce sugar and grain intake.

7. Sweat Out Toxins

Saunas are a great way to eliminate toxins by sweating. Far-infrared (FIR) saunas are safe and effective for this purpose. FIR saunas were used initially in Japan and entered the U.S. market in the early 1980s. They induce three times the sweat volume as a traditional sauna at a far more tolerable temperature. The sauna is ideal for detoxifying and has many other beneficial properties.

8. Exercise Regularly

Besides being important for weight maintenance, exercise is another way to sweat out toxins. Yoga and massage can also help move toxins out of your system. Bouncing on a trampoline (rebounding) is especially good at stimulating lymphatic drainage.

9. Enhance Digestion with Enzymes and Probiotics

If you suffer from chronic digestive problems, such as acid reflux, irritable bowel, or constipation, I suggest adding digestive enzymes and probiotics (friendly bacteria that can help re-balance your intestinal ecology).

10. Detoxify Your Body

The average man uses a fragrant shampoo, conditioner, mousse, shaving cream, toothpaste, aftershave, deodorant, and skin lotions, all containing chemical fragrances, colors, cleaning agents, and petrocarbon additives. Clothes contain odors from detergents and fabric softeners, not to mention formaldehyde and other chemicals to make them color-fast and wrinkle resistant. Chemicals in dry cleaning fluid, moth balls, and shoe polish can harm the brain.

11. Detoxify Your Mind

A toxic mind filled with grief, fear, sadness, anger, and jealousy can hurt you just as quickly as DDT. Relaxation, laughter, joy, and gratitude are great detoxifiers.

12. Add Nutraceuticals

Take a good multivitamin/multimineral as well as anti-inflammatory nutraceuticals to help you detoxify. In addition consider synolytics, NAD, resveratrol, etc.

13. Enjoy a Daily "Detox Cocktail"

There are several supplements that help detoxify the body, such as lipoic acid and milk thistle. Taking these types of nutraceuticals provide a cocktail that helps both Phase I and II detoxification.

14. Take Fiber Each Day

A good fiber intake (35 grams daily) is important to help cleanse the bowel. Both soluble and insoluble fiber help detoxify you. Eating healthy 'real food' will ensure a healthy intestinal transit time (bowel regularity).

15. Consider Removing Your Dental Amalgams

Before removing your silver amalgams, contact Doctors Data and have a provocative heavy metal test done to check if you are mercury toxic. Mercury is especially toxic to the brain and heart. Oral chelators are powerful and inexpensive. Non-prescription alternatives are also excellent for the removal of mercury, lead, cadmium, aluminum, tin, arsenic, antimony, and more.

16. Avoid All Drugs

Try to avoid not only recreational drugs but all pharmaceutical drugs and the many over-the-counter drugs.

17. Take Omega-3 Fish Oils Daily

Omega-3 fish oils are one of the most important supplements you can take. Always be sure to use pharmaceutical grade fish oil to minimize mercury and other pollutants. It is essential for controlling silent inflammation.

18. Consider Colon Hydrotherapy

Colon hydrotherapy (using water to flush the colon) was used in ancient Egypt and in most cultures. There is no odor or risk if a licensed colon therapist is selected. The International Association for Colon Therapy (IACT) in San Antonio, Texas, is the worldwide licensing body for colon therapists; contact them at 210-366-2888.

19. Relaxation, Meditation, and Sleep

Healthy sleep patterns, making time to relax, and developing a meditation ritual will help detoxify the mind and energize your spirit.

20. Don't Forget to Breathe

Diaphragmatic breathing can be an exercise for relaxation and meditation in itself. The act of deep breathing will also stimulate lymphatic flow and help eliminate toxins.

21. Ground Yourself

In his new book, *Earthing*, my colleague Dr. Stephen Sinatra explains how simply using a "silver" impregnated bedsheet will help you sleep better, lower your cortisol, help thin your blood, and offer a host of other health benefits.

Summary

Ninety-eight percent of the atoms in your body are replaced each year. We have a remarkable ability to rejuvenate ourselves when properly detoxified and nourished. In order to achieve optimal results, we need to pay attention to all our channels of elimination. These include the liver, gastrointestinal tract, lungs, kidneys, the skin, the blood, and the lymph.

CHAPTER 11: ALTERED INTERCELLULAR COMMUNICATION

In order to grow and function normally, our cells must constantly transfer information to each other, secreting signaling molecules to their neighboring cells or even sending molecular messengers through the bloodstream to affect cells and tissues far away. Aging changes not only the signals that are sent by cells, but also the ability of receiving cells to respond to such signals. This **dysfunctional communication** leads to issues like chronic tissue inflammation, as well as failure of the immune system to recognize and clear pathogens or dysfunctional cells, increasing susceptibility to infection and cancer.

What is Intercellular Communication?

Intercellular communication can be defined as the conversation between two cells. It is studied under the branch of cell biology, which encompasses the study of cellular organelles and cell signaling. Intercellular as well as intracellular communication both come under cell signaling. Intracellular communication can be defined as the communication that takes place within the cell, for example, the cellular response that occurs in response to molecules present inside the cell.

Cells communicate through chemical signals, these chemical signals are known as ligands. These ligands can only interact with the cell that has the receptor for the particular ligand, this ligand-receptor association provides the specificity to the cell signaling or intracellular communication. These are the following types of intercellular communication that occur between the cell, paracrine, autocrine, endocrine, and cell-to-cell contact signaling.

Feature of Cell Signaling

According to the intercellular communication definition, there are the following characteristic features that define intracellular communication.

1. **Specificity**- It is attributed to the high affinity of the signaling molecule (ligand) and the complementary receptor. The complementarity of structure be-

tween ligand and receptor binding contributes to the high specificity of the signaling pathway.

2. **Amplification**- During intracellular communication, the signal amplifies several fold to generate the response, amplification can be attributed to the cooperative nature of the receptor-ligand association.

3. **Desensitization**- Also known as adaption, it is the condition that arises due to the continuous binding of the ligand to the receptor. It can result in a lack of response by the cell. To avoid such conditions cells follow feedback regulation, which allows removal of ligand and receptor when needed.

4. **Integration**- It can be defined as the ability of the system to receive multiple signals and produce a unified response appropriate to the needs of the cell.

Stages of Intercellular Communication

There are three main stages or steps of communication, they are as follows-

1. **Reception**- It refers to receiving the signal via ligand molecule binding to the receptor. Receptor proteins are the molecules that spans through the plasma membrane, this receptor provides a specific binding site for the ligand. The ligand generally undergoes a conformational change, leading to the sequential activation of the protein cascade. Another common method is phosphorylation and dephosphorylation of the intracellular protein.

2. **Transduction**- It refers to the transfer of the signal from the cell surface to the interior of the cell, it is achieved by activating several proteins via phosphorylation, dephosphorylation. A common method is the production of the secondary messenger. This ensures the amplification of the signal received.

3. **Response**- A cell generates a varying type of response according to the need, it includes transcription and translation of protein or inhibits the synthesis of a certain protein, succession, or inhibition of cell cycle. The result is the change in the metabolic activity of the cell.

Example of Signals to Which Cells Respond

These are examples of the ligand to which a cell responds

1. Antigens

2. Cell surface glycoprotein
3. Developmental signals
4. Growth factors
5. Hormones
6. Neurotransmitter
7. Pheromones
8. Nutrients
9. Mechanical touch
10. Light

Examples of Intercellular Communication

Six basic receptor types can be used as an example of intercellular communication, they are as follows,

1. G-protein coupled receptor, used in vision transmission, epinephrine metabolism.
2. Receptor tyrosine kinase, used in cell division and glucose metabolism
3. Receptor guanylyl cyclase, used in the metabolism of nitric oxide and ROS
4. Gated ion channels, used in the transmission of nerve impulse
5. Adhesion receptors used to maintain integrity and development in embryonic stages
6. Nuclear receptors (steroid receptors), used inactivation and inhibition of transcription of certain proteins.

Types of Intercellular Communication

The intercellular communication types can be categorized into three types: autocrine, paracrine, endocrine signaling, and cell-to-cell contact signaling. This signaling mechanism is used according to the ligand and need of the cell.

Paracrine Signaling

It is the signaling pathway that has ligand molecules traveling a short distance to bind to its receptor. It can be defined as the signaling pathway in which cells communicate over a relatively short distance. The important feature of such a signaling pathway is that it allows the cell to be in coordination with other cells neighboring it. One of the most important roles of paracrine signaling is in embryonic development, it is through the pluripotent cell that decides its cell lineage, which it follows to develop specific organs and tissues.

Another most widely studied example is synaptic signaling, which comes under as a type of paracrine signaling.

Synaptic signaling is the method used by nerves to transmit their impulse or action potential across one nerve to another. The name is derived from the synapse. Synapses are the junction between two nerves. It contains a neurotransmitter that acts as a ligand, which then binds to the receptor present on the membrane of the second nerve. The common ligand that is used is acetylcholine, and the gated ion channel receptor mediates the signal transduction. The binding of a neurotransmitter opens the gated ion channel, which changes the electrical potential of the cell, and thus travels from one nerve to another.

Autocrine Signaling

Autocrine signaling is a type of signaling where the cell releases a chemical molecule, which acts as a ligand that binds to the receptor on the cell that produces it. This type of signaling is generally observed in the self-activatory molecules and as part of the immune response. The most important example of autocrine signaling is apoptosis, it can be defined as programmed cell death. In this case phosphatidylserine, a molecule present on the inner leaflet of the plasma membrane moves towards the extracellular side, acting as a ligand for apoptosis. It also plays an important role in immune response cytokine production and regulation is mediated by the autocrine signaling pathway.

Endocrine Signaling

It is a long-distance signaling pathway, and a ligand molecule is transported over a long distance to which it binds to the receptor. The best example of this type of signaling is hormones, hormones from various glands are poured into the bloodstream and they travel along with it. When they reach the target cell, they bind to receptors generating the appropriate response.

Cell to Cell Contact Signaling

It occurs when two cells are connected through gap junctions or plasmodesmata in the case of plants, these junctions provide a channel through which ligand molecules can travel. Ligand in this case is known as intracellular mediators, which brings the response.

Why We Age

Altered intercellular communication, as described in the Hallmarks of Aging is the change in signals between cells that can lead to some of the diseases and disabilities of aging. It is also one of 10 reasons we age.

Inflammation and hormonal imbalance

As we age, the signaling environment of chemical messages across the whole body tends to become more inflammatory, inhibiting the immune system and potentially causing muscle wasting, bone loss and other harmful effects in a process known as inflammaging.

Multiple different factors cause this inflammaging, one of which is the senescence-associated secretory phenotype (SASP) – is directly caused by another hallmark of aging, cellular senescence. Senescent cells are known to secrete an inflammatory, immunosuppressive, and harmful mixture that has been shown to encourage neighboring cells to become senescent and may contribute to multiple age-related diseases. This mixture is known as the senescence-associated secretory phenotype.

Beyond the SASP, senescent cells have been shown to encourage senescence in nearby cells through so-called bystander effects, including the secretion of DNA-damaging chemicals known as reactive oxygen species (ROS) and the leakage of chemicals from senescent cells into neighboring cells through gap junctions, which are holes between their surfaces.

The smoldering, consistent growth in inflammation across the body leads to cells increasingly activating a chemical in their nuclei, nuclear factor kappa-light-chain-enhancer of activated B cells (NF-kB), which regulates inflammation. NF-kB is a protein complex that regulates the production of proteins, enzymes, and local signals (cytokines). It is present in almost all cell types and is involved in cellular responses to stimuli such as diabesity, stress, cytokines, free radicals, heavy metals, radiation, oxidized LDL cholesterol, and bacterial or viral antigens. NF-kB can be considered a master regulator of cell activity, and its increase can lead to harmful consequences.

Beyond its association with other diseases, when NF-kB is activated in te hypothalamus, a region of the brain dedicated to maintaining normal bodily function, it has been shown to inhibit the production of gonadotropin-releasing hormone (GnRH). This hormone is used to signal other bodily systems, and its reduction may contribute to bone fragility, muscle weakness, skin degradation, and other harmful effects with age.

NF-kB, inflammation and metabolic diseases

Metabolic disorders including obesity, type 2 diabetes and atherosclerosis have been viewed historically as lipid storage disorders brought about by overnutrition. It is now widely appreciated that chronic low-grade inflammation plays a key role in the initiation, propagation and development of metabolic diseases. Consistent with its central role in coordinating inflammatory responses, numerous recent studies have implicated the transcription factor NF-kB in the development of such diseases, thereby further establishing inflammation as a critical factor in their etiology and offering hope for the development of new therapeutic approaches for their treatment.

The competing need to protect the body from infection while maintaining proper energy metabolism represents a fundamental physiological change. Mounting an immune response to infection is energy intensive, but essential for life. Both immunity to disease and economical use of energy reserves have been heavily favored throughout human evolution. Yet in the modern era, when overnutrition is more common than starvation, metabolic diseases have become the leading cause of death in the United States, with an incidence skyrocketing worldwide. Furthermore, as the risk of infectious diseases recedes, an immune system poised to respond vigorously to all inflammatory challenges has itself become a threat. Indeed, inappropriate triggering of such responses may account for the prevalence of inflammatory diseases such as allergy, asthma, diabetes, and cancer.

Metabolic syndrome encompasses a cluster of conditions that result from nutrient excess, hyperglycemia, hyperlipidemia, insulin resistance, obesity, and hepatic steatosis, which together affect a quarter of American adults and over a million children. Metabolic diseases track together, and obese patients are at increased risk for type-2 diabetes, while insulin-resistant patients frequently suffer from cardiovascular diseases such as atherosclerosis. The NF-kB pathway unites the inflammatory and metabolic responses, and as a well-studied mediator of inflammation and immunity, represents an entry point for better understanding metabolic diseases with an eye towards developing novel treatment strategies.

Therapy To Improve Intercellular Communication

1. Nutrition

A major approach used in lab animals to try and treat this hallmark involves decreasing energy intake through food while maintaining nutrient intake, which is known as caloric restriction (CR). CR has been shown to significantly increase lifespan in a variety of animals, including mice and a species of worm called C. Elegans, and a number of approaches are being tested to try and replicate this effect without requiring a strict diet. However, while it has been shown to be very effective in short-lived creatures, longer-lived creatures seem to receive smaller gains in lifespan from CR.

A WFKD is much more sustainable than CR. I especially like the 20/4 i.e. only eating once a day in a 4 hour window. It is easier than you think and helps increase apoptosis and increases stem cells.

2. Senolytics

Since cellular senescence plays a large role in altered cellular communication different senolytics can be used. (See Chapter 13)

3. Kisspeptin-10

An effective alternative to HCG- both stimulate gonadotropin release in both males and females and will help counteract NF-kB.

4. Parabiosis or Apheresis

Another approach to treating this hallmark is based on parabiosis – the merging of the circulatory systems of two individuals. This has been shown to have beneficial impacts on various aging-associated factors in mice, but the method of the benefits is unclear.

According to a paper co-authored by Irina Conboy, a member of LEAF's scientific advisory board, blood from older creatures can be harmful to younger creatures, perhaps due to signaling molecules used for intercellular communications within the old blood. This could suggest that at least part of the benefit of parabiosis is due to the dilution of the harmful signals.

As she explained in an interview with LEAF, a route that is being explored to treat this hallmark is apheresis, in which blood is removed from the body, the pro-aging signaling molecules are removed, and the blood is reintroduced; this is an attempt at mimicking the effect of parabiosis.

5. Nutraceuticals

Curcumin and Resveratrol inhibit NF-kB and can likely improve intercellular communicator.

6. Stress Management

Stress induces an increase in NF-kB that increases expression of mRNA of pre-inflammatory cytokines interfering with cellular communication.

7. Sleep

Lack of sleep activates NF-kB and can aggravate abnormal signaling causing inflammatory related diseases.

8. Pharmaceuticals

Most NF-kb drugs found to inhibit NF-kB have increased cytotoxic effects and are not recommended for anti-aging (clients taking digoxin can experience a decrease in NF-kB).

9. Hormones

As hormones are critical for long-distance signaling and communication it is essential to restore all hormones to optimal levels.

CHAPTER 12: EPIGENETIC-ALTERATIONS

You may wonder how our various tissues and organs can appear so different from one another, since the genetic information encoded in our DNA is exactly the same in all cells in our body. In fact, DNA is modified with epigenetic information that enhances or suppresses the expression of particular genes as required by different tissue types. For example, if a cell should develop into a liver cell, epigenetic modifications will ensure that the parts of the genome specific to liver cells are expressed, while the parts specific to other cell types are ignored. The aging process often involves changes in our epigenetic code, which can lead to changes in gene expression that affect normal cellular function. In the immune system, for example, this could shift the balance between activating and suppressing immune cells, causing our bodies to be less resilient to pathogens.

What we measure is DNA **methylation,** and this is the silencing of gene transcription, so at the beginning of your genes we notice those with essentially decreased expression of that gene. The converse process is called **acetylation**, which is a changed molecule which can open up these proteins to allow your genes to be transcribed i.e. we measure just the negative regulatory process, the DNA methylation. TruDiagnostics measures over 900,000 CPG locations as mentioned in Chapter 1. That is out of 26 million approximately. Most of TruDiagnostics competitors only measure 100,000 locations.

In the LB100 program in addition to the TruDiagnostic Biological Age and Pace of Aging (See Chapter 1). We know that the lower your Pace of Aging is overtime we can see improved healthspan with less sarcopenia and more muscle mass. We also see better cognition and IQ. There is also less visible facial aging.

I have included my first TruDiagnostic test to give the reader a sample of this powerful diagnostic tool that I would encourage all to use. The 3 reports here include:

1. Epigenetic Age
2. Pace of Aging
3. Telomere Length

Although my Intrinsic Epigenetic Age has met the magic 7 years lower than my chronological age you can see I need to improve my Extrinsic Epigenetic Age. Likewise I need to slow my Pace of Aging and improve my telomere length!

With the LB100 program we send additional 1-2 reports to clients each month to help with improving Healthspan and Lifespan.

Although I have no chronic disease and take no medications I have embarked on LB100 to improve my methylation data markers.

YOUR BIOLOGICAL AGE
vs Chronological Age

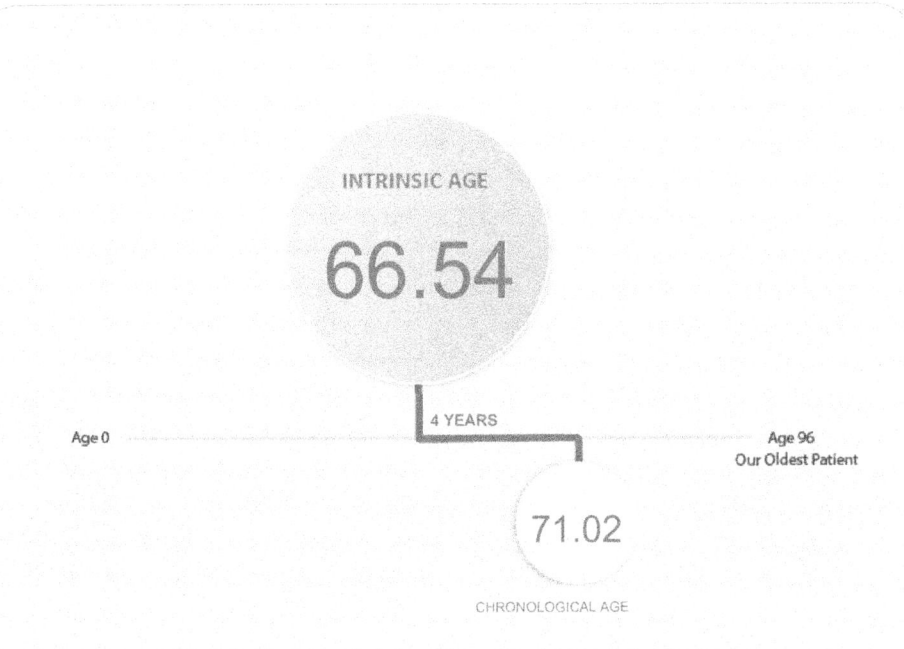

INTRINSIC AGE

66.54

Age 0 — 4 YEARS — Age 96 Our Oldest Patient

71.02

CHRONOLOGICAL AGE

Your biological age is lower than your chronological age.

This is the first of hopefully many tests to measure the status of your DNA. You are older than your DNA. While tests like 23andMe might predict risk of certain diseases, TruAge can see how much your DNA can be changed through proper lifestyle changes.

If your intrinsic age is much higher than your chronological age, don't worry. There are plenty of things you can do to slow your aging. If your intrinsic age is under your chronological age, don't stop doing what you are doing, but implemebt additional benefits.

YOUR EPIGENETIC AGE
Summary

INTRINSIC AGE

66.54

Age 0 — 4 YEARS — Age 100

71.02

CHRONOLOGICAL AGE

TruAge IEAA=2.96

You versus the Population

[Scatter plot of Intrinsic Age vs Chronological Age]

66.78 — This is your Intrinsic Epigenetic Age using our previous (not Principle Component Analysis corrected) algorithm.

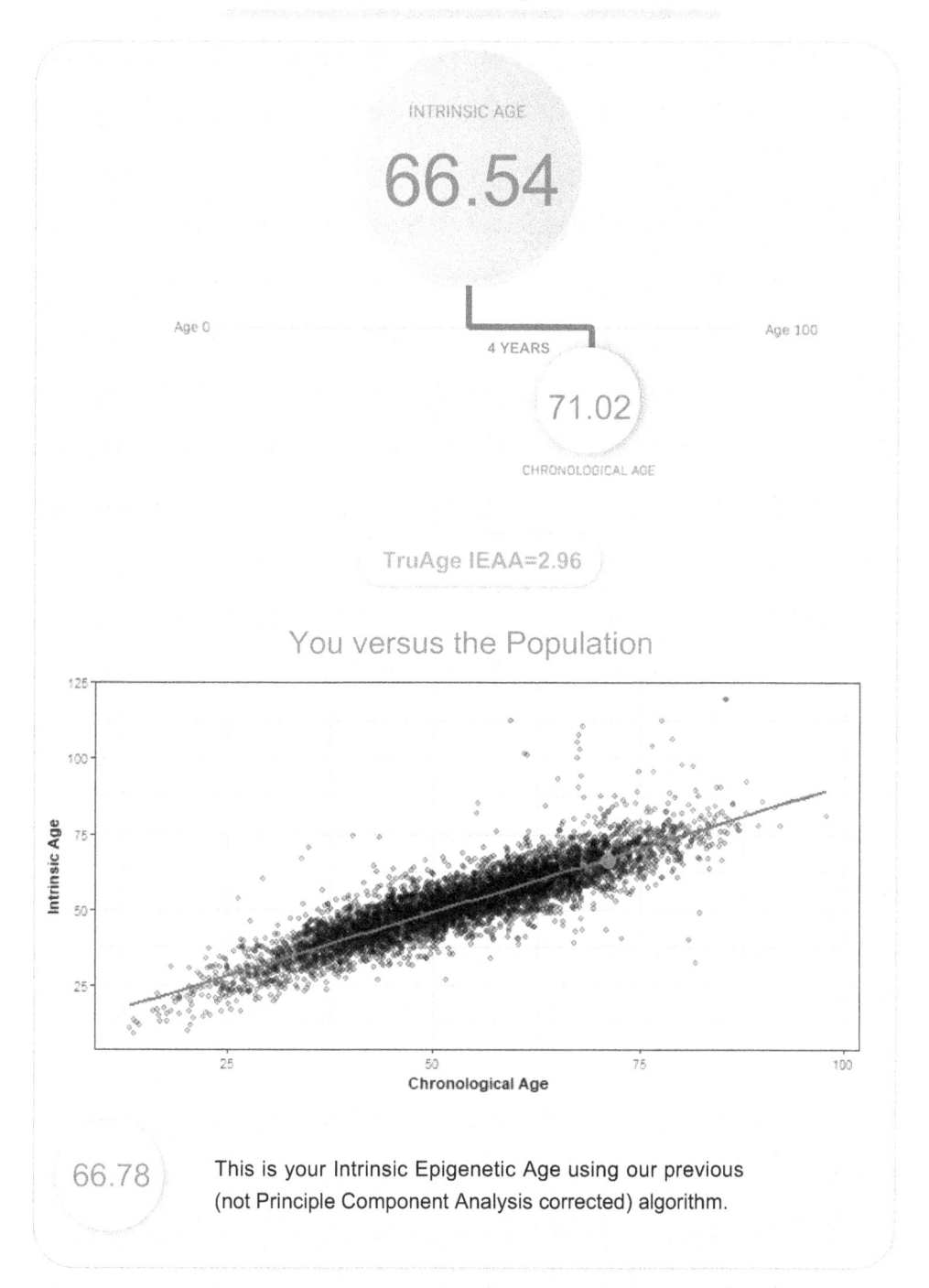

HOW DO YOU COMPARE
to the general population?

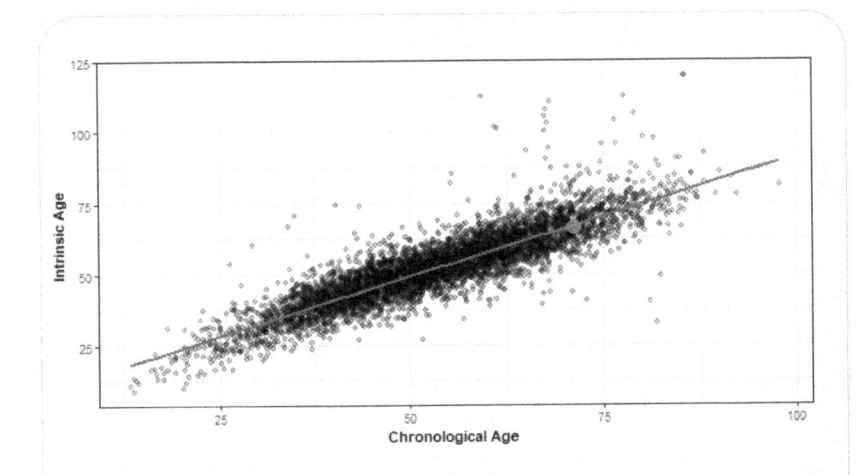

Your Biological Age Compared to the General Population

This graph shows you where most people would range when comparing their chronological age versus their biological age.

One thing to remember is that a majority of our patient population are receiving this test in a preventative, integrative, functional medical community. As a result, our population metrics might be slightly different than those of the true general population. That is because often, the individuals who are being tested can afford the test and are most likely interested in aging in a healthy manner. In order to avoid this bias, TruDiagnostic actively recruits participants outside of this population to make sure we have a good snapshot of all variables such as socioeconomic status, race, gender, nationality and many others. If you have a connection to a under represented group who would like to be involved in this research, please let us know.

DUNEDINPACE REPORT
The Study Explained & Where You Land

TruDiagnostic™
The Epigenetic Company

Summary of this Report:

- This report is able to tell you how many biological years you are aging per year at the precise moment.
- It separates what you are doing now from markers you've accumulated from your past, or inherited from your ancestry.
- You want your rate of aging to be below 1.
- Fastest rate of aging has been 1.4 biological years/1.0 year of chronological aging.
- Slowest rate of aging has been 0.6 biological years/1.0 year of chronological aging.
- The average person will age at a rate of 1.0 biological years/1.0 year of chronological aging
- Dietary interventions like fasting have been shown to decrease the aging rate.
- This algorithm was created by Duke and Columbia via a longitudinal study. This means the researchers followed the same individuals over time which is different from other algorithms of aging.

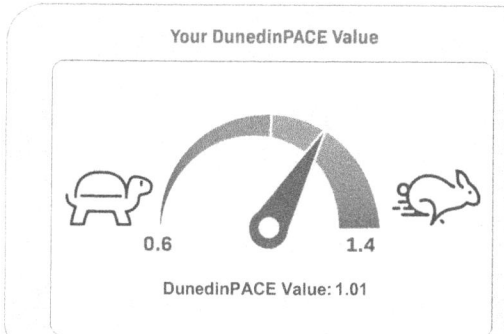

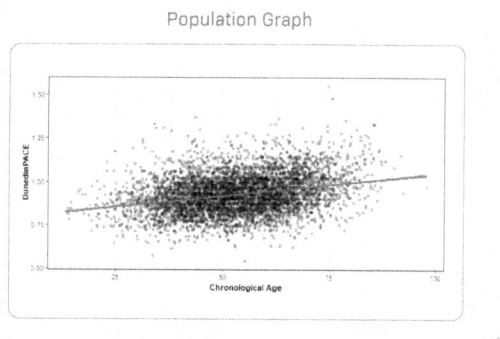

Your DunedinPACE Value

0.6 — 1.4

DunedinPACE Value: 1.01

Population Graph

Methylation based biological aging clocks changed the way we look at aging and preventive medicine!
Aging is the number one risk factor for most chronic diseases. Unfortunately, traditional determinants of age (the number of years since birth) don't always match up with how each individual ages. Some people in their 70s look and feel like they are 50, and then there are some 70-year-olds that look like they could be 90. This is called **phenotypic variation**, and as a result, people have been searching for objective markers to measure the aging process. Thankfully, a highly accurate one was created by measuring epigenetic biomarkers.

Having an objective biological age measurement has massive implications for preventative health and future investigations. However, if we can combine this with an instantaneous rate of aging, we can learn even more about our aging process, our individual aging biology, and the interventions for better preventative health when we combine these two metrics.

YOUR PACE OF AGING VALUE:

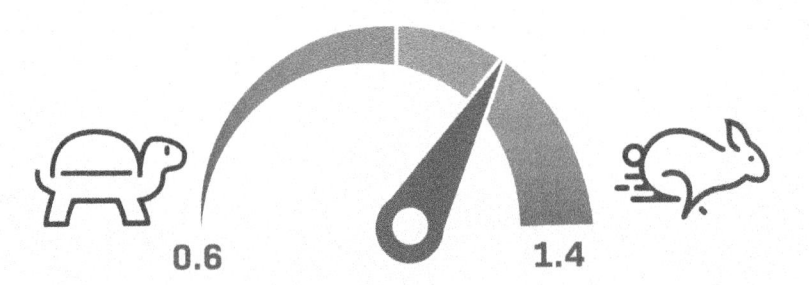

DunedinPACE Value: 1.01

What Does Your Rate of Aging Mean?

You want your rate of aging to be below one; this means you would have a slowed pace of aging. An average pace of aging would be a rate of 1 biological year for every chronological year aged.

DunedinPACE is associated with chronic disease morbidity and mortality. *Within 7 years from testing those with a faster pace of aging are at a **56% increased risk of death and a 54% increased risk for diagnosis of a chronic disease.***

Mortality

Those with faster DunedinPACE levels, which indicates faster aging, at baseline were at increased risk of death having a hazard ratio of 1.29. Hazard ratio represents an instantaneous risk, it is the relationship between the instantaneous hazards between accelerated DunedinPACE and mortality.

Morbidity

Those with a faster DunedinPACE baseline were at an increased risk for a new chronic disease, putting them at a hazard ratio of 1.19. Individuals with faster DunedinPACE experienced higher levels of chronic disease morbidity, which was measured as the count of diagnosed diseases (hypertension, type-2 diabetes, cardiovascular disease, chronic obstructive pulmonary disease, chronic kidney disease, and cancer).

Accelerated Aging Influences

Pace of aging typically increases across much of the adult lifespan. A faster DunedinPACE is the result of a lifetime of accumulated stress to the methylome. Childhood exposure to poverty and victimization is associated with faster DunedinPACE. Adolescents who grew up in families of lower socioeconomic-status and adolescents with exposure to multiple types of victimization exhibited faster DunedinPACE.

GRAHAM SIMPSON
TELOMERE LENGTH REPORT
And How Their Length Affects You

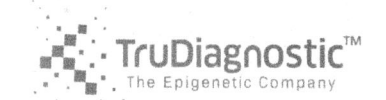

TruDiagnostic™
The Epigenetic Company

YOUR RESULTS:

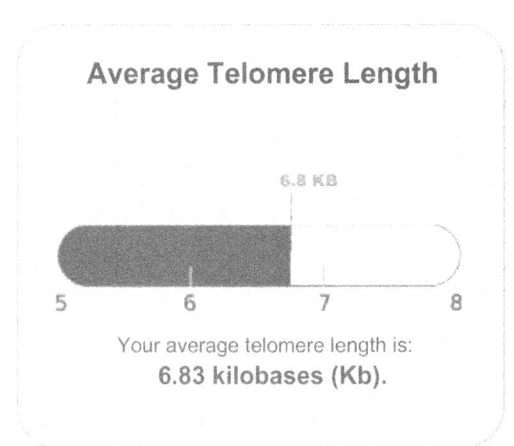

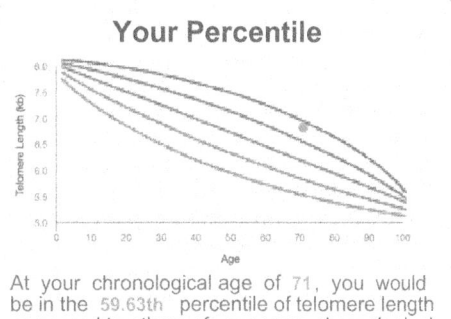

Average Telomere Length

6.8 KB

Your average telomere length is:
6.83 kilobases (Kb).

Your Percentile

At your chronological age of 71, you would be in the 59.63th percentile of telomere length compared to others of your same chronological age. This means that your telomeres are longer than 59.63% of people your age

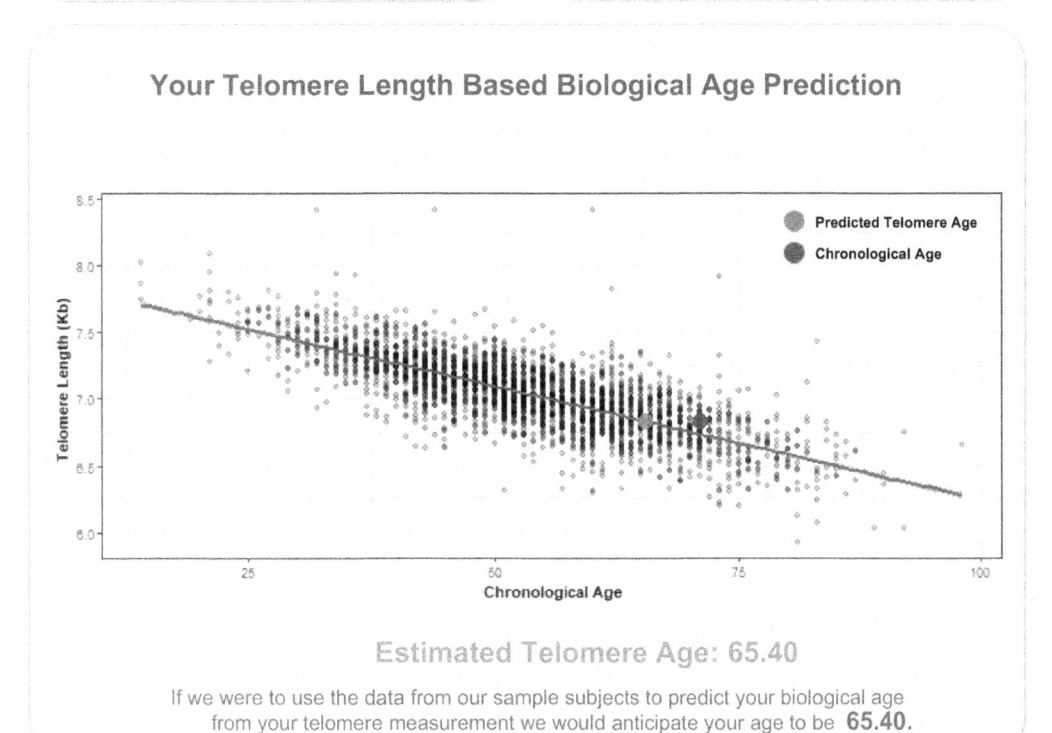

Your Telomere Length Based Biological Age Prediction

- Predicted Telomere Age
- Chronological Age

Estimated Telomere Age: 65.40

If we were to use the data from our sample subjects to predict your biological age from your telomere measurement we would anticipate your age to be **65.40.**

Therapy To Improve Epigenetics

I have used the INTEGRAL HEALTH Model on thousands of clients over the past 20 years with great success.

The INTEGRAL HEALTH Model

What is Proactive Health?

We have a broken-sick care system when what we really need is a whole integrated health system. The focus should be as much on predicting and preventing disease rather than **treating disease. Our approach addresses the complete picture of someone's health.** We embrace 4P medicine.

Personalized: Everyone has a unique set of genes and presentations and that we take into account with each client.

Predictive: We can predict with a few simple tests and questionnaires what you may be predisposed to and therefore what we can prevent.

Preventive: This is where the mainstream medical system is failing; we test to look into your future to prevent disease.

Participatory: It is critical to your health that not only we, but you, participate in taking control of your health.

The 4P Proactive Health approach is gaining traction in the healthcare industry. The essence of 4P medicine is the quantification of wellness and the demystification of disease. 4P medicine will cause every single sector of the healthcare community to rewrite their business plans, and many will be unable to do so due to their conservative traditional outlook.

Proactive Medicine uses the new genomic and epigenetic testing to personalize our approach – as mentioned previously chronic disease develops over time and using imaging and advanced labs we can predict what will likely happen and thus we can often prevent disease, especially if your health professional develops a strong participatory relationship with you.

We assess your current level of health and collectively we will develop a set of **specific goals and follow you through a whole person I.N.T.E.G.R.A.L.** approach.

1. **Inflammation Control**

The underlying root cause of many cardio-metabolic disease. Inflammation is now understood to be at the center of a wide range of chronic conditions from heart disease and hypertension to obesity and diabetes. Even aging itself appears to result from the cumulative effects of silent inflammation (Inflam-Aging).

2. **Nutrition and Metabolic Balance**

Accounts for 70% of your health and wellness. You will be introduced to the original human Keto/Paleo diets whether you are a meat or plant based eater. We will help you **balance your 'sugar' and insulin levels which are critical** for good health and show you how to incorporate proteins and healthy fats into your diet. Remember, Food is Medicine.

3. **Toxin and Cancer Reduction**

Cancer is becoming the number one killer in America. Our ancestors lived in a cleaner environment than we are faced with today. Environmental exposure to heavy metals and other toxins in our environment have become a major issue affecting our health. The gut and mitochondria – **the little 'energy furnaces' in all our cells** - are most damaged, leaving you tired and run down. We will help you decrease your toxic load by simple home-based elimination methods, detoxes and adequate supplementation.

4. **Exercise, Rest and Sleep**

Critical for rejuvenation and longevity. Our primitive ancestors used to move up to 20 miles a day for survival and we are mandated to sit for prolonged periods in awkward unnatural postures. Sitting has been shown to be more of a cardio-metabolic risk factor than smoking and is partly why we are experiencing an epidemic of back pain. We will develop a personalized exercise program to achieve your goals that best suits your lifestyle. We will also include methods to improve the length and quality of your sleep – a critical part of daily rejuvenation and optimal health.

5. **Gut Microbiome**

You have 30 trillion human cells but 100 trillion "bugs", most of them living in your gut. 80% of our immune system surrounds our gut. Remember your gut bacteria known as your 'microbiome' can live without you, but you can't live for one day without them. Your Microbiome is critical to your health. They process your food, boost immunity, fight infections and improve mood, skin and energy levels. Stress and poor nutrition can lead to an imbalance in your microbiome. We will assess and integrate specific foods and supplements into your diet to promote healthy gut flora as needed.

6. Restoration of Hormones

Imbalanced hormones can be the single biggest reason you can't lose weight. Because our primal ancestors were so active, their hormones levels were much healthier right through to late life. Hormones are the **'juice of life,'** they promote hair and skin development, growth, metabolism, sex drive and much more. Without correcting your hormone levels to that of a healthy 30-35 year old you cannot enjoy optimum health and prevent chronic disease.

7. Adequate Supplements

As food sources become less nutritious, supplements become critical. Our body is becoming nutrient depleted from poor quality soil and therefore we are becoming deficient in nutrients that are essential to prevent disease and maintain health. Good quality targeted supplements are essential to protect and optimize your health. We can perform simple tests to see if you are deficient in any vitamins or minerals critical for mental and physical health.

8. Lifetime Mindfulness and Stress Reduction

Stress kills full stop! Relaxation techniques have been used for centuries with significant health benefits. With the constant societal pressures we need to give our mind a chance to **'unplug.'** We will teach you different mindful techniques to manage your stress – the key to feeling energized, looking younger, feeling calmer, staying healthy and avoiding burnout. As your mind becomes sharper it will also help you understand your own unique talents, passions and life purpose.

Personal, Family, Ssocial relationships and Spirituality are all essential for mental wellbeing.

Note: We now have more than 20 methylation reports that cover these 8 INTEGRAL dimensions so we can track how successful our interventions are!

CHAPTER 13: CELLULAR SENESCENCE

Once cells are subjected to enough stress, DNA damage and telomere shortening, they enter a state growth arrest called cellular senescence. This is a protective measure to prevent cells with genomic damage from becoming cancerous, but it **also prevents old, worn out tissues from being replenished.** Senescent cells change dramatically in their function, most importantly in the molecules they secrete, often pro-inflammatory molecules that damage the environment of the cells. **This leads to chronic tissue inflammation** that probably contributes to a variety of geriatric conditions like osteoarthritis, kidney dysfunction and dementia.

Cellular Senescence is defined as irreversible cell cycle arrest driven by a variety of mechanisms, including telomere shortening, other forms of genotoxic stress, or mitogens (substance that trigger cell division), diabesity, or inflammation cytokines, that culminate in the activation of the p53 tumor suppressor and/or the cyclin-dependent kinase inhibitor p16.

Professor James Kirkland at the Mayo Clinic is spearheading multiple senolytic studies. On December 9,2021, Dr. Kirkland described a clinical trial where he had to complete a 450-page detailed Investigational New Drug application. Dr. Kirkland then had to do preclinical (animal and pharmacology) studies before the FDA "allowed" a human senolytic clinical trial to commence. Total time spent to initiate this study was 2.5 years.

What's irrational about this delay is the compound being studied is fisetin, a flavonoid found in some fruits and vegetables.

Fisetin has been used for years as a dietary supplement.

Bureaucratic barriers like this impede rapid testing to repurpose medications (like rapamycin) on aging people.

The Metabolic Roots Of Senescence

What follows is adapted from an excellent review by Christopher Wiley and Judith Campisi published in Nature Metabolism in 2021.

As these authors write: -

"Cellular senescence entails a permanent proliferative arrest, coupled to multiple phenotypic changes. Among these changes is the release of numerous biologically active molecules collectively known as the senescence-associated secretory phenotype, or SASP. A growing body of literature indicates that both senescence and the SASP are sensitive to cellular and organismal metabolic states, which in turn can drive phenotypes associated with metabolic dysfunction. Here, we review the current literature linking senescence and metabolism, with an eye toward findings at the cellular level, including both metabolic inducers of senescence and alterations in cellular metabolism associated with senescence. Additionally, we consider how interventions that target either metabolism or senescent cells might influence each other and mitigate some of the pro-aging effects of cellular senescence. We conclude that the most effective interventions will likely break a degenerative feedback cycle by which cellular senescence promotes metabolic diseases, which in turn promote senescence."

Historic perspective on cellular senescence.

Cellular senescence, the non-dividing altered state into which many vertebrate cells enter when stressed, was first formally described by Hayflick and Moorhead in the early 1960s. Their finding–that normal cells eventually cease dividing (in culture)–challenged the long-held idea initiated by Alexis Carrel in the early 1900s that normal cells were intrinsically 'immortal' (in culture). And, whereas Carrel suggested that organismal mortality might be a consequence of multi-cellularity, Hayflick and Moorhead suggested that the eventual cessation of cell division (subsequently termed cellular senescence) reflected organismal aging. They also noted that cells derived from malignant tumors did not undergo this form of senescence, suggesting that the senescent state existed to suppress the development of cancer. Many years later, Sager and colleagues showed that cellular senescence was a response to potential tumor-inducing stimuli, and thus formally postulated that the senescence response was a potent anti-cancer mechanism. Since the 1960s, our understanding of cellular senescence, including its physiological and pathological roles, has exploded. In addition, it is now apparent that senescent cells both experience and cause many aspects of metabolic reprogramming.

All senescent cells thus far examined develop a complex, multi-component senescent-associated secretory phenotype (SASP). The SASP acts cell non-autonomously to alter the behavior of neighboring cells and the tissue microenvironment. The SASP is strikingly variable and plastic. It depends on the cell type and senescence inducer, and is dynamic, changing characteristics over time. A striking, but not sole, feature of the SASP is the preponderance of pro-inflammatory molecules, including cytokines, chemokines, bioactive lipids and damage-associated molecular patterns (DAMPs; also termed Alarmins). Chronic inflammation is, of course, a major risk factor for many age-related diseases, including late-life cancer; hence the term 'inflammaging' has been used to describe the chronic inflammation that is a common attribute of aged tissues and might be at least partially due to the accumulation of senescent cells in aged tissues.

Adaptive vs maladaptive effects of senescent cells

The senescence response can be beneficial or deleterious, depending on the physiological context. This dualism is consistent with the evolutionary theory of antagonistic pleiotropy. Antagonistic pleiotropy postulates that traits selected to ensure the survival of young organisms in natural environments, in which life spans are short, can become deleterious in modern protected environments, in which life spans are significantly longer. Thus, aging is likely a consequence of the declining force of natural selection with age.

With regard to the beneficial effects of cellular senescence, as noted above, the senescence growth arrest protects young organisms from developing cancer. In addition, SASP factors can optimize the morphogenesis of certain structures in the embryo and initiate parturition in the placenta. Finally, senescent cells occur transiently at sites of tissue damage where they contribute to wound healing, tissue repair and regeneration, most likely through specific SASP factors.

In contrast, senescent cells increase with age in most mammalian tissues, where they appear to persist. Whether this increase is due to increased production or decreased clearance, for example by the immune system, is unclear. More importantly, experiments using human cells and tissues, transgenic mouse models and pharmacological interventions in cells and mice strongly implicate senescent cells in a large number of age-related pathologies, ranging from neurodegeneration to, ironically, age-related cancer. Most of the detrimental effects of senescent cells can be attributed to the SASP, which, as noted above, is rich in pro-inflammatory molecules.

What initiates a senescence response? Little is known about how senescent cells are induced in vivo, particularly during aging. Known inducers of senescence responses–at least in cultured cells and mouse models–include, among others, DNA damage, activated oncogenes and mitochondrial dysfunction (discussed below). Because senescent cells are rare, even in old and diseased tissue, it has been difficult to determine how they were induced to senesce in vivo. However, single-cell profiling, at both the trandriptomic and proteomic levels, promises to help identify the major drivers of senescence during natural aging and in age-related pathologies. In all cases, senescent cells must undergo metabolic reprogramming in order to maintain their viable growth-arrested state and express the genes and proteins needed to sustain the highly complex, dynamic and heterogenous SASP. The causes and consequences of these metabolic shifts are discussed below.

Metabolic drivers of senescence

Several forms of metabolic stress can both drive senescence and influence the SASP (Fig. 1). Here we describe some of these and discuss them in the context of aging and disease.

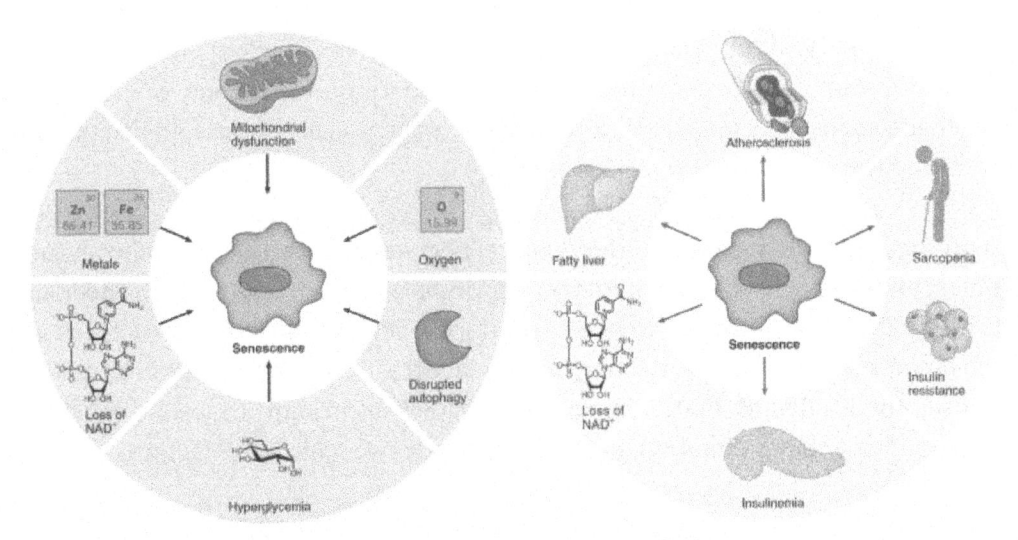

Fig. 1 | Relationships between metabolism and cellular senescence.

Left: Metabolic drivers of senescence. Mitochondrial dysfunction can drive senescence through disruption of cytosolic NAD+/NADH ratios, production of reactive oxygen species, and potentially other mechanisms. Accumulation of excess metals (especially transition metals) also promotes senescence. Loss of NAD+ results in senescence through loss of sirtuin or PARP activities and changes in cellular redox states. Hyperglycemia can drive senescence, although mechanistic detail is still needed. Disrupted autophagy can drive senescence in some contexts, but also prevent it in others. Non-physiological oxygen levels influence the development of senescent cells, with higher oxygen generally favoring senescence. **Right: Senescent cells as drivers of metabolic disease.** Senescent cells and/or the SASP can drive both formation of atherosclerotic plaques as well as plaque instability. In the liver, senescent cells can promote steatosis. The SASP also activates macrophages, which elevate CD38 and lower tissue NAD+ evels. In the pancreas, senescent β-cells promote hyperinsulinemia, but as β-cells are attacked by the immune system, this can become hypoinsulinemia. In peripheral tissues (for example, fat) senescent cells can promote insulin resistance—so senescent cells can drive diabetes and metabolic disease in multiple ways. Finally, senescent cells promote sarcopenia in muscle tissue, which can influence basal metabolism, activity levels, and frailty.

Mitochondrial dysfunction

Mitochondria are major regulators of age-related pathology. Mice that accumulate mitochondrial DNA (mtDNA) mutations at an accelerated rate age prematurely, whereas overexpression of mitochondrially-targeted catalase (mCAT) preserves mitochondrial function and extends lifespan in mice. It is therefore not surprising that senescence and the SASP are similarly responsive to the function of mitochondria within the cell.

Many drivers of mitochondrial dysfunction also result in cellular senescence. For example the lowering of the NAD+/NADH ratio inhibits the key glycolytic enzyme, GAPDH, resulting in ATP depletion, AMPK activation and cell cycle arrest.

Additionally, mitochondria are a source of reactive oxygen species (ROS). Loss of mitochondrial superoxide dismutase (SOD2) in mice drives cellular senescence.

Oxygen

Phenotypes of cellular senescence are highly dependent on the levels of oxygen available to the cell. This dependence is often inversely correlated, as more oxygen tends to accelerate senescence. With over 60 oxygen-consuming enzymes in the mammalian genome, it is not surprising that oxygen levels are a key modulator of many biological processes, including senescence. Sub-physiological levels of oxygen (that is, hypoxia) can also activate AMPK, which can suppress the SASP by mTOR inhibition. Unfortunately, hyperoxia is a medical necessity under certain conditions.

Treatment of fetal human airway smooth muscle cells and lung fibroblasts with moderate hyperoxia (40% O2) increased markersof senescence in as short as 7 days, suggesting that senescent cells may play a role in these disorders. Conversely, hyperbaric 100% oxygen was recently found to lower markers of senescence in specific populations of peripheral blood mononuclear cells, so cell type may play an important role in senescent cell responses to oxygen.

Disrupted NAD+ metabolism

NAD+ plays a major role in the regulation of both the cell cycle arrest and the SASP during senescence (Fig. 2). NAD+ is a major cofactor for both poly-ADP-ribose polymerase (PARP) and sirtuin family proteins (SIRTs). PARP antagonizes senescence by protecting against genotoxic stress, but also promotes NF-kB activation and secretory phenotypes in senescent cells. Importantly, NAD+ levels decline with age in many tissues, and this decline is associated with multiple degenerative conditions, including age-related muscle loss and diabetes.

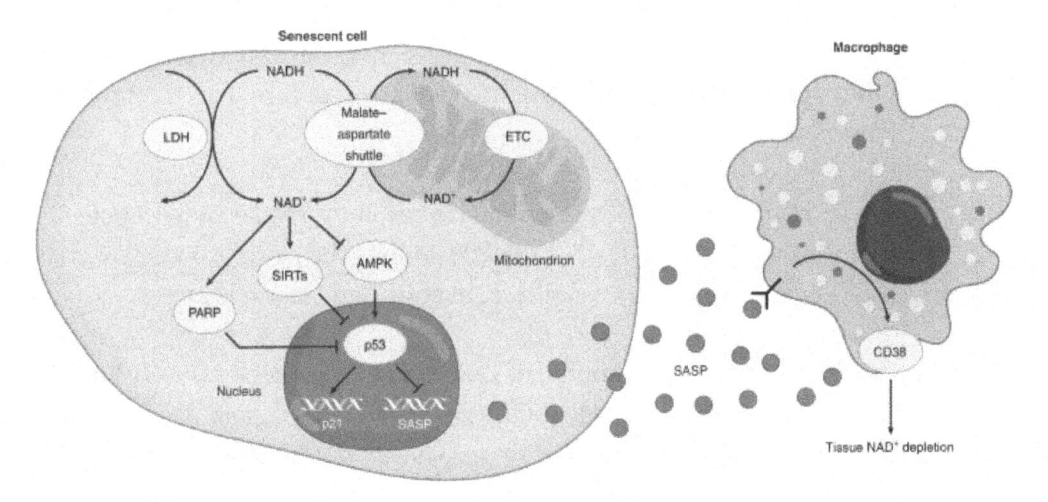

Several sirtuins play key roles in senescence response and the SASP. Beyond SIRT3 and SIRT5, which antagonize MiDAS43, SIRTs 1, 2 and 6 have known roles in senescence. SIRT2 deacetylates and stabilizes the mitotic checkpoint kinase BUBR1, which declines during aging, and protects against aneuploidy—a potent driver of senescence. Notably, supplementation with the NAD+ precursor nicotinamide mononucleotide (NMN) extends the median lifespan of progeric BUBR1 hypomorphic mice. SIRT6 knockout mice show premature aging and a hyperinflammatory state that is driven at least in part by de-repression of retrotransposons, which also occurs with senescence88. Furthermore, overexpression of SIRT6 prevents the loss of homologous recombination observed during senescence. Finally, SIRT1 is degraded by autophagy during senescence. Loss of SIRT1 activity is associated with multiple aspects of senescence, including SASP activation and cell cycle arrest, as well as several senescence-associated degenerative pathologies including neurodegeneration, cachexia, fatty liver and atherosclerosis. Together, the sirtuins and PARP demonstrate the importance of NAD+-consuming enzymes in senescence and help explain why loss of NAD+ levels with age can be deleterious to a tissue.

Hyperglycemia

Numerous studies demonstrate that culturing cells in high levels of glucose accelerates cellular senescence. However, because multiple pathways by which this acceleration occurs have been identified, no unifying model currently explains all forms of hyperglycemia-associated senescence. Most studies focus on endothelial cells, including retinal endothelial cells, but fibroblasts and renal epithelial cells have also been studied. Nonetheless, the few mechanisms ascribed to senescence induction seem unlikely to be common to multiple cell lineages.

High glucose also drives senescence in fibroblasts, and glucose restriction can extend replicative lifespan. Hyperglycemia can also result in the formation of advanced glycation end-products (AGEs), which can drive senescence in some models.

More research is therefore required to fully elucidate the relationship between AGEs and cellular senescence. Furthermore, studies linking high glucose to senescence have not addressed the SASP, and therefore the consequences of this form of senescence are still somewhat unclear. Despite these needs, the links between diabetes and senescence are growing, and increases in senescent cells at sites of diabetic complications indicate that this is an important area for future research.

Lysosomes and autophagy.

Autophagy, the process by which a cell breaks down its organelles and macromolecules, is dysregulated in senescent cells. Specific factors show selective microautophagic degradation in senescent cells, whereas macroautophagy appears to be less active in senescent cells. Many senescent cells have dysfunctional lysosomes. The complex nature of the relationship between senescence and autophagy are exciting areas of research at this time.

Therapy To Decrease Cellular Senescence

1. Dietary interventions and senescence.

Multiple dietary interventions can limit the accumulation of senescent cells with age. Calorie restriction (CR) was one of the first lifespan-extending interventions to be identified. Thus, when it was found that senescent cells can limit lifespan, it seemed that links between CR and senescence were likely. CR lowers markers of senescence in the colons of mice and humans and in inguinal white adipose tissue. CR prevents the development of senescence in the kidney of aged animals, whereas high-calorie diets increase senescence.

Other dietary interventions can similarly extend health span and either or both median and maximum lifespan. These interventions include methionine restriction and ketogenic diets. Methionine restriction lowers markers of senescence and the SASP, while injection of mice with β-hydroxybutyrate, a major ketone body produced by ketogenic diets, lowers markers of senescence in vascular smooth muscle and endothelial cells. These results indicate that dietary interventions that create a favorable metabolic state that can limit the accumulation of senescent cells.

Metabolic interventions that influence senescent cells

As described above, hyperglycemia induces senescence. It therefore reasons that diabetes could be pro-senescence, and interventions that lower blood sugar should antagonize the formation of senescent cells. Indeed, kidney proximal tubule cells become senescent within 4 weeks of induction of diabetes in mice, and this rise in senescent cells can be prevented by lowering glucose levels with insulin or inhibiting glucose transport into the cells by inhibiting the activity of the sodium-glucose co-transporter SGLT2. Similarly, acarbose—which lowers blood sugar by antagonizing intestinal carbohydrate absorption—extends lifespan in mice and prevents diet-induced atherosclerosis-associated senescence in rabbits.

Another antidiabetic medication, metformin, extends both lifespan and health span in mice, and is a drug being studied for the first clinical trial to monitor general aspects of aging. Metformin antagonizes the development of senescence in response to ceramide in immortal mouse myoblast cells and extends the replicative lifespan of human fibroblasts and mesenchymal stem cells. Additionally, metformin lowers several SASP factor levels, including many proinflammatory cytokines, by interfering with NF-kB activation.

Furthermore, metformin protects against the development of senescence in murine models of intervertebral disc degeneration and chronic kidney disease. Metformin therefore interferes with senescence at several levels and is perhaps the best-characterized metabolic intervention that antagonizes senescence and the SASP.

2. Exercise as an intervention for senescence

While numerous studies highlight the health benefits of exercise and its improvement of health span with age, few studies to date have demonstrated lifespan extension due to exercise in mice; just one late-life exercise study showed lifespan extension. There is evidence that exercise can prevent senescence and segments of the proinflammatory SASP in the sera and hearts of aged mice. More notably, exercise offsets diet-induced senescence and the SASP in mouse adipose and liver tissues, suggesting that the most beneficial aspects of exercise may not pertain to already healthy animals, but rather those likely to develop metabolic disease. In humans, exercise and activity are associated with reduced markers of endothelial and leukocyte cell senescence. These data suggest that exercise can offset deleterious aspects of senescence brought about by poor diet and sedentary lifestyles.

3. Multiple roles for senescence in diabetes and its complications

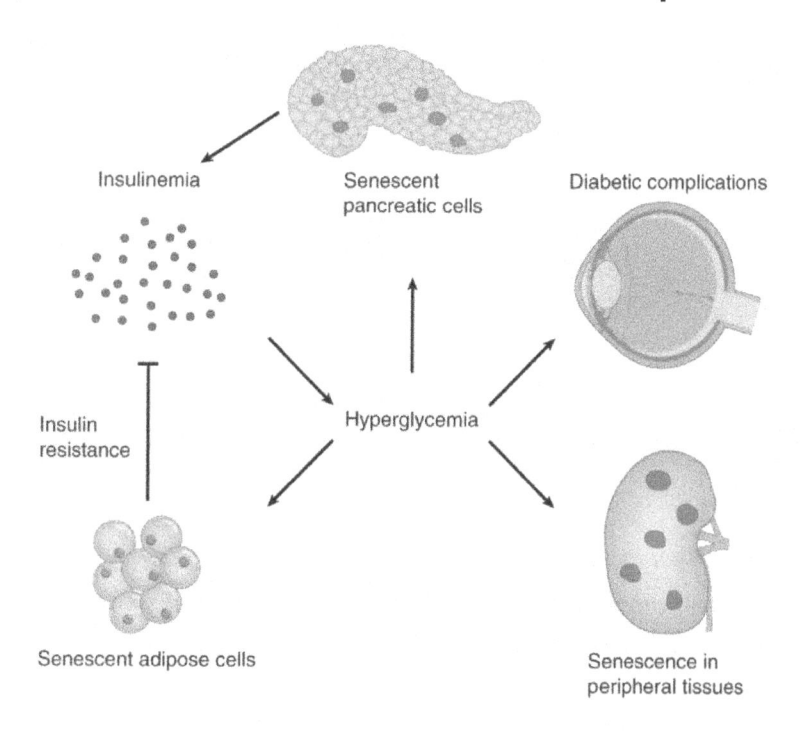

Senescent adipose cells can result in insulin resistance, which results in hyperglycemia, which can in turn promote additional adipose tissue senescence. Hyperglycemia also forces pancreatic β-cells to over-produce insulin. This stress results in β-cell senescence, leading to insulinemia, resulting in further hyperglycemia. Hyperglycemia also results in senescence in peripheral tissues such as the retina and the kidney, fueling diabetic complications.

There are three types of interventions that target senescent cells and their degenerative pathologies. First, we can slow the formation of senescent cells, as observed during dietary restriction and similar interventions. Second, we can allow senescent cells to accumulate, but prevent them from causing harm, as observed during metformin-mediated SASP suppression or after CD38 inhibition.

Finally, we can use senolysis to remove senescent cells. Unlike the first two interventions, senolysis can be used intermittently—allowing for a 'hit and run' approach that might be easier to implement in humans—whereas dietary and suppressive drug regimens require regular adherence to maintain benefits.

4. Senolytic Fisetin

Fisetin is a flavonoid molecule found in fruits and vegetables. There are over 6,000 flavonoids found in vegetables, fruits, herbs and medicinal plants.

Flavonoid components are well known for their antioxidant, anti-inflammatory, anti-carcinogenic and anti-mutagenic properties.

The foods highest in fisetin are strawberries although you have to eat at least 37 to get its benefits.

Food	Fisetin in mgm/gm
Strawberry	160
Apple	26.9
Persimmon	10.6
Lotus Root	5.8
Onion	4.8

Until recently, the only senolytic therapy that had demonstrated effectiveness in humans use a combination of quercetin and dasatinib (SPYRCEL). There are currently more than 20 ongoing studies on synolytics.

Researchers have found higher number of senescent cells in older adults with chronic disease. The study that used a combination of dasatanib and quercetin was performed in Rochester, Minnesota, by the Mayo Clinic researchers.

The team engaged participants who had diabetes-related kidney disease. James Kirkland, Ph.D., was the senior author. He talked about senescent cells and the importance of the research on a range of human illness.

"Senescent cells can develop in all mammals in response to disease, injury, or cancerous mutations. Senolytic drugs do not interfere with generation of senescent cells, which could lead to cancer. However, once formed, senescent cells can contribute to developing cancers, multiple other diseases, and consequences of aging.

By targeting senescent cells with senolytics in mice, we can delay, prevent, or treat multiple diseases and increase health and independence during remaining years of life. As we increase our understanding of these drugs and their effects, we hope there may be benefits for a range of human diseases and disorders."

5. Senolytic Dasatinib

Dasatinib, sold under the brand name Sprycel among others, is a targeted therapy medication used to treat certain cases of chronic myelogenous leukemia and acute lymphoblastic leukemia.

Specifically it is used to treat cases that are Philadelphia chromosome-positive. It is taken by mouth. Common adverse effects include low white blood cells, low blood platelets, anemia, swelling, rash, and diarrhea.

6. Environmental Mitochondrial Toxicants

Although environmental contaminants have in general been less well studied than drugs from the mitochondrial toxicity perspective. There are a number of toxins that damage and may well hasten senescence. They include: -

- Paraquat
- Rotenone
- Carbon monoxide
- Arsenic
- Lead
- Cadmium
- Copper
- Particulate matter
- Lipopolysaccharide
- Perflourinated compound
- Cigarette smoke
- Dioxin
- Manganese

Mitochondrial dysfunction can drive senescence through multiple pathways.

7. Micronutrients

At the recent 14th Clinical Trials on Alzheimer's disease taking a daily supplement for three years was associated with a 60% slowing of cognitive aging. In our LB5/LB100 program we use Telovite that has been shown to stabilize telomere length.

Finally, age is a major outcome of human nutrition, while nutritional interventions can prevent many age-associated diseases. Much is known about the role of macronutrient stress in longevity and senescence, but less is known about how malnutrition of key micronutrients controls the development of senescence. For example, choline deficiency is common in the elderly in the United States, and is a driver of hepatic steatosis—a condition also promoted during age by senescent cells. The relationship between nutrition and senescence is therefore fertile ground for future exploration and will undoubtedly be the subject of multiple studies moving forward.

8. Spermidene and Autophagy

As discussed before, overtime cells fatigue and become damaged. Old cellular matter that accumulates begins to degrade cell functionality. This leads to a variety of health problems and age – related diseases.

Thankfully, our bodies have an answer for the cellular renewal processes. It's called autophagy.

Autophagy is typically induced during situations of energy deficiency when the body needs more resources. Our cells switch from building mode to an equally important "breakdown mode" - an emergency and cleaning all-in-one program that solves the body's energy needs while using up unnecessary parts of our own cells. This revitalizing power of autophagy can be triggered by fasting, exercise and spermidine.

Spermidine intake is associated with multiple benefits including:

Cellular processes – DNA stability, cellular growth, cellular differentiation, apoptosis (cell death)

Reduces inflammation – and removes toxic protein, aggregates from cells which cause neurodegeneration. It also increases cortical thickness and hippocampal volume.

Increase – Healthspan and Lifespan – in animal studies spermidine not only improves healthspan but can prolong life by 25%.

Reduces Mortality – Humans in a 20-year epidemiological study in humans, higher consumption of spermidine rich food correlates with reduced mortality and life expectancy was prolonged by 5 years.

Heart Function – spermidine supports cellular respiration which leads to increased mitochondrial content in heart cells and acting through autophagy prevents age-associated cardiovascular diseases.

Did you know?

Since Dr.Madeo discovered that spermidine triggers autophagy over a decade ago over 100 international research teams are investigating its health benefits.

Research shows that spermidine levels start to decrease at age 25 –30 years.

Interestingly, in a recent study in one of the "Blue Zones", spermidine levels in 90 and 100 year old mirror that of a young person's body.

Although the phenomenon of autophagy was first described in 1963 only in 1990 was the underlying mechanism fully decoded by the Japanese researcher Yoshinori Ohsumi. He was awarded the Nobel Prize for Medicine in 2016 for uncovering the genetic basis for autophagy'

Spermidine is a unique naturally occurring molecule, part of a group of polyamines. It is found in all plants and animals in nearly every cell in the body. Spermidine comes from the food we eat and is synthesized in the gut microbiome or synthesized in cells.

Nine Spermidine Rich Foods include the following:
1) Wheat and whole grains (30%)
2) Soybeans and soy products
3) Aged Cheese (Cheddar, Brie, Parmesan etc.)
4) Mushrooms (Maitake/Oyster and Snow mushrooms)
5) Green Peas
6) Rice and rice bran oil
7) Mangos
8) Chickpeas (Garbanzo Beans)
9) Cauliflower and Broccoli

CHAPTER 14: STEM CELL EXHAUSTION

One of the most obvious consequences of growing old is worse recovery from injury, caused by a decline in the ability of our stem cells to replenish damaged tissues. Your stem cells spend most of their time dormant in a niche, but as they are activated to heal wounds and restore tissues, **they are also susceptible to telomere shortening, DNA damage and cellular senescence.** Over time this results in stem cell exhaustion.

One of the important contributions to the aging process is a **progressive reduction in stem cell activity.** The majority of tissues in the body are in a constant process of turnover. The **somatic cells** making up the bulk of all tissues reach the **Hayflick limit** on replication and self-destruct, and are replaced by new cells generated by tissue-specific **stem cell** population. With age, these stem cells spend even more time quiescent and thus the supply of new somatic cells declines, causing tissues and organs to deteriorate and ultimately fail. This loss of stem cell support is thought to have evolved as part of a balance between risk of death by cancer versus risk of death through failing tissues. As cells become more damaged with age, the risk of cancer with cell activity increases. Lower levels of stem cell activity dampen that risk somewhat, at the cost of a slower decline into frailty and disease. Still, restoration of youthful stem cell activity is one necessary component of any future toolkit of rejuvenation therapies. To the degree that this raises cancer risk that is an additional challenge to overcome along the way, not a reason to stand back and do nothing.

As explained previously epigenetic alterations, while every cell in your body has the same genetic code, regions of DNA are turned off and on in each one, allowing us to have many unique cell types. While normal cells cannot change their epigenetic settings very easily, stem cells have greater freedom, allowing them, in some cases, to turn into effectively any cell type in the body.

Stem cells perform a wide range of functions, including beneficial signaling that improves tissue function, regulation and health as well as the replacement of damaged or lost red blood cells, white blood cells, and solid tissues.

Because of the importance of these functions, a reduction in stem cell activity, also known as stem cell exhaustion, can lead to many diseases and general issues, such as immunosuppression through reduced production of bacteria-killing and virus-killing white blood cells, muscle loss, frailty, and effect many Hallmarks of Aging.

What causes stem cell exhaustion?

As we age, the activity of our stem cells slowly decreases for multiple reasons. For instance, senescent cells constantly secrete a mixture of pro-inflammatory, immunosuppressive chemicals known collectively as the senescence-associated secretory phenotype (SASP), which reduces stem cell activity, contributing to immune senescence and loss of tissue regeneration.

The SASP is part of a wider inflammatory phenomenon known as "inflammaging," which comes from a range of sources and creates a smoldering background of chronic low-grade inflammation that disrupts stem cell function and tissue repair. Inflammaging is caused by senescent cells, cell debris, crosslinks, immunosenescence, and age-related changes to the gut microbiome.

Stem cells are also not immune to direct damage and destruction: telomere shortening, for instance can lead to stem cells losing function and becoming senescent and while numerous quality control mechanisms are in place, their DNA can slowly mutate to the point of causing senescence or cancer.

Therefore, while the pool of stem cells can regenerate itself, it does so with lower quality and speed over time, eventually contributing to chronic diseases.

Adult stem cells lose their ability to repopulate tissues with fresh functional cells. The result is systemic deterioration of tissues throughout our aging bodies. Treatments that are currently being used to slow aging, such as boosting AMPK and sirtuins, appear likely to facilitate stem cell rejuvenation. Regulation of mTOR enhances the regenerative capacity of hematopoietic stem cells in aged mice.

Factors that Confer Stem Cell Health

As it relates to stem cell regeneration, the following processes are intimately involved:

1. **DNA repair** pathways affected by:
2. **SIRT1 NAD+ FoXO**
3. **Protein synthesis** affected by:

4. **AMPK mTOR FoXO**
5. **Mitochondrial function** affected by:
6. **SIRT1 NAD+ FoXO**

Hallmarks of degenerative aging include dysregulation of AMPK, FoxO and SIRT1, depletion of NAD+, and excessive activation of mTOR.

In what may be a unified approach to living healthier, the ability to reactivate aged stem cells is already being practiced by some enlightened people today.

This includes those who take steps to balance AMPK, SIRT1, FoxO and NAD+ while normalizing excess mTOR.

Therapy for Stem Cell Exhaustion

1. **Induced Pluripotent Stem Cells (IPSCs)**

In the early days of stem cell research, the most versatile stem cells were collected from early-stage embryos. However, a lot has changed in the last decade, and we have found ways to turn adult cells back into stem cells and re-inject them back into the body. We call these reprogrammed adult stem cells induced pluripotent stem cells (iPSCs).

iPSCs were first created by Shinya Yamanaka, who was later awarded the Nobel Prize for this accomplishment when he discovered a set of signaling chemicals that influenced ordinary cells into becoming stem cells. These chemicals were later named Yamanaka factors, and they also appear to reverse another cause of aging, epigenetic alterations, to some extent.

Thanks to the widespread use of iPSCs, novel stem cell therapies should not need to use embryonic cells; therefore, there are no longer any related ethical issues surrounding their use.

2. **Stem Cells**

Stem cell research is perhaps the most mainstream of research topics in the aging field, and it attracts a vast amount of funding. In general, stem cell research has made rapid progress in the last decade and is a well-funded area of regenerative medicine. There are already multiple stem cell therapies already in clinical use, and many others are currently in clinical trials. Some of them attempt to replace our current stem cell compartments, and others seek to repair the cells that are already there. In addition, NAD+ therapy has been shown to fight stem cell senescence.

I advise holding off on most stem cell infusions until more is known about safety and efficacy for example very small embryonic like (VSEL) stem cells. As many as 80% of embryonic stem cells have gross chromosomal abnormalities.

3. Removing Senescent Cells

Removing senescent cells and their secreted SASP may also potentially have a positive impact on stem cell function; the removal of some inflammatory sources would likely reduce the overall burden of inflammaging and could plausibly reduce stem cell inhibition and keep our tissues much healthier for longer.

4. Combating Telomere Loss

The same can be said for combating telomere loss, the decline in proteosis, and all of the other Hallmarks of Aging.

5. Plant Based Nutrients

Although stem cells have the power to reproduce themselves (self-renew) so they can replace aging cells they are also adversely impacted by aging. Stem cells can be improved by many nutrients like curcumin, resveratrol, gynostemma, pentaphyllum, NAD precursors along with a low carb healthy eating pattern.

These plant nutrients can help protect and revitalize stem cells. The stem cells acts a reservoir to replace old damaged or dying cells. When specialized cells in tissues stop working or are impaired by injury or disease, stem cells have the ability to develop into the needed cell type which helps rejuvenate the cells.

To work properly stem cells must perform these two functions: -
1. Self-renewal
2. Differentiation

However as mentioned, advancing age takes its toll on them as well. As this damage accumulates over time, stem cells stop dividing and lose their ability to replace old and damaged tissue cells and begin to die. Physical frailty advances, cognition declines, metabolism slows and the body become more susceptible to age-related disease and dysfunction.

6. Key Ways To Keep Stem Cells Young and Healthy

a. The Role of mTOR in Obesity and Aging

Inhibiting mTOR (an enzyme that regulates protein synthesis and cell growth) and activating FoxO (a protein that regulates the expression of genes) that limit the buildup of toxins and enhances autophagy, cellular 'housekeeping' that keeps stem cells running smoothly.

"mTOR" stands for the mechanistic target of rapamycin. It is a protein found inside most cells and is responsible for regulating cellular growth by sensing and integrating diverse nutritional and environmental cues. Excessive activation of cellular mTOR is involved in diseases plaguing aging populations, such as cancer, type II diabetes, and obesity. Regulating mTOR activity extends lifespan in laboratory models by delaying the development of chronic diseases, including cancer. Maintenance of stem cell pools requires a finely tuned balance between stem cell renewal and differentiation. When mTOR is excessively activated in certain stem cell lineages, the pool of stem cells becomes exhausted. This diminishes our ability to regenerate our tissues with fresh functional cells. When properly balanced, mTOR will not adversely impact cellular aging. Enhancing autophagy in hematopoietic stem cells improves their regenerative capacity. One way of inducing autophagy is suppression of excess mTOR via AMPK activation.

Most people need lower mTOR. Regulation of mTOR represents a viable approach to preserve the stem cell pool. This, in turn, would help maintain functionality of our tissues and organs over time. When calorie intake is reduced, mTOR activity diminishes, and autophagy is beneficially activated.

This process (autophagy) cleans up accumulated cellular waste products and preserves cell function. The autophagy-regulating signaling network that includes AMPK and mTOR serves to maintain this delicate autophagy balance. Interventions that activate AMPK serve to balance mTOR and enable optimal levels of cellular autophagy.

b. AMPK activation to lower mTOR

Activating the enzyme AMPK – considered the 'master regulator' of metabolism in the body. This improves energy balance in stem cells and leads to replacement of old, damaged proteins. AMPK was first identified in 1973 for its role in fat metabolism. Based on evidence from pre-clinical studies, it is expected that when people practice severe calorie restriction, AMPK activity increases, which confers protective effects. One of AMPK's benefits is to signal cells to consume stored fat. One way that AMPK performs this fat-removing process is by down-regulating mTOR. AMPK is a master energy sensor in cells. When AMPK is activated by compounds like metformin or Gynostemma pentaphyllum, cells think they are energy deprived. The desired effect for most aging people is to prompt cells to turn down excess mTOR and utilize fat stores for energy production. Balancing mTOR activity and autophagy can be achieved via increasing cellular AMPK in the following six ways:

1. Reduce calorie intake and more specifically, avoid sugars and simple carbohydrates. High blood levels of glucose (and insulin) fuel excess mTOR activity.

2. Brief periods (3-5 days) of calorie restriction per month have shown great benefits indicative of balanced mTOR, but compliance is difficult.

3. Consider 'intermittent fasting' for 14-18 hours five days a week, based on voluminous data, including a fascinating report published in the December 26, 2019 issue of the New England Journal of Medicine.

4. Preclinical studies show that calorie restriction mimetics such as resveratrol and NAD can be used to support SIRT1 and FoxO function.

5. AMPK activators such as the drug metformin and/or nutrients such as Gynostemma pentaphyllum extract, berberine and hesperidin help support mTOR activity and autophagy.

6. Increased physical activity can meaningfully boost AMPK.

The impact of boosting AMPK and lowering excess mTOR may enable rejuvenation of aging bone marrow (hematopoietic) stem cells. A safe way of balancing mTOR is to boost cellular AMPK activity. Increasing AMPK regulates mTOR, which facilitates removal of cellular debris (via autophagy). As it relates to combating aging, activating autophagy appears to be a critical factor for the rejuvenation of aged hematopoietic stem cells. Hematopoietic stem cells are crucial for producing new immune cells, platelets and red blood cells. Middle aged and elderly people today have ready access to low-cost approaches to help preserve their bone marrow stem cell pools. When the bone marrow stem cell niche becomes exhausted, life can no longer be sustained. That's because oxygen carrying red blood cells, immune-protecting white cells and hemorrhage-guarding platelets must to be continually produced in the bone marrow for systemic existence.

c. **Activating Sirtuins**

Activating sirtuins, proteins that regulate cellular health, and protect and repair DNA. Resveratrol activates SIRT1 inside cells, which is linked to many of the same longevity-enhancing benefits as calorie restriction. Based on our interpretation of emerging evidence, age control could be enhanced by modest doses of resveratrol, with adequate NAD replenishment to ensure sirtuin functionality.

Most people over age 40 should initiate supplementation with the oral NAD precursor (nicotinamide riboside) in the daily dose of 300mg to 600mg, along with 100mg to 300mg of resveratrol and AMPK-activating compounds. By targeting known regulators of stem cell self-renewal and differentiation, we are proposing a unique protocol to rejuvenate your own stem cells.

Sirtuins are dependent on NAD to interact with FoxO, a beneficial transcription factor, to promote healthy gene expression. The cellular enzyme AMPK has a dynamic interaction with sirtuin 1 (SIRT1). The potential combined benefit of boosting AMPK, NAD, SIRT1 and FoxO is the favorable impact this might have in promoting stem cell health. Moreover, AMPK activity helps to normalize excess mTOR, which can impede stem cell functionality.

d. **NAD**

Increasing NAD is a promising way to self-renew existing stem cells in order to extend lifespan and prevent disease. A study published in June 2019 shows a NAD boosting supplement called nicotinamide riboside increased stem cell colonies by 75% in the gut of aging mice.

The most critical role of NAD is DNA repair. Each day, our DNA sustains numerous breaks that are repaired by NAD dependent enzymes. With age, NAD levels plummet. Another study published in 2019 showed that a modest dose of nicotinamide riboside boosted NAD levels by 51% in overweight humans.

Nicotinic Riboside (NR) → Nicotinamide Mononucleotide (NMN) → Nicotinamide adenine dinucleotide (NAD)

Other studies point to the role of NAD in restoring circadian rhythms needed for restorative sleep. Age-related sleep deterioration and digestive disorders adversely impact quality of life and accelerate degenerative processes in older individuals. New data reveal how NAD improves functionality of existing stem cells and replenishes mitochondria in cells throughout the body.

What is NAD?

Nicotinamide adenine dinucleotide (NAD) is a compound found in every living cell. It is critical for cell energy production. Recent research shows NAD does much more. Hundreds of different proteins in each cell require NAD to work properly. The most important proteins are the sirtuins, cellular guardians that protect against DNA damage that leads to many age-related ailments.

Sirtuins are an important target for anti-aging interventions. Multiple animal studies have demonstrated that increasing sirtuin activity leads to longer life and reduction in age-related loss of function. As NAD levels decline with aging, there is reduced sirtuin activity. Boosting NAD helps ramp up sirtuin activity. Increasing NAD levels can bring additional benefits tied to healthy longevity including:

- Promoting AMPK activity, an enzyme that improves metabolism and helps protect against obesity and diabetes,

- Modulating p53, a tumor suppressor gene that repairs damaged DNA and protects against cancer initiation,

- Inhibiting NF-kB (nuclear factor-kappa B), a protein that induces the chronic inflammation tied to many diseases and premature aging, and

- Inhibiting mTOR, a molecular complex whose abnormal activation contributes to many chronic diseases of aging.

NAD and Resveratrol A Powerful Anti-Aging Duo

Resveratrol a plant compound found in red grapes, red wine, and other darkly colored fruits. Among its many benefits, it activates sirtuins, the key defender proteins linked to longer, healthier life.

But resveratrol can't do this if cells are low in NAD. That's because NAD is required for sirtuins to work properly. It would be like pressing the accelerator in your car when your gas tank is empty.

The solution is to increase intake of nicotinamide riboside to boost NAD levels at the same time as promoting sirtuin activity with resveratrol. This combination ensures that the enhanced sirtuin activity can have its maximum beneficial effect on health and aging.

Higher levels of NAD correlate with improved health and a lower occurrence of age-related disorders. Lower NAD levels contribute to many diseases of older age, including sleep disturbances, metabolic disorders, diabetes, cardiovascular disease, and cognitive decline.

An easy way to boost NAD levels is with nicotinamide riboside, which converts to NAD in your body. In human subjects, a 300mg dose of nicotinamide riboside increased cellular NAD levels by 51%. Nicotinamide riboside is highly absorbable or bioavailable when taken orally.

Recent studies of NAD and nicotinamide riboside have shown two primary ways in which they improve health.

1. **Replacing Old Mitochondria and Improving Mitochondrial Function**

Mitochondria are the power suppliers of every cell, breaking down nutrients like sugars and fats into energy the cell can use to do work. When mitochondria age, they become dysfunctional, contributing to many illnesses.

Evidence indicates that sirtuins perform cellular housekeeping that includes replacing old and damaged mitochondria with healthy, new ones. This process rejuvenates cells and improves their metabolism while maintaining their optimal function.

Because sirtuin activity is dependent on NAD (which plummets with age), supplementation with nicotinamide riboside can help preserve cellular functions. Replenishing NAD levels with nicotinamide riboside resulted in enhanced mitochondrial function that: -

- Rejuvenated aging bone marrow cells, helping to maintain immune function and prevent bone marrow failure and related diseases,

- Improved muscle function and reduced muscle pathology in an animal model of muscular dystrophy, and

- Lessened liver inflammation and induced mitochondrial biogenesis, the formation of new mitochondria, in mice liver cells.

2. Rejuvenating Stem Cells

Healthy stem cells in tissues are needed to replace dead or dying functional cells with new ones. But stem tissues age and become dysfunctional over time, causing tissues to deteriorate and increasing risk for disease.

Nicotinamide riboside intake can help prevent this. In a study on elderly mice, nicotinamide riboside replenished NAD levels, which improved mitochondrial function that rejuvenated stem cells in muscles. It also prevented the deterioration of muscle, skin and certain stem cells.

This prolonged the lifespan of old mice by approximately 5%. Though this number may not seem huge, the supplementation only began when the mice were already two years old, the equivalent of about 80 years in humans.

Boosting NAD levels can have positive impact on multiple areas.

Longevity

Studying the effect of a supplement on human longevity is difficult, because of the long average lifespan of humans. But many studies show that increasing NAD prolongs the life of a variety of organisms.

In yeast, a single-cell organism with a short lifespan, nicotinamide riboside increased lifespan demonstrated by improved cell replicated capacity. Studies of worms show that nicotinamide riboside can prolong their life by at least 10%. These effects extend to mammals as well.

Physical Performance

In a recent study of older men, levels of NADH, the reduced form of NAD were significantly increased by 59% only two hours after taking one dose of nicotinamide riboside, while markers of oxidative stress were decreased.

The men in this study had an 8% improvement peak in isometric muscle torque (a measure of muscle force) and a 15% improvement in fatigue associated with exercise.

Brain Health

Studies of mouse models of Alzheimer's disease have shown improvements with nicotinamide riboside supplementation.

In the most recent study, it reversed the cognitive deficits in mice, improving memory. The pathology observed in the brains of Alzheimer's disease patients amyloid plaques, was also reduced in the brains of these animals. A previous study had similar findings.

Obesity and Metabolic Disorders

Sirtuins improve metabolism and can be helpful guardians against weight gain, metabolic syndrome and type II diabetes.

By boosting sirtuin activity, nicotinamide riboside enhanced metabolism and prevented excessive weight gain in mice.

In animal models of type II diabetes, this improved metabolism helped control blood sugar levels and protected against the damage done by high blood glucose.

Cardiovascular Health

Improved metabolism and lower body weight helps reduce risk for cardiovascular disease. But nicotinamide riboside does even more to help the cardiovascular system.

One recent study focused on mice with heart disease that had a 30% reduction in NAD levels. Untreated, they typically developed heart disease. But nicotinamide riboside attenuated the decline in cardiac function.

People aged 50 have about 40% less NAD whereas 80-year old people can have 90-98% lower levels of NAD compared to 21-years old.

Heart failure risk increases as people grow older. Recent studies show that nicotinamide riboside protects the organs of the cardiovascular system and protects other tissues from the effects of cardiovascular disease.

Normally, if blood flow to a tissue is compromised due to disease, the tissue dies, as happens in myocardial infarction or a stroke. Preclinical studies show that nicotinamide riboside improves the response of tissues to this type of injury, reducing damage and encouraging recovery of the tissue.

NAD is a critical component for a healthy aging program. Every cell requires it for hundreds of processes. These include activity of sirtuins, cellular guardians linked to prolonged lifespan and healthspan. NAD levels and sirtuin expression diminish with advancing age, accelerating aging processes and degenerative disease risk.

Nicotinamide riboside is a compound that increases cellular NAD levels, enhancing sirtuin activity. New research has found that maintaining more youthful NAD levels can slow certain aspects of biological aging. NAD also improves the health of stem cells that can replace dead and dying cells and keep vital tissue functioning. This not only extends lifespan, but also helps reduce the risk for metabolic disease, obesity, cardiovascular disease, cognitive dysfunction and more.

e. How FoxO Enhances Stem Cell Health

Bone-marrow-derived stem cells are termed hematopoietic stem cells and are essential to sustaining life processes.

FoxO (Forkhead Box) are cell proteins that play an important role in stem cell biology. FoxO help regulate the expression of genes involved in cell growth, proliferation, differentiation, insulin regulation, and longevity.

During aging, the removal and regeneration of functional cells becomes disturbed mainly due to a decrease in the regenerative potential of adult stem cells.

Deletion of FoxO1/3a/4 in the bone marrow of mice leads to apoptosis (death) of hematopoietic stem cells. This prevents the re-population of critical bone-marrow-derived stem cells. Aged mice in which FoxOa was deleted display reduced regenerative potential and depletion of stem cell pool. Treatment of FoxO-deficient mice with N-acetylcysteine restored the hematopoietic stem cell compartment. These observations correlate with the idea that decreased function of adult stem cells is involved in the onset of age-related diseases. Current evidence favorably implicates FoxO transcription factors in longer human lifespans. You can learn technical details about FoxO by searching Google: "FoxO and aging."

For simplicity's sake, it's good to know that boosting NAD and sirtuin expression (with resveratrol) promotes favorable FoxO genetic transcription.

Multi-Modal Approach to Stem Cell Renewal

We know now of several factors involved in the maintenance and potential rejuvenation of our aging stem cells.

The encouraging aspect of all this is we can target these stem cell renewal processes today via:

1. AMPK activation
2. Sirtuin activation
3. FoxO activation
4. NAD replenishment
5. mTOR regulation (via AMPK activation)

This approach may enable elderly individuals to rejuvenate their aged stem cells, which could then repopulate senile tissues with fresh, functional (somatic) cells.

CHAPTER 15: TELOMERE ATTRITION

Similar to the plastic tips of shoelaces protecting their braided ends, telomeres protect the terminal ends of our chromosomes from deterioration. The normal DNA replication mechanisms in most of our cells are not able to copy the ends of our DNA completely, so the repetitive DNA sequences of the telomere region shorten with each cell division. After a number of replications, this leads to cell growth arrest, limiting the ability of tissue to regenerate as we age.

Telomeres shorten each time a cell divides, which, over time, leaves the genetic DNA unprotected and allows cellular function to be compromised – like a shoelace that loses its plastic end cap and becomes frayed.

Telomere – a compound structure of repetitive DNA nucleotides (TTAGGG) that acts as a protective cap at the end of each strand of DNA shortens over time due to aging and lifestyle factors (poor nutrition, psychological stress, lack of exercise, etc.) leaving the DNA that makes up our genes vulnerable to damage.

Telomerase – an enzyme made only inside cells that is responsible for telomere growth. Telomerase stabilizes telomere length by adding DNA nucleotides (TTAGGG) onto the telomeric ends of the chromosomes.

TA-65 - a patented, all-natural plant-derived product has been proven in double-blind placebo controlled human studies to help maintain or rebuild telomeres by activating telomerase.

Hayflick Limit – a scientific theorem which explains that cells have a finite ability to divide. Cells stop replicating and no longer function properly when they reach the Hayflick Limit. Named after Leonard Hayflick, Ph.D., who determined this limit to be about 50 divisions.

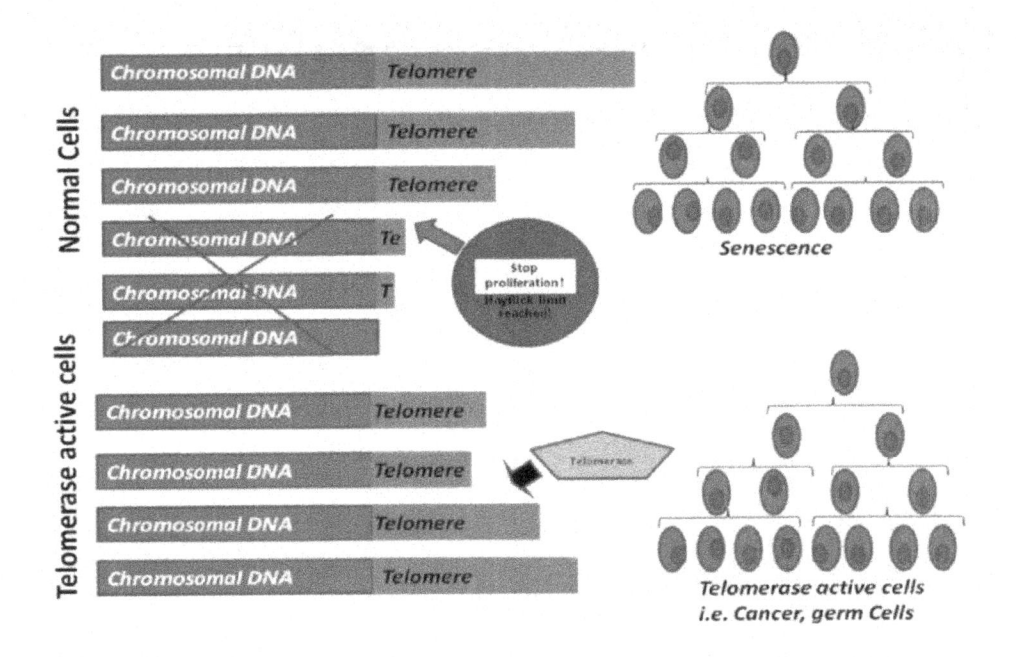

What We Lose With Age

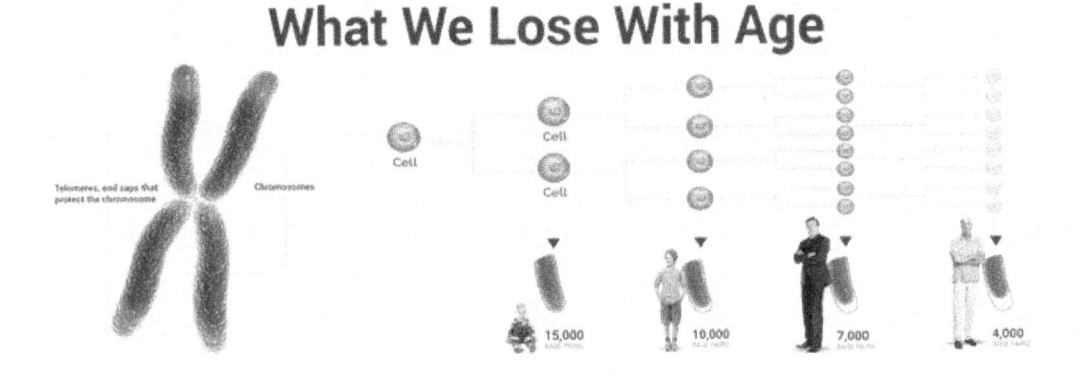

Every time cells divide, telomeres shorten.

Telomeres protect chromosomes. Over time, repeated cellular replication results in shortening of the telomere end caps. Eventually, this leaves the genetic DNA vulnerable to damage and mutations. In response to telomere shortening, cells are programmed to take one of two paths: -

Apoptosis – programmed cell death; the cell naturally self-destructs.

Senescence – a state where the cell can no longer replicate. Not only does the cell no longer function properly, it can secrete inflammatory cytokines that damage other cells. Generally, apoptosis is better than senescence. The body disposes of dead cells, but senescent cells are still partly alive. Zombie cells crowding out healthy ones and damaging neighboring cells and tissue.

Both apoptosis and senescence can result in poor cellular function. Compromised cellular function begins to occur before the telomeres are critically short. Think of shortening telomeres as the cellular aging clock their decreasing length is a countdown to natural cell death.

Shortening telomeres signal changes in gene expression to an older phenotype. Telomerase Activation can maintain telomere length – and slow down the speed of that cellular aging clock.

IT ONLY TAKES ONE WEAK LINK IN THE CHAIN

There are 23 pairs of chromosomes in each cell – that's 48 DNA strands. Telomeres are located at both ends of these DNA strands. This means there are 92 telomere end caps in every cell. It only takes one critically short telomere to affect the function of that cell. Think of a chain with 91 strong links and only one week link. It only takes that one weak link to break the chain.

The body has its own mechanism to protect telomere length: the enzyme telomerase. Telomerase is an enzyme that adds nucleotides to telomeres, extending these DNA end caps, and thereby extending the Hayflick Limit. In germ (reproductive) cells, a protein-coding gene that activates telomerase, Telomerase Reverse Transcriptase (TERT), is permanently switched on. Stem cells and some rapidly dividing cells also have telomerase, but unlike germ cells, the gene is not turned on permanently and the amount of telomerase declines with age. The vast majority of somatic (body) cells have the TERT gene turned off. As cells lose their ability to make enough telomerase, they cannot replenish worn out cells.

In the 1980s, scientists studying telomeres (caps at the end of each strand of DNA) discovered telomerase (the enzyme that maintains telomere length). The research of these scientists revolutionized our understanding of cellular aging. This pioneering research was so important that the Nobel Prize in Physiology/Medicine was awarded in October 2009 for the discovery of how chromosomes are protected by telomeres and the enzyme telomerase.

In early genetic research, nucleotide molecules found at the ends of the chromosomes were regarded as non-functioning 'garbage DNA.' We now know that's hardly the case. Shortening of these DNA sequences, acts as an aging clock and explains the Hayflick Limit – the number of times cells can divide before becoming non-functioning (senescence) or die (apoptosis).

The Effects of Telomere Shortening

There are now more than 24,000 published studies on telomeres. Some important findings include:

- Key scientists now believe that short telomeres are the root cause of cellular aging.

- Apoptosis or cellular senescence is triggered when too many critically short or "uncapped" telomeres accumulate in a cell.

- Named by Nobel Prize Laureate Elizabeth Blackburn, 'Telomere Syndromes' refer to a whole class of problems associated with cellular aging caused by short telomeres.

Telomeres acts as a clock within our cells, representing their age and how well they function. As they shorten, they signal changes in gene expression, changing the cells phenotype to that of an older cell. When telomeres become critically short the cell will either die or become senescent. Senescent cells as mentioned can crowd out healthy ones and damage neighboring cells and tissues because they secrete toxic inflammatory cytokines.

In their book 'The Telomere Effect' Elizabeth Blackburn, Ph.D. and Elissa Epel Ph.D., demonstrate that how we live each day has a profound effect not just on our health and well-being, but how we age as well. Dr. Blackburn's discovery that the length of our chromosomes can determine how fast our cells age and die can have a direct effect on our Healthspan and Lifespan.

Increase your lifespan by increasing your healthspan

Aging begins at the age of 25 for most of us. It is only a decade or two later that we begin to notice the effects.

JOE	HEALTHSPAN		DISEASESPAN		EARLY DEATH	
DYLAN		HEALTHSPAN			LONG LIFE	
BIRTH	20	40	60	80		DEATH

Our **healthspan** is the number of years of our healthy life, free of disease.

Our **diseasespan** are the years we live with noticeable disease that interferes with our quality of living (obesity, diabetes, heart disease, cancer, Alzheimer's, ED, autoimmune disease, etc.).

Our **lifespan** is the total number of years we live.

In the above diagram, Joe has developed one or more diseases in his 40s and has a short lifespan, while Dylan remains free of disease and lives to a hundred.

Why do people age differently? As the obesity researcher George Bray said, "Genes load the gun and our lifestyle (environment) pulls the trigger." Your lifestyle will mostly determine your healthspan, diseasespan and lifespan.

Today with Proactive Medicine, we can easily recognize biomarkers before functional and structural changes occur and thus predict the onset of chronic disease and thus prevent disease from occurring.

This book is written for you to help guide you how to evaluate and quantify your own health and make the necessary lifestyle changes that will dramatically improve not only your Healthspan but also your Lifespan.

With this proactive, preventive health approach and a simple digital platform, you can track your progress over time with a specificity that is unprecedented.

I firmly believe that the two major factors that cause chronic disease and aging, that shortens our lives, are metabolic stress (insulin resistance) and psychological stress.

I say this from my experience as a practicing physician for more than 40 years. I believe this is validated by looking at the data from the 'Blue Zones' where the longest lived people on the planet live. Researchers found that all these Blue Zone long lived people all demonstrated 9 common denominators. Interestingly 5 of the 9 were Psychological and 4 of the 9 were related to Metabolic Stress.

What all these Blue Zone long-lived people demonstrated were 9 common denominators they all shared: -

1. **The 80% Rule** – they stopped eating when their stomach is 80% full.
2. **Eat Mostly Plants** – this is the cornerstone of most centenarian diets.
3. **Drink Alcohol Moderately** – often wine later in the day.
4. **They Move Naturally** – throughout much of the day.
5. **They Find Purpose** – "why they wake up each day."
6. **Downshift** – they have routines to shed stress.
7. **Find Belonging** – faith based services 4x/month adds 14yrs of life.
8. **Put Love Ones First** – centenarians put their family first.
9. **Find The Right Community** – social circles that support healthy behavior.

#1-4 are all about **Metabolic Stress** and #5-9 are to do with **Psychological Stress.**

These are the key lifestyle factors that influence the Hallmarks of Aging.

As Dr. Elissa Epel writes, "Your cells are listening to Your Thoughts" – and shows in The Telomere Effect how you experience stress shortens your telomeres and how you can shift that stress to improve your telomeres and become healthier.

People who respond to stress by feeling overly threatened have shorter telomeres than people who face stress with a rousing sense of challenge.

A small dose of stress does not endanger your telomere. Epel shows however that caregivers for example, a daughter looking after a parent with Alzheimer's have a far stronger threat response. The chronic stress of being a caregiver made them more vulnerable and the ones with the strongest threat response had the shortest telomeres. It's not just from experiencing a stressful event, it's also from feeling threatened by it, even if the stressful event hasn't happened yet. This "Toxic Stress" is severe stress that lasts for years. Short telomeres create sluggish immune function and make you more vulnerable to even catching a common cold or Covid-19. Short telomeres also promote inflammation that causes chronic disease and aging. A stressful childhood can also shape your telomeres for life.

Therapy to Prevent Short Telomeres

1. **Reduce Metabolic Stress**
- Anti-inflammatory Diet (Mediterranean/Keto)
- Consume Omega-3's – plenty of fresh ocean fish
- Moderate meat consumption
- Plenty of plant foods
- Intermittent Fasting – try eating once a day only
- Avoid grains, sugar and most plant oils
- Get to your ideal body fat (Men <20%) (Women <28%)
- Decrease all toxins in your environment
- Balance your hormones
- Aim for 7-8 hours of good sleep each night
- Add plenty fermented food in your diet (microbiome)
- Moderate exercise
- Metformin and Rapamycin etc

2. **Reduce Psychological Stress**
- Stress Reduction – Mindfulness Meditation/ Braintap.com/ Yoga etc.
- "Why do you get out of bed each day?" – find a purpose
- Focus on family/loved ones
- Find 4 close friends and commit to each other for life
- Resilient Thinking VS Negative Thinking
- Lighten up on yourself (self-compassion)
- Expand healthy social networks
- Find ways to enhance your relationship with your significant other
- Forgive yourself and others
- Find something larger than yourself
- Practice gratitude
- Braintap.com

CHAPTER 16: TEMPORAL HIERARCHY OF THE METRICS OF AGING

The study of aging relates to changes in physical and functional dimensions that occur over time in living organisms. Yet, a model that establishes the hierarchical relationship and interlaced time courses of molecular, phenotypic, and functional hierarchical domains of aging in humans has not been established. We propose that studying the mechanisms and consequences of aging through the lens of these hierarchical domains and their connections will provide clarity in semantics and enhance a translational perspective. The study of human aging would be the most informative from a life course, longitudinal perspective, given that manifestations of aging are already detectable early in life at the molecular level, yet the phenotypic responses remain masked by compensatory/resiliency mechanisms. Understanding the nature of these mechanisms is paramount for developing interventions that reduce the burden of disease and disability in older people.

Dr. Luigi Ferrucci

As Dr. Ferrucci writes, "It is customary to think about human aging as a set of characteristics that change over time and signify someone as older or younger."

We can conceptually define these hierarchical levels as the metrics of aging and, for the purpose of these discussion, describe them (Figure 1) as follows: **biological aging,** the changes that occur with aging at the molecular, cellular, and intracellular levels; **phenotypic aging**, the interconnected changes in body structure/composition, energetics, homeostatic control mechanisms, and neuronal function/plasticity that occur in all aging individuals over time and may contribute to clinical diseases; **functional aging,** the age-associated decline in physical, cognitive, emotional, and social functions that may be either so subtle as to be evident only under challenge or so severe that they curtail performance of basic activities of daily living and contribute to loss of independence.

The Metrics of Aging

Functional Aging (impact on daily life)

- Cognitive Function
- Physical Function
- Mood
- Mental Health

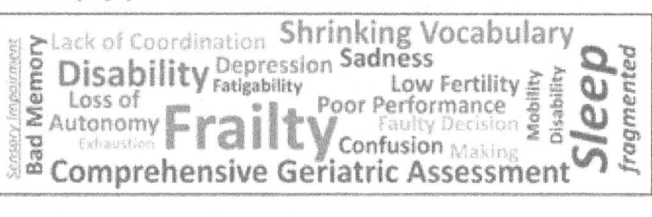

> Lack of Coordination, Shrinking Vocabulary, Disability, Depression, Sadness, Fatigability, Low Fertility, Loss of Autonomy, Poor Performance, Mobility Disability, Sensory Impairment, Bad Memory, Frailty, Faulty Decision Making, Confusion, Exhaustion, Comprehensive Geriatric Assessment, Sleep fragmented

Phenotypic Aging (phenotypes that change)

- Body Composition
- Energetics
- Homeostatic Mechanisms
- Brain health

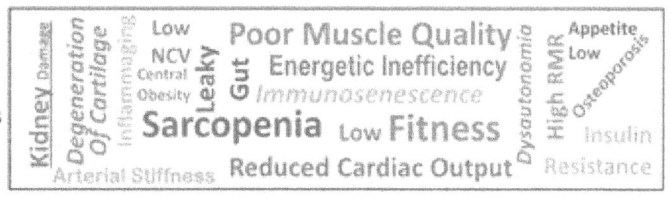

> Kidney Damage, Degeneration Of Cartilage, Inflammaging, Low NCV, Central Obesity, Leaky Gut, Poor Muscle Quality, Energetic Inefficiency, Dysautonomia, High RMR, Appetite Low, Osteoporosis, Sarcopenia, Low Fitness, Immunosenescence, Insulin Resistance, Arterial Stiffness, Reduced Cardiac Output

Biological Aging (root mechanisms)

- Molecular Damage
- Defective Repair
- Energy Exhaustion
- Signal/Noise Reduction

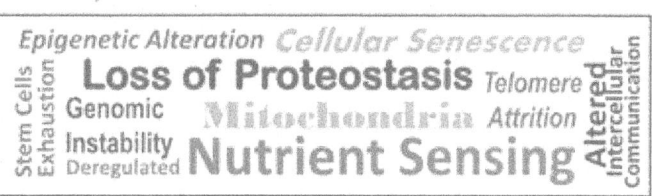

> Epigenetic Alteration, Cellular Senescence, Stem Cells Exhaustion, Loss of Proteostasis, Telomere Attrition, Genomic Instability, Mitochondria, Deregulated Nutrient Sensing, Altered Intercellular Communication

To understand aging biology it is important to understand the connections between biological mechanisms of aging, aging phenotypes, chronic disease and functional limitations.

The hallmarks of aging in the article published in 2013 by Carlos Lopez-Otin provides evidence that these mechanisms contribute to the development of aging phenotypes, age related diseases and functional limitations.

My belief is that these hallmarks did not evolve independently but rather represent the same underlying mechanism from Metabolic and Psychological stress on the organism.

Figure 2 represents a life course that represents the anatomic and physiological change that occur during a person's lifespan.

Until early adulthood there is stability, freedom form disease with only subtle declines in health as well as diminished physical and mental function that becomes evident only if elicited by extreme stress or challenge.

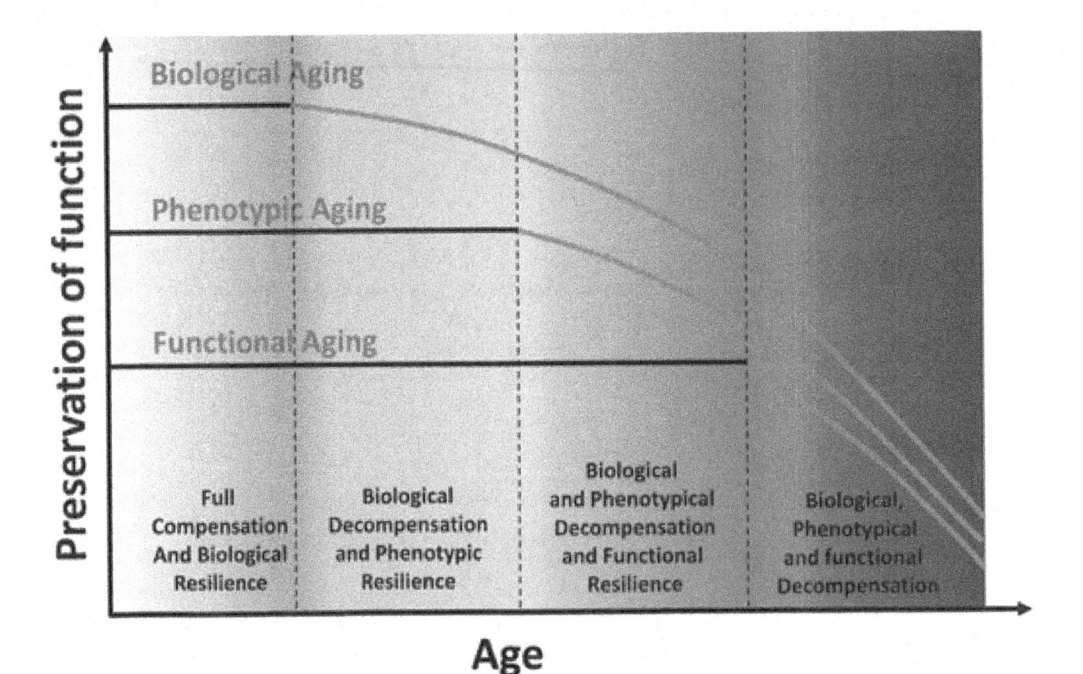

[Figure: Graph showing Preservation of function vs Age, with three declining curves labeled Biological Aging, Phenotypic Aging, and Functional Aging. The x-axis is divided into four stages: Full Compensation And Biological Resilience; Biological Decompensation and Phenotypic Resilience; Biological and Phenotypical Decompensation and Functional Resilience; Biological, Phenotypical and functional Decompensation.]

The intensity of the challenge required to detect this decline progressively decreases over time until functional impairment becomes evident, even in the absence of a challenge.

Dr.Ferrucci continues, "Some individuals show signs of aging earlier than others. Conceptually, the global rate of aging can be imagined as a dynamic equilibrium between entropic stresses (red arrows in Figure 2) and homeostatic mechanisms that constantly restore order (green arrows). The resilience mechanisms that constantly perform maintenance and repair are evolutionarily conserved and allow humans to maintain health and function for many years. However, their efficiency eventually fades and allows entropy to result in frailty and death. The nature of these compensatory mechanisms must be understood to develop effective therapies in slowing aging, thereby preventing or delaying the burden of disease and disability that comes with it. This approach is a drastic departure from the traditional model of medicine, which is based on measuring damage and risk factors, in contrast to assessing functional reserve and boosting resiliency."

Functional Aging occurs only when all resilience mechanisms of the biological and phenotypic aging domains are exhausted.

Environment, behavioral and societal compensatory mechanisms play important roles buffering the effect of underlying declines in functional aging. There is overwhelming evidence that frailty and disability are powerful risk factors for multiple adverse health outcomes, such as nursing home admission, disability and mortality.

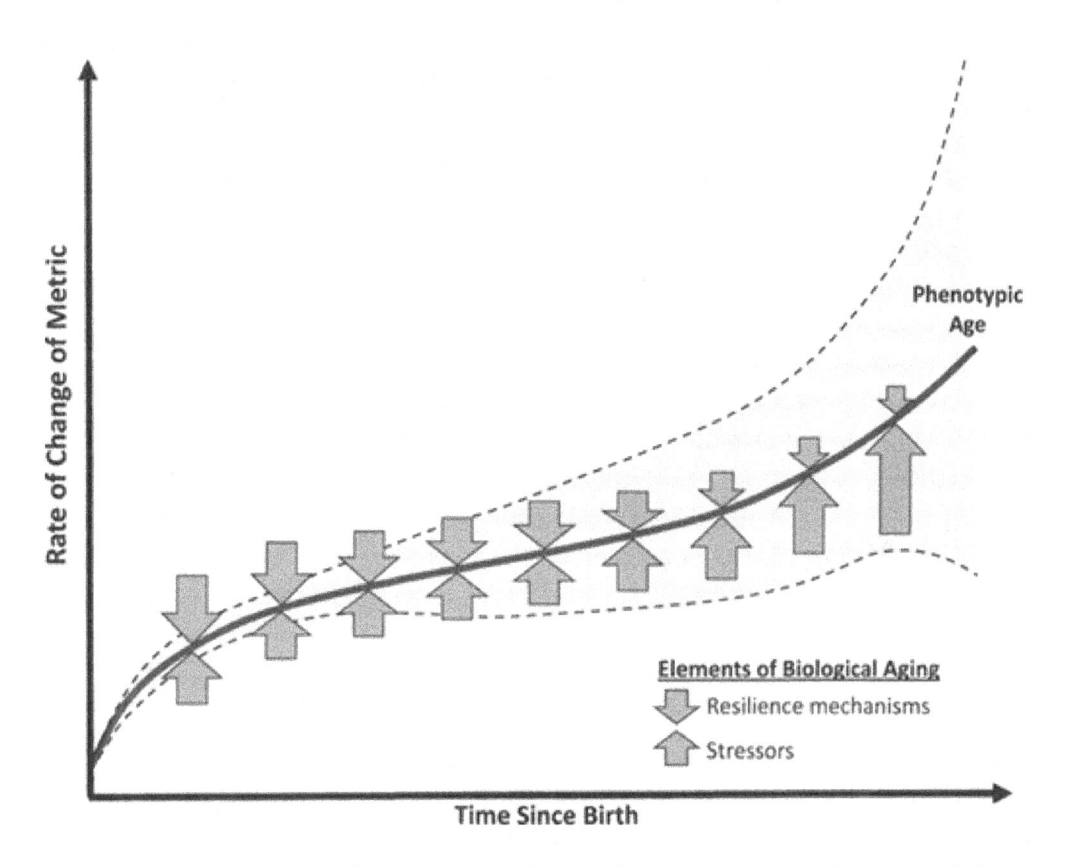

Figure: Rate of Change of Metric vs. Time Since Birth, showing Phenotypic Age curve with Elements of Biological Aging — Resilience mechanisms (down arrows) and Stressors (up arrows).

Dr. Ferrucci ends the Metrics Of Aging with the following insight, "In spite of their success as prognostic indicators, frailty and other measures of functional aging are still rarely used in day-to-day medical practice, mostly because of inadequate evidence that frailty can be prevented or reversed. Developing methods to measure the biological mechanisms of aging in humans may enable identification of individuals on a trajectory of accelerated aging early in the process, who then can be screened for subclinical diseases and thereby targeted for future interventions that globally affect the aging rate and effectively delay frailty. Ultimately, interventions that effectively slow or delay the mechanisms of aging in subjects diagnosed with accelerated aging will need to be identified and properly tested."

An article by Jose Lara et al was published in 2013 titled, "Towards Measurement of the Healthy Aging Phenotype in Lifestyle-based intervention studies." The author recognized that given the biological complexity of the aging process there is no single, simple and reliable measure of how healthily someone is aging. Intervention studies need a panel of measures which can capture key features of healthy aging. Their study adopted the concept of the "Healthy Aging Phenotype" (HAP) and was focused on (1) identifying the most important features of the HAP and (2) identifying the key tools.

They selected a panel of biomarkers of physiological and metabolic health, physical capability, cognitive function, social wellbeing and psychological wellbeing which they proposed may be useful in characterizing the HAP and which could have the ability as outcome measures in intervention studies.

There is very good evidence that behavioral factors (notably smoking, diet, alcohol consumption, and physical activity) and social factors (including roles, relationships and support) are strongly associated with health and wellbeing in later life. However, there is very little evidence about the long-term efficacy of practical, lifestyle-based interventions to change these factors and thereby promote health and wellbeing in later life. In addition, evaluating the efficacy of such interventions is limited by the lack of appropriate outcome measures. Most of the existing tools for measuring changes in health and wellbeing in response to interventions have not been developed or validated for use in older individuals and many are focused on disease or disability rather than on healthy aging.

The HAP provides some insight as to how we must shift our focus away from traditional medicine which simply measures risk factors and damage to a more proactive model to assess functional reserve and boost resiliency. We can identify individuals now on a trajectory of accelerated aging early in the process and with tools used in the HAP, methylation data, mobile monitoring devices and AI we can diagnose subclinical disease and intervene early to affect the Pace of Aging and effectively delay frailty.

CHAPTER 17: WHAT THE BLUE ZONES TELL US ABOUT LONGEVITY?

More than 20 years ago Giovanni Mario Pes and Michel Poulain who had been studying longevity in Sardinia (the region of the world with the highest concentration of male centenarians) introduced the term Blue Zone and subsequently published an article in the Journal of Experimental Gerontology in 2004.

Previously, in 2000, Dan Buettner launched a program aimed at identifying all the world's longest-lived people and identifying their common denomination. He first used the term Blue Zones as an international certification and is largely responsible for articulating the common traits.

BLUE ZONES is a brand and certification mark developed by Michel Poulain, Dan Buettner, and Giovanni Mario Pes when investigating people around the world living longer and better. BLUE ZONES is now a registered trademark owned by BLUE ZONES, LLC, and used by Mssrs. Poulain, Buettner and Pes under license.

Centenarians exist worldwide but there are only a few areas where their concentration is exceptional so that the population could be considered as living longer. The interest to find such areas and populations is not recent. In the 70's, an article in *National Geographic* mentioned longevity hotspots in Vilcabamba (Ecuador), Abkasia and Georgia (Caucasia) and for the Hunzas (Pakistan). However, after a strict validation of the alleged age of the oldest old in these areas, these three longevity hotspots were dismissed. This is because age exaggeration is still often found among the oldest in numerous countries around the world.

Later, under the aegis of National Geographic research expedition lead by Dan Buettner, Michel Poulain certified potential BLUE ZONES in Nicoya, Costa Rica (2007) and Ikaria, Greece (2008) and later in Okinawa (Japan) and Loma Linda (California). Together with Giovanni Mario Pes, they certified these populations as meeting BLUE ZONES™ criteria and investigated their exceptional characteristics. The identification and certification of a BLUE ZONES™ area or group is based on demographic criteria that are country-specific and depending on available documentation and its reliability. The population of a BLUE ZONES certified area should show a statistically significant higher longevity compared to national levels and display various features related to their lifestyle, nutrition, genetics and both human and physical environmental conditions that might be considered in determinants for living longer and better.

Considering that the paradigm of BLUE ZONES gets more and more interest from scientists, media and the general audience and that the lessons transferred from the BLUE ZONES might contribute merely to improve the wellbeing of our aging societies, the three undersigning founders insist upon strict respect of the criteria used when identifying or certifying new BLUE ZONES areas and such validation can only be based on thoroughly validated data, not on opinion or specific point of view.

Dan Buettner's goal was to reverse engineer longevity. As he describes this: - "Since only about 20% of the average person's life span is dictated by genes, I reasoned that if I could find the common denominators among people who've achieved the health outcomes we want, I might distill some pretty good lessons for the rest of us to follow. I discovered nine powerful lessons – the power nine – that underpin all five Blue Zones. Here they are:"

1. **Move Naturally (M)**

The world's longest-lived people don't pump iron, run marathons, or join gyms. Instead, they live in environments that constantly nudge them into moving without thinking about it. They grow gardens and don't have mechanical conveniences for house and yard work.

2. **Find Purpose (P)**

The Okinawans call it *ikagai* and the Nicoyans call it *plan de vida;* for both it translates to "why I wake up in the morning." Knowing your sense of purpose is worth up to seven years of extra life expectancy.

3. **Downshift (P)**

Even people in the Blue Zones experience stress. Stress leads to chronic inflammation, associated with every major age-related disease. What the world's longest-lived people have that we don't are routines to shed that stress. Okinawans take a few moments each day to remember their ancestors. Adventists pray, Ikarians take a nap, and Sardinians do happy hour.

4. Follow the 80% rule (M)

Hara hachi bu, the Okinawan, 2,500 year-old Confucian mantra said before meals, reminds them to stop eating when their stomachs are 80% full. The 20% gap between not being hungry and feeling full could be the difference between losing weight and gaining it. People in the Blue Zones eat their smallest meal in the late afternoon or early evening, and then they don't eat any more for the rest of the day.

5. Eat mostly plants (M)

Beans, including fava, black soy, and lentils, are the cornerstone of most centenarian diets. Meat-mostly pork- is eaten on average only five times per month. Serving sizes are 3 to 4 ounces, about the size of a deck of cards.

6. Drink wine at 5 (M)

People in all Blue Zones (except Adventists) drink alcohol moderately and regularly. **Moderate drinkers outlive non-drinkers.** The trick is to drink one to two glasses per day (preferably Sardinian Cannonau wine) with friends and/or with food. And no, you can't save up all week and have 14 drinks on Saturday.

7. Find belonging (P)

All but five of the 263 centenarians we interviewed belonged to some faith-based community. Denomination doesn't seem to matter. Research shows that attending **faith-based services four times per month** will add four to 14 years of life expectancy.

8. Put love ones first (P)

Successful centenarians on the Blue Zones put their families first. This means keeping aging parents and grandparents nearby or in the home. (It lowers disease and mortality rates of children in the home too.) They commit to a **life partner** (which can add up to three years of life expectancy) and invest in their children with time and love (and they'll be more likely to care for you when the time comes).

9. Find the right community (P)

The world's longest-lived people chose-or were born into-**social circles that support healthy behaviors.** For example, Okinawans created moais – **groups of five friends that committed to each other for life.** Research from the Framingham Studies shows that smoking, obesity, happiness, and even loneliness are contagious. So the social networks of long-lived people have favorably shaped their health behaviors.

What exactly is research on the Blue Zones telling us? Firstly, the data collected on these long-lived people (for example in Ikaria 1 in 3 citizens reach 90) is very well documented and validated. Second, is that each of these Blue Zones share the same 9 key lifestyle denominators – 5 are Psychological factors and 4 are Metabolic. Third, although it is my opinion, having seen clients for more than 40 years, that the large majority of my vibrant, active elder clients share many of these same traits. Finally, each of the hallmarks of Aging shows that Metabolic and Psychological Stress are involved in the aging process.

In summary, what follows are several key thoughts to reduce both metabolic and psychologic stress that the Blue Zones have proven will shorten both your healthspan and lifespan if not controlled.

In 1800, the world's average life expectancy was only about 30 years. The typical person in the USA now lives to age 79. Once we make it to 65, statistics show we can look forward to another 19 years, on average. A healty 80 year old, free of chronic illness, has a good shot to make it to 90 years plus!

Most of us, 99.98% to be precise, are dead before 100. There is no biological law that says we must age. We now recognize aging as a disease – the most common disease – one that not only can but should be treated aggressively.

For the first time we now have therapies that can slow, stop and even reverse aging. The new methylation clocks show that we might be able to slow Biological Aging up to 20 years in a persons life. The older we get, the more important our personal lifestyles become. The older we get, the more important our personal lifestyles become.

Researchers agree that if you address the hallmarks of aging, you can slow down aging. Slow down aging you can forestall disease. Forestall disease you can push back death. We know that slowing any one of these hallmarks may add several years of healthy living. It is important also to remember that each hallmark is connected to the others – a change in one will effect the others.

Although genetics plays a role, the major player is epigenetics – our lifestyle and environment ultimately determine how we age.

My firm conviction is that Metabolic and Psychological Stress are the primary determinants of longevity. I would like to end this chapter with some thoughts on Metabolic Stress by Dr. Rober Lustig and on Psychological Stress by Dr. Patrick Porter as these both form the foundation of the LB100 program.

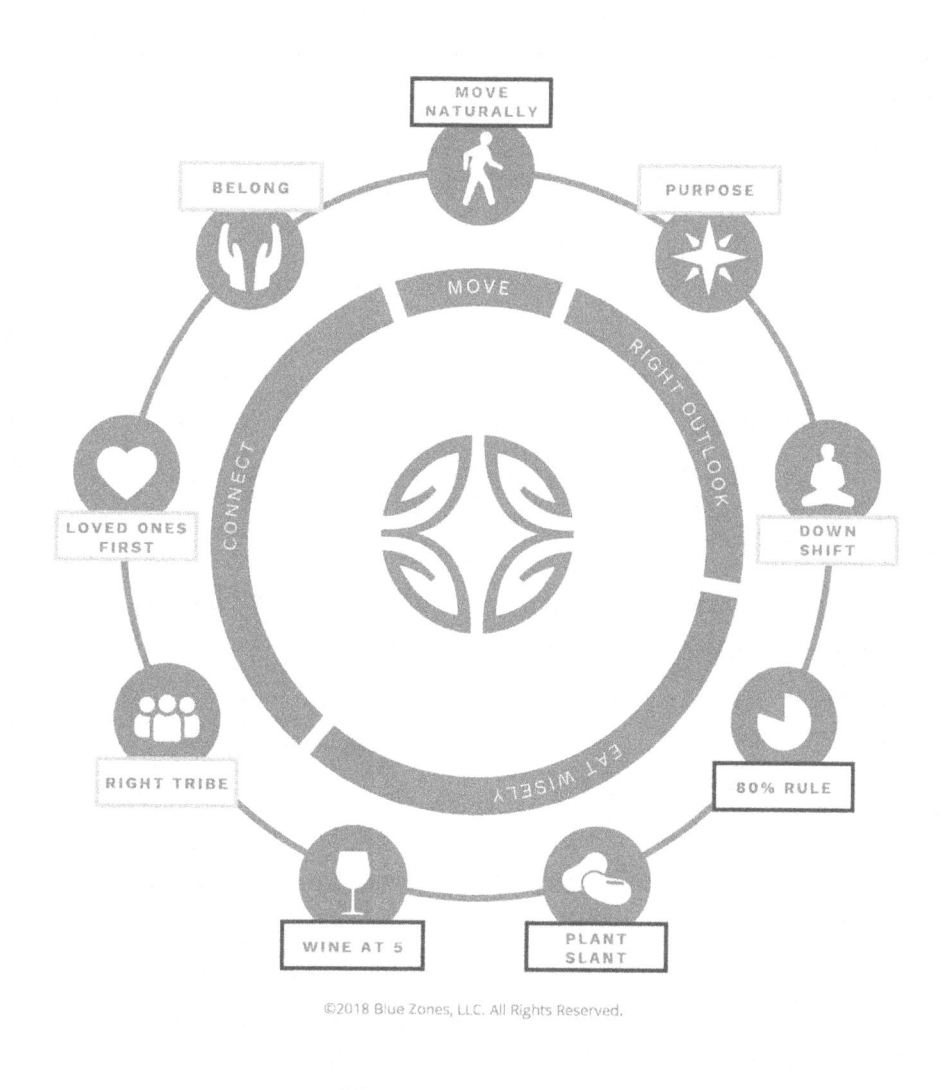

©2018 Blue Zones, LLC. All Rights Reserved.

METABOLIC STRESS

PSYCHOLOGICAL STRESS

The Prime Hidden Drivers of Metabolic Stress

Most American adults have not understood the recent science that not all foods are equal in causing cardio-metabolic disease as they are still stuck in the "calorie mode" and have not yet transitioned to "insulin mode."

A low carb high fat diet that reduces insulin improves "insulin sensitivity" reducing the burden of metabolic disease and helps fat cells give up their stored fat and promotes weight loss. This diet also improves "leptin sensitivity" at the brain level resulting in you feeling full and reducing your total food intake.

On the other hand, all calorie restricting diets lead to lower leptin levels within 18 hours signaling brain starvation and increase fat cells to store food. Remember high insulin levels makes you fat and keeps you fat!

The cell is the basic building block of life. In order to stay alive a cell has to burn energy. Most cells burn glucose a simple sugar and the building block of starch. The liver and fat cells need insulin to open the cell membrane to let the glucose in, other organs don't need insulin for glucose entry.

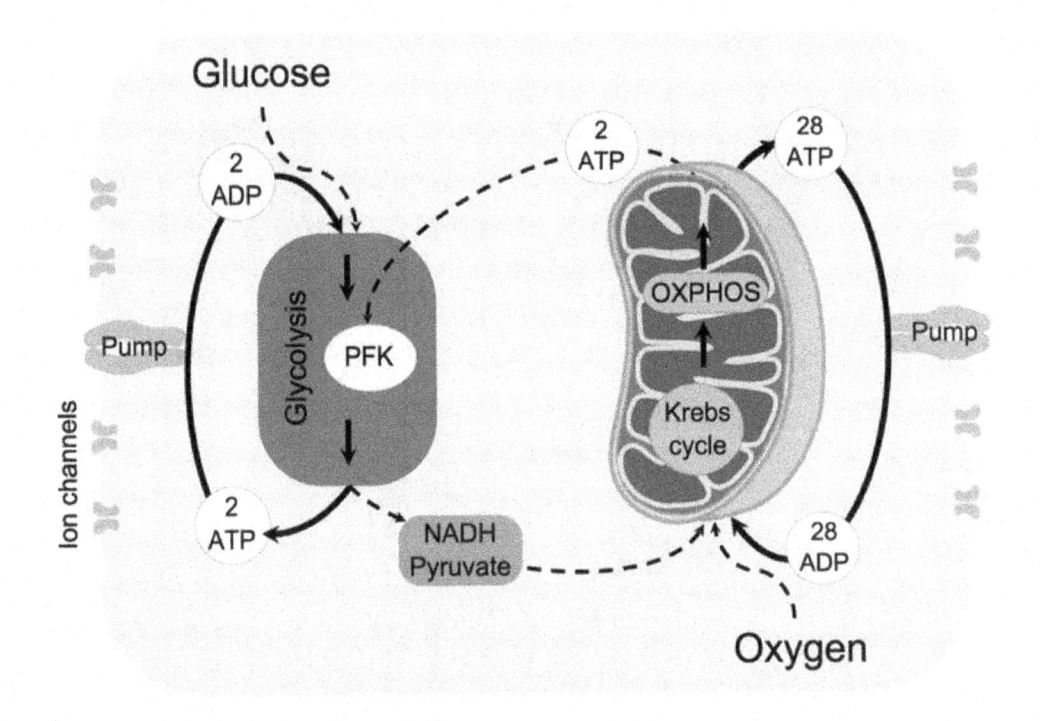

But if glucose is in short supply and insulin levels are low, then the fat tissue will give up some of its fatty acids to enter the bloodstream, and the liver will turn those fatty acids into ketones, which then seep back into the bloodstream, so that any cell can burn those ketones instead, even without insulin.

Cells are magicians. They either make glucose disappear of it there's too much they turn glucose into fat, which wreaks havoc on metabolism.

Energy Metabolism. The cell imports glucose and converts it into pyruvic acid (glycolysis left side), yielding two ATPs. If the mitochondria are functioning, the pyruvic acid is metabolized by the Krebs cycle (right side), yielding twenty-eight ATPs and carbon dioxide.

If the mitochondria are busy or dysfunctional the pyruvic acid diverts into a process called de novo lipogenesis (new fat making) to turn into fatty acid called palmitic acid, which is then bound to a glycerol molecule and exported out of the liver as a triglyceride particle.

Both pathways, especially within the mitochondria release toxic by products called oxygen radicals. If the cell is not detoxified these free radicals can cause the cell to die. Fortunately cells have organelles called a "peroxisome" that store various antioxidants to neutralize the oxygen radicals. What follows are "eight processes" that if working right contribute to longevity and good health. But if some of these are not working right you get chronic cardio-metabolic disease, a shorter healthspan and die early. These are the true diseases (mostly hidden) all due to **processed food!**

1. **Glycation**

The Maillard reaction only needs 2 molecules to occur fructose or glucose, and an amino acid (protein) - put them together the protein starts to "brown" and become less flexible. The faster the Maillard reaction occurs the faster we age.

2. **Oxidative Stress**

If there are more oxygen radicals than antioxidants we get **oxidative stress** that causes cellular dysfunction and in some cases cell death.

3. **Mitochondrial Dysfunction**

When glucose and oxygen and mitochondrial capacity are all matched everything runs smoothly. When glucose comes in faster than the mitochondria can process we get de novo lipogenesis and a fatty liver which leads to **insulin resistance.** If this happens in the pancreas you get a fatty pancreas and insulin deficiency. The sicker your mitochondria, the earlier you die.

4. **Insulin Resistance**

As mentioned just two organs in your body need insulin to function: the liver and adipose tissue. When the other cells in your body are not responding to the insulin in your bloodstream – this is called **insulin resistance.**

When glucose can't get into certain cells those cells starve which leads to organ dysfunction. Insulin resistance isn't due to low insulin but high insulin levels because the cell is not responding to the insulin signal. Various problems lead to defective insulin signaling including genetics, obesity, chronic stress, lack of sleep, obesogens like estrogen, BPA, phthalates and mostly by processed food. High insulin levels cause cellular dysfunction, leading to chronic disease, morbidity and early death. Processed food is the biggest problem.

5. **Membrane Integrity**

Membranes are damaged through two mechanisms: the lipids in the cell membrane themselves are changed by toxins or oxidative stress or the lipids are inflexible. Saturated fatty acids are flexible. Unsaturated fats are usually better for you but beware in heating these as if they have a low smoke point they cause oxidative stress and you now have a "transfat."

6. **Inflammation**

Processed food causes inflammation and can also damage the gut microbiome causing a "leaky gut" that can produce a low grade inflammatory response to lipo-polysaccharides (LPS) from gram negative bugs. Also excess sugar produces palmitic acid that causes further inflammation. Many people are lectin sensitive that can also cause further inflammation in the gut.

7. Epigenetics

Processed food is a primary driver of altered epigenetics turning on killer genes. Methylation problems also cause epigenetic changes that can alter epigenetics as can endocrine disrupting chemicals and nutritional deficiencies for example folic acid.

8. Autophagy

All organs do better with autophagy which is an essential process that maintains healthy cells by removing damaged proteins and malfunctioning organelles especially mitochondria. Vitamin D plays an important role in autophagy. A ketone diet and intermittent fasting can increase autophagy and the stem cell population.

Adapted From Metabolical by Robert Lusting, MD

The Prime Hidden Drivers of Psychological Stress

The Universal Laws That Can Change Your Life

We are beings of energy, and every good scientist knows that universal laws and principles govern energy. When your energy is in harmony with universal law, you feel harmonious. When your energy is out of sync with universal law, you feel disharmonious. Universal laws are what dictate the results of our thoughts and actions. It's that simple.

These universal laws govern us at each level of our being – spiritual, physical, and emotional. Stress happens when our egos try to control these laws. In other words, when we express a desire, or take an action, we attempt to direct the outcome. When you are in the flow and live in harmony with universal laws, you gain health, happiness, and prosperity. Therefore, doesn't it make good sense to ride, rather than fight, the current of energy that builds and maintains all of creation?

How much easier would life be if we simply made decisions with good conscience and then left it up to the universal principles to provide the result? I think it would feel something like a juggler, who has held dozens of balls in the air for years, finally letting them fall where they may.

1. Law of Acceptance

If something in your life isn't working, chances are good you aren't accepting that you have a problem. Until you reach a state of acceptance by being one hundred percent honest with yourself, your mind will simple give you the status quo. This is why the twelve-step program includes this law.

The Serenity Prayer

God grant me the serenity to accept the things I cannot change, courage to change the things I can; and the wisdom to know the difference.

2. Law of Attraction

Any time you find yourself describing experiences in terms such as coincidence, serendipity, good luck, bad luck, fluke, fate, chance, good fortune, bad fortune or destiny you are likely on the receiving end of the Law of Attraction.

3. Law of Cause and Effect

What you sow, you reap. This law can work in either a positive or negative way. Your job is to figure out how to use the Law of Cause and Effect to create the life you want.

4. Law of Forgiveness

Buddha said, "He who angers you conquers you" when we think negative thoughts the brain spews out a cascade of chemicals that have the potential to destroy the body. However, if we forgive the people that hurt us, then the body responds with the right elixir of hormones that create health, harmony and vitality.

5. Law of Abundance

One needs to understand that everything in the universe is connected by energy. Energy is the driving force behind all life. Thus the energy coming from our own minds directs what happens in our bodies and what we attract to ourselves.

6. Law of Non-attachment

Attachment to the end result of any goal causes stress. Again Buddha said, "desire is the root cause of suffering."

These universal laws dictate our thoughts and actions. Stress results when our egos try to control these laws. Stress can manifest in a myriad of ways. I commonly see anxiety, depression, and problems with sleep and hypervigilance. Often difficulty concentrating, feelings of being overwhelmed and memory issues are the result.

Getting out of the fight or flight response and into the relaxation response is the best step you can take to overcome stress. The relaxation response can't happen if you are generating high beta brain wave activity. Your brain wave activity must dip into alpha (intuitive mind) or theta (inventive mind).

How is technology changing the way we use our brain?

Light and sound technology, also known as *visual/auditory* entrainment, is introduced to the brain through the ears and optic nerve using computerized technology emitted through headphones and especially designed glasses equipped by light-emitting bodies (LEDs). The lights flash at predetermined frequencies and are coupled with binaural beats, which are heard at a low level through the headphones. The visual/auditory entrainment is typically synchronized, but can be varied depending on the desired effect.

The flickering light patterns and binaural beats reach the brain by way of the optic nerve and inner ear respectively. Within minutes the brain begins to match the frequencies of the light pulses and sound beats. The method by which this entrainment occurs is known as *frequency following response*. Unlike biofeedback, where the user attempts to consciously change brainwave activity, light and sound induced entrainment influences the brain without any conscious effort.

The frequency following response stimulates the relaxed brainwave frequencies known as *alpha and theta*. This is the state in which the individual relaxes and the mind develops focus. Listeners experience a reduction in inner chatter and improved concentration. Because frequency following response is a learned response, the effect is cumulative. After a few weeks of regular use, users gain a sense of balance and inner calm. Most people report feeling serene, focused, and alert even when faced with high-pressure situations. Furthermore, most users report experiencing enhanced creativity and feeling more rested with less sleep.

What is Creative Visualization?

Creative Visualization, otherwise known as guided imagery, uses language to transport individuals out of their current space and into a new space of inner calm, peace, and tranquility. A natural byproduct of creative visualization occurs when the muscles go loose and limp, thereby creating the relaxation response.

What is the Relaxation Response?

Once the relaxation response is triggered, the brain sends out neurochemicals that virtually neutralize the effects of the fight-or-flight response. We immediately notice the physical benefits such as a decrease in blood pressure, a lower respiratory rate, a slower pulse, relaxed muscles, and an increase in alpha brain-wave activity. Alpha brainwaves are associated with deep relaxation and being in this state allows for greater access to what I call the *intuitive mind,* which is where healing is most likely to take place.

Because the relaxation response is hard-wired, you do not have to believe it will work for you to experience the benefits. The relaxation response happens in the body and not in the mind. You will learn in detail how to turn on the relaxation response, which naturally turns off the harmful fight-or-flight response, so you can easily transform your life and your world. The relaxation response is the perfect state for learning, healing, or focusing on goals.

"Repeated activation of the relaxation response can reverse sustained problems in the body and mend the internal wear and tear brought on by stress."

-Herbert Benson, MD
Timeless Healing, 1996

Why use Creative Visualization and Guided Relaxation Together? (CVR)

We all have an inner critic, a part of our mind that, based on past experience, will reject new information without proper evaluation. This is known as the *critical factor*. Relaxation techniques subdue the critical factor of the mind. In other words, the part of the mind that might reject unfamiliar information is put on hold during the relaxation response.

Everyone possesses a right-brain and a left-brain. These two parts of the brain play a role in the critical factor, are essential components in the magic elixir, and perform different tasks.

Relaxation can only happen when you release control and allow the left brain to rest for a while.

How will CVR Help You Reduce Stress?

CVR can help you change the way you see yourself and your life. Once you have a new image of yourself – as a healthy, happy, optimistic person – your fears and frustrations fade away, your anxiety vanishes, and you no longer let small things stress you.

In other words, CVR makes sure you are focusing on everything that makes you feel positive and optimistic. When your perception of yourself changes from *stressed person to easygoing person,* you no longer will have tension and doubt. If this happens, can you imagine how motivated and energetic you would feel?

Dr. Porter has made a more than two-decade study of people who are naturally easygoing and resilient. He knew that the key to permanent success was hidden in their underlying psychology. By talking with these people, he discovered a common thread that included a positive self-image, a relaxed, easygoing demeanor, the capacity for *seeing* the future as bright and full of opportunity, and the ability to leave the past in the past.

What is this Magic Elixir that Can Transform Your Life and the World?

The magic elixir resides right there in your brain. It's the miraculous mixture of chemicals in your brain that cascade through your body whenever you're relaxed, or think a positive thought, or have a happy experience – or whenever you visualize these things. It's the miraculous power within each of us to eliminate the effects of stress, heal our bodies, and enjoy life to its fullest. The magic elixir is created through the power of your other-than-conscious mind and activated by CVR to bring you health, vitality, and anything and everything you desire for your life.

People who dare to relax with CVR enjoy all of these benefits and more:

- The Relaxation Response replaces the Fight or Flight Response.

- The right and left hemispheres of the brain become more balanced.

- Blood flow to the brain increases, resulting in clearer thinking, better concentrate, improved memory, and enhanced creativity.

- Serotonin levels increase by up to twenty-one percent, which calms the mind and body and creates an overall sense of wellbeing.

- Endorphin levels increase by up to twenty-five percent. These are the hormones that flow through the body when we feel happy. Endorphins provide the brain with alertness, are a natural anti-depressants, provide relief from pain, and create pleasurable and loving feelings.

- Twenty minutes of CVR can be equivalent to three to four hours of sleep. Consequently, you may find yourself sleeping less, feeling more rested, accomplishing more, and basically enjoying life more fully.

- Energy levels soar.

- Relationships become more fulfilling.

- Career satisfaction improves.

- A sense of purpose develops.

- The ability to make personal changes, such as losing weight, quitting smoking, ending nail biting or other nervous habits happens faster and easier.

- And last, but certainly not least, one gains a seemingly effortless ability to handle and manage stress.

Adapted From Thrive in Overdrive by Patrick Porter, PhD

I would like to end this chapter with some thoughts from Tony Robbins latest book Life Force. Robbins is arguably the most well known motivational speaker on the planet.

Robbins in chapter one writes: "nothing matters more than our mindset and the power of our mind and emotions to heal every facet of our being. Why? Because whatever we do with our bodies, if we don't manage our minds and emotions, we will never experience the quality of life we truly desire and deserve.

By liberating yourself from fear, you'll be free to live more, love more, achieve more , and share more - to experience at a higher level the astounding Miracle of being alive."

In the last chapter of the book he describes the secret of his success that he learned painfully as a young boy and later in life - that the quality of our life is the quality of our habitual emotions. Where you live emotionally determines what your life is really like. Negative emotions can become a persons go-to pattern.

Robbins realized that our lives are controlled by just three decisions:

1. What we decide to focus on?

Whatever you focus on you are going to feel. Wherever focus goes, energy flows.

2. What does this mean?

As Robbins writes -"As soon as we focus on something, our brain has to make another decision, and that is: What does it mean? This choice directly controls your quality of life. Whether that meaning is positive or negative it completely shapes our life. In the end, our life is controlled by what we focus on and the meaning we give it. Meaning equals emotions, and your emotions equal the quality of your life."

3. What am I going to do?

"Every moment we are making those first two decisions: What am I going to focus on, and what does it mean? Again, meaning creates emotions, and our emotions shape the third and the most important decision: What am I going to do? This is the make -or-break choice that defines your life, the now that leads either to massive action or accepting life as it is. But remember, actions don't happen in a vacuum. They're shaped by those first two decisions, on focus and meaning. The emotions that grow out of meaning powerfully affect what action we take. If one person is infuriated by an incident at their job, and someone else is inspired by the very same situation, how do you think they'll respond - the same way, or different ways? So these are decisions we're literally making moment-to-moment. The problem is that most people make them unconsciously, and so our life becomes a habit of failure or success depending on what type of habits we have in this area.

When life gives you pain and suffering, will you just suffer? Or will you find the way to grow and use it to find a way to serve others?

My core belief is that life is always happening for us, not to us, but it is our job to find benefits in the challenge"

Remember genetics loads the gun, but epigenetics - our lifestyle(metabolic and psychological stress) pulls the trigger!

Ray Kurzweil the well known futurist wrote: "No matter what quandaries we face - business problems, health issues, relationship difficulties, the great social and cultural challenges of our time - there exists an idea that will enable us to prevail. We can and must find that idea. And when we find it we need to implement it"

I believe that the "idea" is our awareness of integral consciousness (Non-local mind) that we can experience and live from. Robbins writes in a similar fashion -"the most important decision that you can make is to decide that life is too short to suffer and that you are going to appreciate and enjoy this gift of life, no matter what happens. Decide to live in a "beautiful state" (integral consciousness) no matter what happens around you. It simply means to find the beauty, find something to be grateful for (One mind), something to appreciate and then solve your problems"

ERA III Medicine (Non-Local)

Integrate Structures of Consciousness (One Mind)

One Mind includes all individual minds. It includes thoughts, emotions and cognition. The One Mind involves a vivid sense of connectedness with all sentient life, and a profound sense of love, caring and compassion. It is the over arching principle that makes individual awareness possible. In other words our mind is not confined to our brain or body, as we have been taught, but it extends infinitely outside them. Having no boundaries or limits, individual minds merge with all other minds to form the One Mind.

Larry Dossey MD

CHAPTER 18: RE-EVALUATING MONOTHEISTIC RELIGIONS

"If the doors of perception were cleansed everything would appear to man as it is, infinite."

- William Blake

Just over 80 years ago, in September 1939, Germany invaded Poland without warning starting WWII – the most cataclysmic conflict in the history of the world thus far.

In 1943, philosopher John Gebser, political historian Eric Voeglin and psychoanalyst Carl Jung each independently recognized that the mounting crisis for Western civilization was in fact a fundamental restructuring of consciousness.

Today we recognize that this is not just a Western Crisis but a crisis of the world and all humankind and appears headed toward an event that can only be described as a "global catastrophe."

Vaclav Havel (1936-2011), the author, poet and playwright who was the first president of the Czech Republic, saw a hell looming in our world and had the guts to say so on the international stage. As an antidote, he endorsed a type of awareness he called "responsibility to something higher." In a speech to a joint meeting of the United States Congress on February 21,1990, he said: Consciousness preceeds Being, and not the other way around…for this reason, the salvation in this human world lies nowhere else than in a human heart…Without a global revolution in the sphere of human consciousness, nothing will change for the better in the sphere of our being as humans, and the catastrophe toward which this world is headed-be it ecological, social, demographic or a general breakdown of civilization-will be unavoidable. If we are no longer threatened by world war or by the danger that the absurd mountains of accumulated nuclear weapons might blow up the world, this does not mean that we have definitely won. We are still capable of understanding that the only genuine backbone of all our actions, if they are to be normal, is responsibility. Responsibility to something higher than my family, my country, my company, my success – responsibility to the order of being where all our actions are indelibly recorded and where and only where they will be properly judged."

In February 2022, Vladimir Putin, like Adolph Hitler before him, invaded the Ukraine without provocation. Thus, the Russian authorities and armed forces have been accused of committing multiple war crimes by carrying out both deliberate attacks against civilian targets and indiscriminate attacks in densely populated areas.

The Russian military allegedly exposed the civilian population to unnecessary and disproportionate harm using cluster munitions - a type of weapon that is prohibited by 110 states because of its immediate and long-term danger to civilians - and by firing other explosive weapons with wide-area effects such as air-dropped bombs, missiles, heavy artillery shells and multiple launch rockets. The result of the Russian forces' attacks was damage or destruction of civilian buildings including houses, hospitals, schools, kindergartens, nuclear power plants, historic buildings, and churches. According to international law experts, evidence points in Russia deliberately targeting Ukrainian hospitals across the country.

It remains to be seen how this war will end.

Larry Dossey, my friend and colleague, in his book One Mind offers us a solution: - "One Mind is a potential way out of the division, bitterness, selfishness, greed and destruction that threaten to engulf our world from which beyond a certain point, there may be no escape."

Before I introduce One Mind I would like to talk about the plight of Christianity which is still the largest theistic religion in the world – approximately 2.38 billion people practice some form of Christianity globally. This means that about 1/3 of the worlds total population is Christian - I believe Christianity in its current form will not be able to sustain us in the years ahead.

What is a theist?

A theist is a person who believes in God. A monotheist is a person who believes in **one** God. Monotheism is accepted by Christianity, Islam and Judaism, although each has a distinct view of God.

In contrast, an **atheist** is the denial of the existence of God. (**Agnosticism** believes the existence of God is uncertain).

I am one of the many modern men and women for whom traditional religions, in my case Christianity, has lost most of its ancient meaning.

John Shelby Spong, an American Bishop of the Episcopal Church of Nework, NJ (1979-2000) feels much the same way when he writes: -

The opening phrase of the Apostles' Creed speaks first of God as the "Father Almighty." Both of these words offend me deeply. Here the mystery that I treasure in God begins to be filled with limiting cultural definitions. The word *Father* is such a human word – so male, so dated. It elicits the traditional God images of the old man who lives just beyond the sky. It shouts of the masculinity of the deity, a concept that has been used for thousands of years to justify the oppression of woman by religious institutions. That history and that practice repel me today. The Christian Church at times has gone so far as to debate whether women actually had souls and whether girl babies ought to be baptized. That Church universally relegated women to clearly defined secondary roles until the latter years of the twentieth century, when that sexist prejudice began to dissipate.

I would like to point out several reasons why it is very difficult for many others and myself to believe several tenets of Christianity.

1. **The Biblical Understanding of Creation:** This creation story dates the world at a point a little more than 6,000 years ago. That was the calculation that Bishop James Ussher of Ireland made from biblical data. We know today that this is simply not the case.

2. **Galileo Galilei** (1564-1642) building on the insights of Nicolaus Copernicus (1473-1543) concluded that the sun did not rotate about the earth but rather that the earth rotated around the sun. As Spong writes, "This meant that the Earth could no longer be envisioned as the center of the Universe and thus God might not be quite so involved in the day-to-day affairs of human beings." the ancient worldview against which the Christian story had been framed had been dealt a mighty blow. Galileo was condemned to death as a heretic. In order to save his life, he was given the opportunity to recant, which he decided to accept."

3. The full acceptance of this idea was not complete until December 28, 1991, when the Vatican finally admitted that Galileo had been right and the Church and Bible had been wrong.

4. **Isaac Newton** (1643-1727). Newton was determined to demonstrate in intimate detail how the world worked and how God worked within the world. Humans gradually learned that the world operated according to fixed laws. The exploration of sickness as a divine affliction, the weather patterns and others worked according to these laws.

5. **Charles Darwin** (1809-1882). A century after Newton, Darwin added enormously to modern knowledge and the myth of creation. This biblical myth suggested that man and woman were made on the final day of God's busy first week. God finished the perfect creation with this majestic act and preceded to take the divine rest on the seventh day, thus creating the Sabbath. Darwin in his book "The Origin of Species," suggested that the world of God creation was not yet finished, directly contradicting the literal biblical text. The world, he said, was still evolving, still being created.

6. **Original Sin.** The climax of the story of creation came when God made man and woman the steward's overall creation in the Garden of Eden. They were given everything they needed save one - they were forbidden to eat the fruits from the tree of knowledge of good and evil (the "forbidden fruit").

Finally, listening to the voice of temptation (incarnate in a wily serpent) they ate the forbidden fruit God had been disobeyed. The perfection of creation had been ruined. Human life had fallen into sin. All life cried out for a savior so they could be redeemed. It was the conviction that humans were sinful and in need of redemption that enabled guilt and religion to be so closely tied in the history of the Western world. As Spong writes - "The power of Western religion has always rested on the ability of religious people to understand and to manipulate the sense of human inadequacy that expresses itself as guilt. Religious leaders learned that controlling peoples behavior rested upon exacerbating these human feelings of guilt. This was even stronger when this was connected to the universal human reality of desire, especially sexual desire. Sex was evil. Sex was universal. So evil was universal. It was said to be the heritage of Adam. We were fallen creatures in need of rescue."

As Bishop Spong points out: -

As this understanding of the redemptive work of Christ was being developed in Christian history, Augustine, the bishop of Hippo (354-430) and one of the premier theological minds of the Western world, set stage for an interpretation of Christ that would last for more than a thousand years. He solidified the relationship between Jesus and the fallen world by making concrete the theory of the atonement accomplished in Jesus. For Augustine, Adam and Eve were quite literally the first human beings. Their banishment from the garden resulted in death being the price that all human beings had to pay for their sin.

Death was not natural, Augustine argued, it was punitive. The sin of Adam had been passed on through the sex act to every other human being. The connection between sin and sex was clearly established. All human beings were lost, incapable of saving themselves, and destined to die in their sin. That universality of sin was what Christ had broken. He had suffered the consequences of sin, had paid the ransom due to either God or the devil, and had broken the power of death over human life. He had taken away the sting of death, which was sin. He had robbed death of its victory. "O death, where is thy victory. O grave, where is thy sting?" Paul continued by saying, "The sting of death is sin" (1 Cor. 15-15-56).

1. The Meaning of the Virgin Birth

As Augustine worked out this theological understanding of life, the virgin birth tradition became very important to him. The virgin birth accounts were literally true for Augustine, and they were absolutely necessary to salvation itself. Indeed, salvation could not have been achieved, for Augustine, apart from the literal virgin birth.

The reasoning behind this was clear. The sin of Adam was passed on sexually from father to son. Human life was born in the sin of Adam, from which no one could escape. A savior required to do the redemptive task could not himself be the victim of Adam's sin. That separating of Jesus from the human sin of the fall was accomplished for Augustine by the virgin birth. The sin of Adam did not corrupt the humanity of Jesus because the Holy Spirit of God was his father. He was thus not a child of Adam at all. At that time it was believed that the woman did not contribute genetically or materially to the birth of the child but merely nurtured the male's "seed" to maturity. So the fallenness of the woman's humanity was not an issue."

2. Why did Theism actually emerge?

As I will point out later in the **Structures of Consciousness** in this monograph, self-consciousness is a relatively late development in mankind's evolution but is the primary reason for man's existential fear. As Bishop Spong also points out - "Our deepening probe suggest that theistic religion was born at the exact moment when human self-consciousness first emerged out of the evolutionary process. Indeed, I would suggest that what we might call human history has never existed without both self-consciousness and theistic religion. I would go further and say that it was the emergence of self-consciousness that demanded the creation of theistic religion. Since religion was conceived in theistic terms at the very moment of the rise of self-consciousness, at the dawn of human history, theism was able to develop its powerful and exclusive lock on the definition of God. That is why the death of theism feels like the death of God. The two have never been separated before. So looking still for clues to help us into some new approach to the divine, we seek to understand what happened at the dawn of human life to make this combination so intense.

We are helped in this pursuit of insight by the great father of the psychoanalytic discipline, Sigmund Freud. In 1927, he sketched out his thoughts on this subject in a book entitled *The Future of an Illusion*. Here Freud probed the origins of human life and the various human creations that enabled human beings to cope with their existence. Religion was, he argued, a major one of those human creations.

The birth of theistic religion, Freud argued, grew out of the trauma of self-consciousness. For billions of years, Freud observed, the creatures who inhabited this earth did not have a sufficient intellectual capacity to raise questions about the meaning of their lives or indeed to ask whether life possessed any ultimate meaning. They simply lived and died in an endless pattern without knowing that this was either their reality or their destiny.

Finally, however, a creature evolved with a brain sufficient to be self-aware, self-conscious, and to have the capacity for self-transcendence. The shock of mortality and meaninglessness entered history at that moment, Freud contended. Now the world possessed a creature who could anticipate dying, who could understand disaster, and who could view its destiny to be nothing more than decay. This was a traumatic realization, and with that realization, definable human existence was born.

If trauma is sufficiently intense, and if it cannot be dealt with adequately in any other way, then the inevitable human response is hysteria. Religion, Freud contended, was the coping mechanism, the human response to the trauma of self-consciousness, and it was designed above all else to keep hysteria under control and to manage for these self-consciousness creatures the shock of existence.

3. Carl Jung (1875-1961)

Jung saw the Christian religion also as part of a historic process necessary for the development of consciousness, but only a fading shadow of religion remained available to the Western world.

4. Albert Einstein (1879-1955)

Einstein established both time and space by seeing them not as external properties, but as significant related aspects of existence. He also introduced relativity as something present in all things, including that which religious human beings had once called "eternal and unchanging truth." The God content of the past no longer sustains the contemporary spirit. There is an increasing sense even among believers that the word God now rings with a hallow emptiness.

5. There was no fall into sin – Bishop Spong writes:

"To ascribe goodness to creation implies that the work of creation is complete. Darwin, however, made us aware that the creation is even now not finished. Galaxies are still being formed. Human life is also still evolving. Suddenly the whole mythological framework in which and by which the Christ figure had been captured came tumbling down. What is sin? It is not and never can be alienation from the perfection for which God in the act of creation had intended us, for there is no such thing as a perfect creation. Thus, there was no fall into sin. Yet there is a sense in which all human beings are still caught in the struggle to become our deepest and truest self. We human beings have emerged slowly but surely out of the evolutionary soup of billions of years. We were not created in God's image in any literal way. We simple evolved out of lower forms of life and ultimately developed a higher consciousness. The purpose of creation was not necessarily fulfilled in the arrival of human life, for human life, as we know it, did not enter history until very recently.

There is also ample reason today to believe that the species of life known as Homo sapiens is not eternal. We have fouled our environmental nest so thoroughly, we have overpopulated our world so irresponsibly, we have developed weapons of mass destruction so totally that human survival faces, at best, long odds. We human beings appear to be incidental, both to the past life and to the future life of this planet. Life seems quite capable of going on with or without human participation."

6. Crucifixion, Resurrection and Ascension

The **crucifixion** of Jesus occurred in the 1st century Judea, most likely in AD 30 or AD 33. Pontius Pilate served as prefect of Judea from 26-36 AD. He convicted Jesus of treason as Jesus had declared himself King of the Jews and the Son of God.

As we will discover when human beings are united with God we become 'one spirit with Him.' It was Paul's radical idea (1 Cor 2:10) that in Jesus, God and human life were now seen to flow together. In the being of Jesus we see a revelation of the Ground of Being. (One Mind)

Transcendence stands for the inexhaustible depths of the divine once the contact is made. Human life is capable of entering the infinity of God because the infinity of God can be found in the heart of every human life. "I am the way, the truth and the life" (John 14:6)

It is my belief that this Ground of Being (One Mind) will be recognized apart from any system of religious thought. Bishop Spong's own teacher Paul Tillich, states there is no imploring an external theistic power to serve our needs. One rather experiences a growing awareness of the Ground of Being and of ones relationship with all those who also share that infinite and inexhaustible ground - "the eternal now." The God of church, synagogue, and mosque is no more. The God who is the Ground of Being cannot be owned by any theistic religion. God is a universal presence undergirding all life. The age of faith is no more. Post modern people can now experience and know the Ground of all Being (One Mind).

Resurrection is an action of God. Jesus was raised into the meaning of God. It therefore cannot be a physical resuscitation occurring inside human history.

Ascension - the story of ascension assumed a three tiered universe and is therefore not capable of being translated into the concepts of a post-Copernican age.

It is important to recognize that all three theistic religions have an 'esoteric tradition' (intended for or likely to be understood by only a small number of people with a specialized knowledge or interest). Just like in **Christianity** the true message of Jesus was that the Ground of all Being (God or One Mind) can flourish in each of us. I briefly discuss how One Mind manifests in a similar manner in Islam and Judaism.

7. Theological Pessimism

As mentioned half the population on the planet are thought to be Christian. Many of this community believe in prophecies such as Damnation, the Rapture, Armageddon and the Apocalypse which engenders a lot of theological pessimism. In most forms of Western Christian belief **Damnation** to hell is what humanity deserves for its sins. The **Rapture** believes the transporting of believers to heaven at the Second Coming of Christ – "people will be raptured from automobiles as they are driving along and float up to heaven". **Armageddon** is the prophesied location of a gathering of armies for a battle between good and evil at the end times while the **Apocalypse** is the complete and final destruction of the world, as described in the biblical book of Revelation - "the bells ringing" are supposed to usher in the Apocalypse. Can we seriously believe in these prophecies in the 21st Century?

How can we resuscitate Optimism in our world today? And why is this important for us?

Optimism is hopefulness and confidence about the future or the successful outcome of something – the exact opposite of pessimism.

This is of vital importance to our health and longevity. We know that perceptions not only control behavior, they control gene activity as well – part of the new science of epigenetics.

An interesting study was done in a nursing home back in the 1970's. One half of a group of patients were given a pot-plant (a small ivy plant) and were instructed to water and care for the plant - the other half continued their usual day to day activities in the nursing home. At the end of 18 months there was a 50% decrease in mortality in those who were looking after the pot-plant.

My friend and colleague Richard Rahe and Thomas Holmes co-created the Social Readjustment Scale that listed the different life stressors people experienced during life. The most stressful event was the death of a spouse. The remaining spouses mortality is 10 times higher then other aged married couples. Let me also remind you that 30-50% of medical treatment (whether from drugs or surgery is due to the placebo effect –these three examples is why Optimism is essential in our lives.

Islam

I would like to give a brief account of Mansour Hallaj and Imadaddin Nasimi who both recognized One Mind and met a similar fate to that of Jesus. As I will show there are many people over the two thousand years who have recognized the reality of One Mind. (See Table on page 322)

Socrates, one of the most pivotal figures in all of Western Culture, was executed by the Athenian court in 399 BC on false charges of impiety and corrupting the youth. The real reason was that he had made many enemies over the years due to his criticism of prominent Athenian politicians and his refusal to acknowledge the Olympian Gods. He was forced to drink Hemlock, a poison reserved for philosophers and desenters; Politics, dogma, control have been with us for over 2,500 years.

Mansour Hallaj (858-922)

A Persian mystic, poet and teacher of Sufism was born in Iran in 858. He is best known for his saying "I am the truth" which many saw as a claim to divinity, while others interpreted it as the diminution of his ego, allowing God to speak through him. He was executed after a long period of confinement on religious and political charges by the Abbasid court in Iraq on March 26,922. He later became a major figure in the Sufi tradition. Sufism is the Islamic belief and practice in which Muslims seek to find the truth of divine love and knowledge through direct personal experience of God and to facilitate the experience of the presence of divine love and wisdom in the world.

His last words were "all that matters for the ecstatic is that the Unique should reduce him to Unity" and he cited Quaranic Verse 42:18 - "Those who do not believe in it seek to hasten it, but the believers stand in awe of it. They know it to be the Truth, those who argue about the Hour are far, far astray."

Imadaddin Nasimi (1369-1417)

An early Persians poet and mystic, believed to have come from Nesim near Baghdad. (Nasimi often known as Nesimi). Nesimi was either of Azerbaijan or Turkish descent. Turkish was as familiar to him as Persian, for he wrote in both languages. Arabic poems are also ascribed to him.

From his poetry, it's evident that Nesimi was an adherent of the Hurufi movement, which was founded by Nesimi's teacher Fazlullah Astarabadi of Astarabad, who was condemned for heresy and executed in Alinja near Nakhchivan. The center of Fazlullah influence was Baku and most of his followers came from Shirvan (present-day Republic of Azerbaijan), then ruled by the Shirvanshahs.

His work consists of two collections of poems, one of which is in Persian and the other in Turkish. One of Nesimi's most famous poems is the 'gazel' with the following:

"Both worlds can fit within me, but in this world I cannot fit I am the placeless essence, but into existence I cannot fit."

The poem serves as an excellent example of Nesimi's poetic brand of Hurufi's mystical form. There is a contrast made between the physical and the spiritual which are seen to be ultimately united in the human being. As such, the human being is seen to partake of the same spiritual essence of God: the phrase la-me-kah or "the placeless," in the second line is a Sufi term used for God. The same term however, can be taken literally as meaning ""without a place," and so Nesimi is also using the term to refer to human physicality. In his poem, Nesimi stresses that understanding God is ultimately not possible in this world, though it is nonetheless the duty of human beings to strive for such an understanding. Moreover, as the poem's constant play with the ideas of the physical and the spiritual underlines. Nesimi calls for this search for understanding to be carried out by people within their own selves.

Interestingly, in the Middle Ages Nasimi was widely popular among Armenians to such an extent that some Armenian sources speak of him as a poet who "accepted Christianity." Researcher Miraly Seyidov explains this by the fact that Nasimi didn't attach importance to difference between religions, judging people not by religious affiliation, but by spiritual qualities: whether he's a Christian or a Muslim, a person is already valuable because he/she is a person.

Nesimi became one of the most influential advocates of the Hurufi doctrine and the movement's ideas where spread to a large extent through his poetry. While Fazlullah believed that he himself was the manifestation of God for Nesimi at the center of Creation there was God, who bestowed His light on man. Through sacrifice and self-perfection, man can become one with God. Around 1417, as a direct result of his beliefs – which were considered blasphemous by contemporary religious authorities – Nesimi was seized and according to most accounts, skinned alive in Aleppo.

Judaism

The esoteric understanding of Judaism is the Kabbalah. The literal translation of the word **Kabbalah** is 'that which is received.' To receive we must be receptive. We must open ourselves, creating a vessel in which to absorb that which we wish to understand or grasp, and in turn become part of Kabbalah. To open the self to a higher reality, to view the spirit within the matter, to raise our consciousness to the point where our perception of reality is completely changed, and the divine within all creation is revealed.

Kabbalah has always been essentially an oral tradition in that initiation into its doctrines and practices is conducted by a personal guide to avoid the dangers inherent in mystical experiences. Esoteric Kabbalah is also "tradition" in as much as it lays claim to secret knowledge of the unwritten Torah (divine revelation) that was communicated by God to Moses and Adam. Though observance of the Law of Moses remained the basic tenet of Judaism, Kabbalah provided a means of approaching God directly. It thus gave Judaism a religious dimension whose mystical approaches to God were viewed by some as dangerously pantheistic and heretical.

Zohar (The Book of Radiance) is perhaps the most important book in Kabbalah – it was composed in Spain in the 13th century and covers the first five books of the bible (Torah) - A 1,900 page text in Aramaic (ancient Hebrew).

Margot Pritzker (her family owns Hilton Hotels) approached Daniel Matt from Berkley to translate the Zohar. It took Matt nearly two decades to translate and is published in 12 volumes. As Matt says, Religious faith is all about repairing the world, not enforcing dogma. The Zohar's final volume arrives at a time when world religion seems increasingly removed from the kind of private, contemplative spirituality evoked by the Zohar (the last three volumes were translated by Nathan Wolski and Joel Hecker).

The Islamic State militant group posts beheadings on YouTube, American evangelicals forsake their Christian convictions for short-term political gains, Jewish settlers in the West Bank take land away from their Palestinian neighbors. In India earlier this spring, Hindus killed a Muslim man who was transporting cows, an animal considered sacred in Hinduism. Whoever your god or gods are, they cannot have had this in mind.

In an age of extremism, Matt's work is a rejoinder that calls for humility, patience and wonderment. This has long been an animating theme. "We have lost our "truth" Matt wrote in his 1996 book, *God & the Big Bang: Discovering Harmony Between Science & Spirituality.*" Many people have shed the security of traditional belief...If they believe in anything, perhaps it's science and technology. And what does science provide in exchange for this belief? Progress in every field except for one: the ultimate meaning of life."

Kabbalah is a spiritual wisdom, it sits diametrically opposed to religion. Kabbalah is original spiritual teaching before religion was on the scene. Its where all monotheistic religions have common ground (One Mind).

Ecological Spirituality

Finally, we also need a reassessment of what Genesis meant when it tells humankind "to subdue the earth and have dominion over all living things on it." In the past, there was no capacity to inflict lasting damage on the balance of nature. During the past century we have found ways in manipulating the very forces that shape nature – gravity, the atom, the gene. The extent of earthly changes – depletion of the ozone, deforestation, global warming, contamination from the toxic chemicals and nuclear waste, the extinction of many species – the masters of a pliant earth – we need to move away from this wanton destruction towards a caring stewardship and a reverence for all life acknowledging the One Mind.

Systems thinking is a general worldview concerning the nature of reality. A systems view of life is an ecological view that is grounded, ultimately, in spiritual awareness. Connectedness, relationship and community are fundamental concepts of ecology: and connectedness, relationship and belonging are the essence of spiritual experience.

In Thinking in Systems: A primer by Donella (Dana) Meadows she does not explicitly address spirituality but provides a careful look at the nature of caring in relationship to systems thinking: -

"Living successfully in a world of complex systems means expanding not only time horizons and thought horizons; above all, it means expanding the horizons of caring. There are moral reasons for doing that of course. And if moral arguments are not sufficient, then systems thinking provides the practical reasons to back up the moral ones...No part of the human race is separate either from other human beings or from the global ecosystem. In a 1993 speech, Meadows made a beautiful statement about her vision for a better world: -

"I call the transformed world toward which we can move 'sustainable,' by which I mean a great deal more than a world that merely sustains itself unchanged. I mean a world that evolves, as life on earth has evolved for three billion years, toward ever great diversity, elegance, beauty, self-awareness, interrelationship, and spiritual realization." ("Beyond the Limits," speech given in Spain, Fall 1993)

I believe in addition to nature we can find the connectedness, relationship and belonging with stories, art and literature – we can appreciate One Mind (God) in all things if we remain open and receptive. The understanding of the psycho-historical development of the 'Structures of Consciousness' is an important context for all of us in the post-modern world that can help us recognize One Mind.

CHAPTER 19. THE STRUCTURES OF CONSCIOUSNESS

In The Great Chain of Being by Arthur Lovejoy he writes the following: -

"Any unit-idea which the historian thus isolates he next seeks to trace through more than one – ultimately, indeed, through all – of the provinces of history in which it figures in any important degree, whether those provinces are called philosophy, science, literature, art, religion or politics. The postulate of such a study is that the working of a given conception, of an explicit or tacit presupposition, of a type of mental habit, or of a specific thesis or argument, needs, if its nature and its historic role are to be fully understood, to be traced connectedly through all the phases of men's reflective life which those workings manifest themselves, or through as many of them as the historian's resources permit."

Without some knowledge of the past, a man or woman cannot be fully human, he or she cannot be truly a person at home in the world.

Human knowledge is growing exponentially – in fact, it is now believed to be doubling every two years. This fact has important implications for all of us. In order to make sense of the vast amount of information coming our way, it is essential to have a context that organizes this information to help order our consciousness and worldview. Historians, psychologists, philosophers, and others have all independently recognized that the mounting crisis for Western civilization is in fact the beginning of a fundamental restructuring of consciousness.

One of the primary ways that humans provide meaning is by telling stories. Joseph Campbell, author of *The Hero with a Thousand Faces* and many other books on mythology, spent his life uncovering the essential stories (myths) that humankind has used to inform their worldview and their actions. Campbell often wondered what the "new story" would be for us in the twenty-first century that would provide us with meaning and a sense of wholeness. I believe that art and literature together with our stories will lead us to One Mind. This is the "new story." We can best accomplish this by understanding the 5 structures of consciousness described by Jean Gebser in his book The Ever Present Origin (1943).

Gebser in the Preface of his Ever Present Origin also provides a chilling warning of this coming global catastrophe.

"We must soberly face the fact that only a few decades separate us from that event. This span of time is determined by an increase in technological feasibility inversely proportional to man's sense of responsibility – that is, unless a new factor were to emerge which would effectively overcome this menacing correlation.

It is the task of the present work to point out and give an account of this new factor, this new possibility. For if we are not successful – if we should not or cannot successfully survive this crisis by our own insight and assure the continuity of our earth and mankind in the short or the long run by a transformation (or a mutation) of consciousness then the crisis will outlive us.

Humanity has evolved from simple consciousness to self-consciousness and is now ready for its next major transition, from self-consciousness to integral consciousness. Integral consciousness is an emergent psycho-historical development. The is the 'new factor' that Gebser believes can help man overcome our current crisis. We live today in what Gebser terms the perspectival era. Priort to this, there was the unperspectival era, consisting of archaic, magical and mythical periods. Gebser clearly articulates the new era now dawning for humanity beyond these four – the aperspectival era and integral consciousness (One Mind) as Gebser states somewhat differently, if we do not overcome the crisis it will overcome us; and only someone who has overcome himself is truly able to overcome. Either we will be disintegrated and dispersed, or we must resolve and effect integrality, in other words, either time is fulfilled in us – and that would mean the end and death of our present earth and (it's) mankind – or we succeed in fulfilling time: and this means integrality and the present, the realization and the reality of origin and presence.

According to Gebser it is the irruption of time into our consciousness that helps transform us from the mental (perspectival era) into our integral (aperspectival era) consciousness. It is a matter of our recognizing time as a quality and intensity, rather than an analytical system and it's perverted form of past, present and future in the perspectival era."

The story of the Cosmos 13-15 billion years ago and the story of the Earth, about 5 billion years ago, I will not discuss here. Rather I will focus on the human story which began about 5 million years ago.

Life on earth is believed to have begun in its most primitive form from 3.7 billion years ago. Here we find a vast empty space where the only living things are bacteria and other single cell organisms that can grow and divide without oxygen (these organisms thrived on hydrogen sulfide).

450 million years ago plants were the only multicellular life forms on earth – they were responsible for the oxygen that replaced the earlier atmosphere of hydrogen sulfide that caused many of the bacteria to hop inside cells of organisms to escape the oxygen. These organisms made a deal to provide food and energy in exchange for a safe home – these engulfed bugs (mitochondria) are the main source of energy for us. About 350 million years ago insects showed up and began eating the plants – plants responded by developing powerful defenses to protect themselves, for example, proteins called lectins.

Fast forward to about 40 million years ago when our early ancestors lived in the trees, where according to Steven Gundry MD, we ate tree leaves and other two-leafed plants (dicots) along with the fruit of those plants. Grazing animals in contrast ate single leaf plants (monocots) such as grasses and their seeds. Our intestines and out gut bacteria within evolved very differently from those grazers and we were able to tolerate the respective plant compounds including lectins.

About 10,000 years ago with the advent of farming all this changed. That's where we began to cultivate grains and other single-leafed plants for the first time since homo habilis (tool making man) two million years ago. Over the last 50 years things have gotten a lot worse with drugs, GMO and processed foods together with pesticides, herbicides, glyphosate, high sugar diets, artificial sweeteners etc. (See Optimizing Men's Health and Longevity (2021). Suffice is to say, that many researches today believe that due to the alteration in our microbiome most of the population have some degree of dysbiosis and leaky gut that may be the primary driver of inflammation and the epidemic of chronic disease we see today.

Life is possible only because the universe is developing in the precise fashion it is. Life demands awareness and it is life that gives rise to consciousness. Here, we will focus on the human story of consciousness.

The details of the evolution of human consciousness, through the five distinct periods are well described by Jean Gebser in his 1943 book *The Ever Present Origin* to which the reader can refer for a more in depth analysis. The following summary of the aforementioned periods is sufficient for our purpose. When reading these summaries, be cognizant that these same stages must be integrated as phases in our own psychological growth. Of central importance for this ordering of consciousness and emergent sense of well-being is *anamnesis,* or the remembering of both our own personal and collective (as a species) psychohistorical development (ontogeny recapitulates phylogeny).

THE STRUCTURES OF CONSCIOUSNESS

Era	Time	Sense Organ	Awareness	Culture	Social	Spirit
Archaic	5 million – 200,000 B.C.	Body-kinesthetic	Visceral	Latent: Egoless	Nomadic hunters	Participation mystique
Magical	200,000 – 10,000 B.C.	Ear	Emotional	Music/Dance; Egoless	Hunter-gatherers	Ritual
Mythical	10,000 – 2,000 B.C.	Mouth	Imagination	Myth; Egoless	Farming; Language	Gods/ symbols
Mental	2,000 B.C. – present	Eye	Reflection; Recognition	Science Art; Egocentric	Industry; Fear/ alienation; Knowledge	God/ dogma
Integral	Future	Meta-sense	Individuation; Concretion/ Verition	Integral Art; Science; Ego-free	Love/ Wholeness; Wisdom	Overself/ Transcendent One Mind

Modified from: Gebser, J. *The Ever Present Origin.* Ohio University Press, 1985. (English Translation)

Archaic Human (5 million to 200,000 B.C.)

Homo habilis ("handy man") appeared about 2 million years ago and had a brain about half the size of our modern brains. The sense organ that predominated in Homo habilis was the body-kinesthetic sense. Although Homo habilis had not developed language, Protolanguage may have started to develop around the fire at night during this period. Homo habilis did, however, develop the ability to make stone tools. This archaic human, although advanced beyond all prior evolutionary stages, was still undifferentiated from the surrounding world and had no sense of self. Thus, Homo habilis did not possess existential fear.

It is believed that our human ancestors learned to control fire toward the end of the Homo habilis epoch or shortly thereafter (approximately 1.4 to 1.8 million years ago). This newfound tool was likely used to begin exploring the environment and in overcoming the continuous problems of locating food and shelter.

What follows is a series of 'art objects' which will help you get a sense of the 5 structures of consciousness that have developed over time and that are also co-present in each of us.

STRUCTURE	SPACE/TIME RELATIONSHIP			SIGN
	DIMENSION	PERSPECTIVE	TIME	
Archaic	Zero-dimensional	None	Prespatial Pretemporal	None
Magical	One-dimensional	Pre-Perspectival	Spaceless Timeless	Point
Mythical	Two-dimensional	Unperspectival	Spaceless Natural Temporicity (Cyclical)	Circle
Mental	Three-dimensional	Perspectival	Spatial Abstractly Temporal (Linear)	Triangle
Integral	Four-dimensional	Aperspectival	Space-free Time-free One Mind	Sphere

I have also included the video found earlier on page 31 I made 20 years ago that will give you a more dynamic view of these structures of consciousness from several film clips.

ARCHAIC STRUCTURE OF CONSCIOUSNESS

SPACE AND TIME RELATIONSHIP			
DIMENSION	PERSPECTIVE	TIME	SYMBOL
Zero	None	Prespatial Pretemporal	None

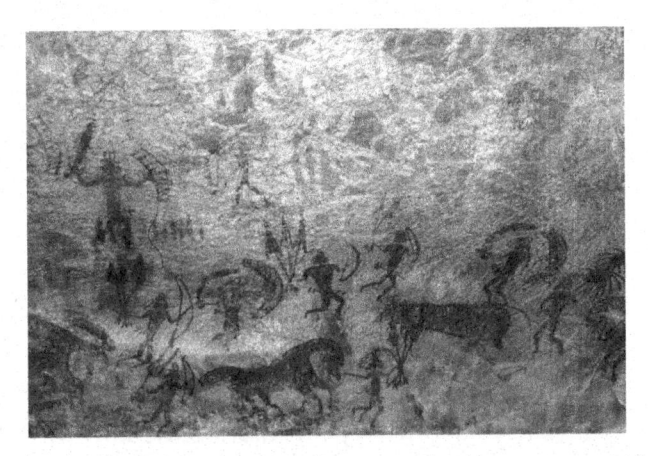

Rock Art from Bhimbetka, India (250,000 BCE)

The oldest known prehistoric art is the series of petroglyphs discovered during the 1990's in two ancient caves in India.

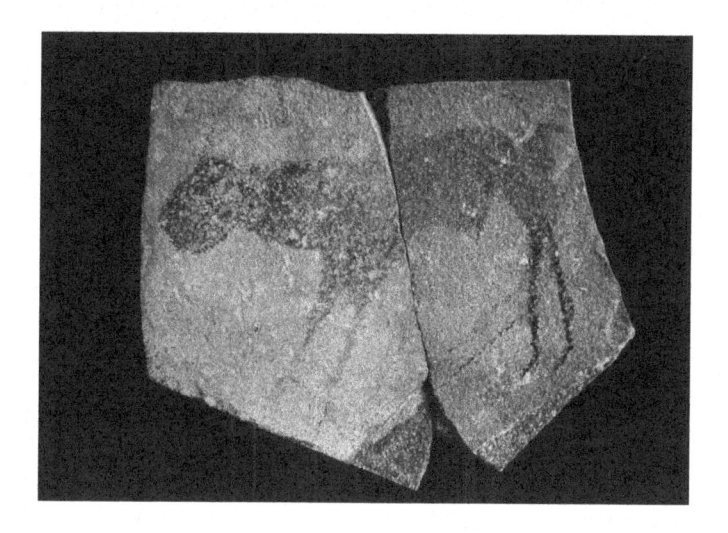

Rock Art from S-W Namibia, Africa

(35,000 years ago)

The oldest known African rock art discovered in the Apollo 11 cave in the Huns Mountains in Namibia. (the discovery occurred at the same time as the Apollo 11 mission to the moon-hence the name of the caves).

Magical Human (200,000 – 10,000 B.C.)

By 45,000 years ago, humans had spread over most of Africa, Europe and Asia and numbered about 1 million. During this period, these hunter-gatherers increased in population and sophistication. They began to use more advanced tools and developed mime and ritual. The voluntary expressive use of the face and voice to transmit emotion began in this mimetic-magical period but advanced significantly in the mythical period with the development of the larynx and the modern vocal apparatus. The magical human begins to awaken to an awareness and knowledge of personal finiteness and vulnerability.

Magical man's reality is at first a system of associations, individual objects, events, deeds, separated from one another like points in the overall unity. In a sense one may say that in this structure consciousness was not yet in man himself, but still resting in the world. Impulse and instinct unfold with a vital consciousness which enabled man, despite his egolessness, to cope with the earth and the world as a group – ego sustained by the clan.

All magic, even today, occurs in the natural vital, egoless, spaceless and timeless sphere. Insight into these realities helps clarify what parapsychology is trying to study – they can become consciously known only if modern man, despite his rational and logical attitude, realizes the power of spacelessness and timelessness and, with that realization, accomplishes what magical man was not able to do because he was still remote from consciousness and deeply emersed in this egoless, timeless, spaceless world of unconscious unity.

The group, beginning to grow dimly conscious of itself as a unity (the group-ego), begins to free itself from its merger with nature, breaking its spell – whoever wishes to prevail over the earth must liberate himself from its power. The ear is the predominant sense of the magical human.

MAGICAL STRUCTURE OF CONSCIOUSNESS

SPACE AND TIME RELATIONSHIP			
DIMENSION	PERSPECTIVE	TIME	SYMBOL
One-dimensional	Pre-Perspectival	Spaceless Timeless	Point

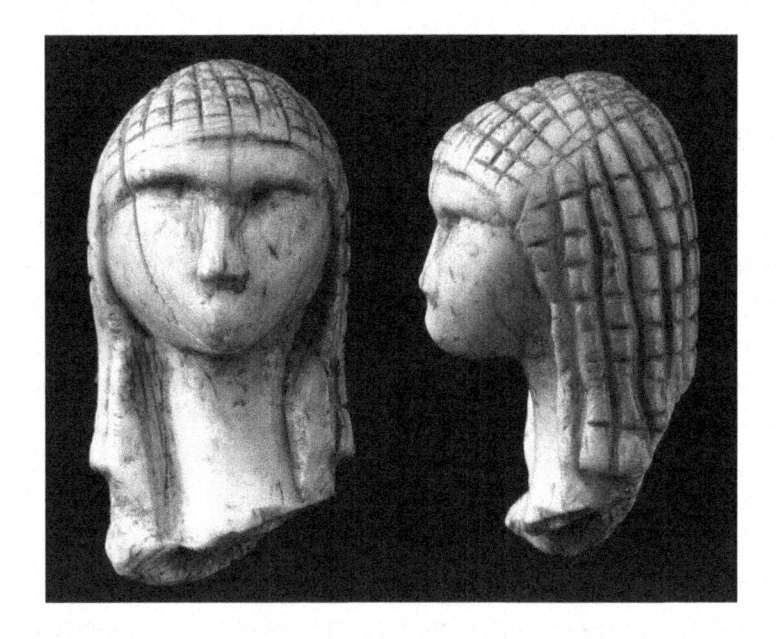

Sculpture Brassempouy, France (23,000 BCE)

Notice: The absence of the mouth. There is no ego. Magical man is in a sleep-like consciousness and merged unity.

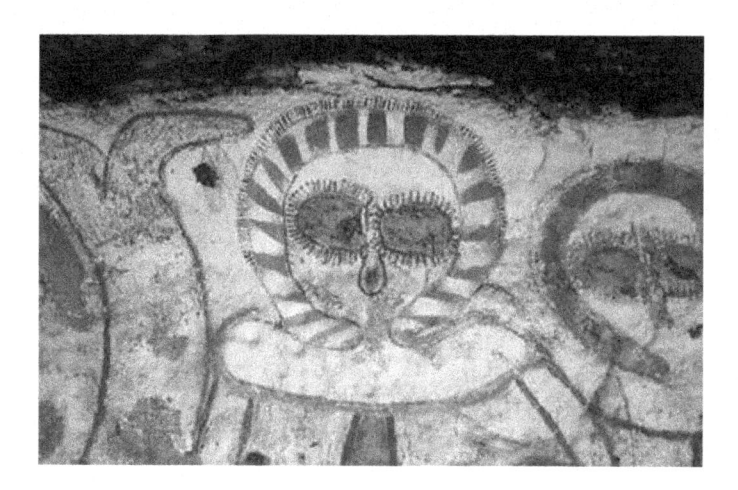

Painting Kimberley, Australia (3,500 BCE)

Again paintings do not emphasize the mouth of the Magical Man. The merging of man with nature with its spaceless/timeless character endowed magical man with telepathy and clairvoyance. This is explained in part by the elimination of consciousness that allows magical man an "unconscious participation" in the group soul (similar to non-locality seen in fish, birds and insects).

The Prince with the Crown of Feathers, Knossos, Crete (500 BC)

Man is extricating himself from the nature bound magical structure standing out in partial relief from the background, his torso against the "sky" simultaneous with the soul. Man's first awareness of mythical consciousness.

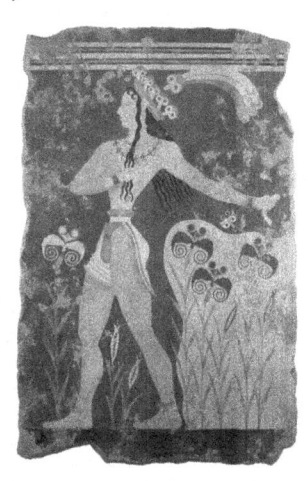

Mythical Human (10,000 – 2,000 B.C.)

The Neolithic age (New Stone Age) began about 10,000 years ago. Neolithic people differentiated themselves from all previous humans by settling in permanent villages. This was the result of two important developments: the growth of agriculture and the later domestication of several kinds of animals. By 8,000 B.C., most of the major institutions of humankind were established. Language is the hallmark of the mythical human, although it is unclear how rapidly speech developed and spread. The most elevated use of language in tribal societies is that of mythic invention, the myth being the prototypical integrative mind tool. The mouth is the dominant sense organ of this mythical human.

Mythic culture tends toward the rapid integration of knowledge. Myth governs the collective mind and a sense of "we" membership prevails. The mythic human was still egoless, lived in a dream state, and used speech to tell stories that explain reality. Language allowed for the integration of knowledge, symbols, imagination, ideals, morality and belief systems into Mythic Culture, which in turn expanded individual and collective consciousness. With this expanded consciousness and the ability to more clearly picture the future, humankind needed to see this unfolding future as a promise that death was in the distance.

MYTHICAL STRUCTURE OF CONSCIOUSNESS

SPACE AND TIME RELATIONSHIP			
DIMENSION	PERSPECTIVE	TIME	SYMBOL
Two-dimensional	Unperspectival	Spaceless Natural Temporicity (Cyclical)	O

Mythic Man's development of Agriculture was a two edged sword however – On the one hand it provided a more stable food supply and moved our hunter-gatherer ancestors into towns and cities increasing population growth. On the other hand it was the beginning of the modern Western diet that kills 80% of us today.

The Muse, Greece (5th Century BCE)

Ever since Homer the muse has been invoked to begin epic songs in which mythic events have their formation in language. In the magical period there is no myth (mouth is related to mythos speech Gk). The mythical structure leads to the emergent awareness of the soul presented by the sea. This structure bears the stamp of the imagination rather than the emotion of magical man dominated by impulse and instinct. Slowly the timelessness of magical man gradually transitions to the circular periodicity of mythical time.

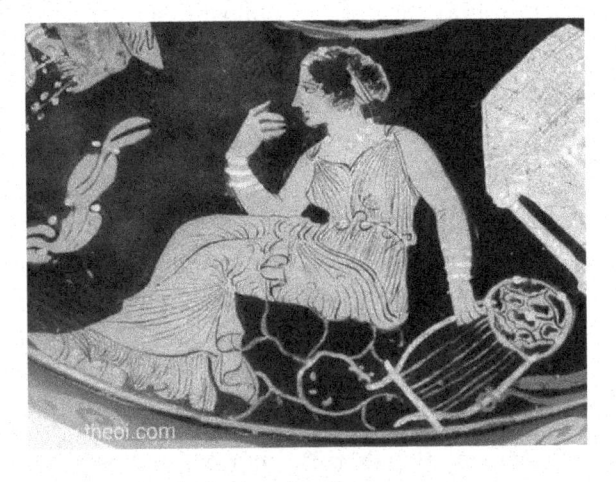

The mythic imaginatory consciousness alternates between the magical timelessness and the dawning awareness of natural cosmic periodicity (cyclical time). The illumination of life coming from myth interpretation is akin to the successful dream interpretation of modern depth psychology.

These mythologemes begin to take shape as man becomes aware of his soul. They are the most visible signs of an emerging consciousness, which of course is also an emergence of the ego often depicted as a sea voyage – such a voyage is a symbol of mans gradual mastery over his soul.

Another significant motif appears at the same time in both east and west: wrath or anger – this is the force which bursts the confines of clan and community to the extent it manifests the "hero" in the individual and spurs him on toward further individuation, self-assertion and consequently ego emergence (examples are found in both the Bhagavadgita and the Iliad). Only in acting or being acted upon does man begin to sense his individuality. Only someone who has rescued himself can rescue others.

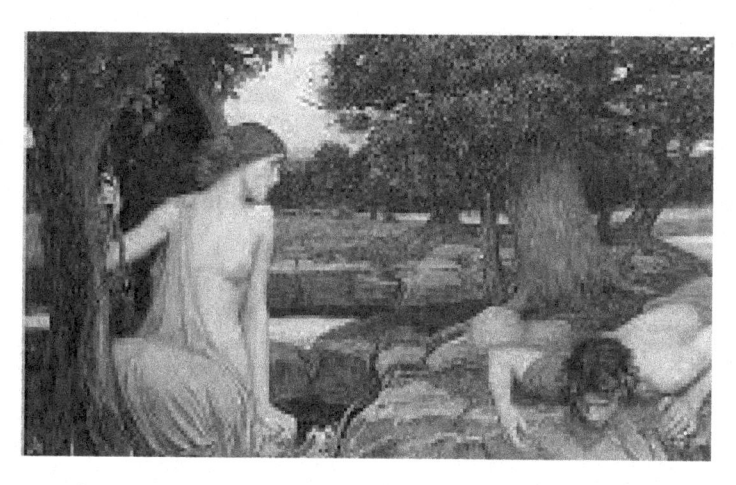

Narcissus – Painted by John William Waterhouse (1903)

The motif of the sea voyage and consciousness is found in all cultures. This same water aspect is also seen in the myth of Narcissus-the water-self symbolism is clear. To look into the mirror of the soul is to become conscious and to apprehend the soul is nothing less than to become conscious of the self.

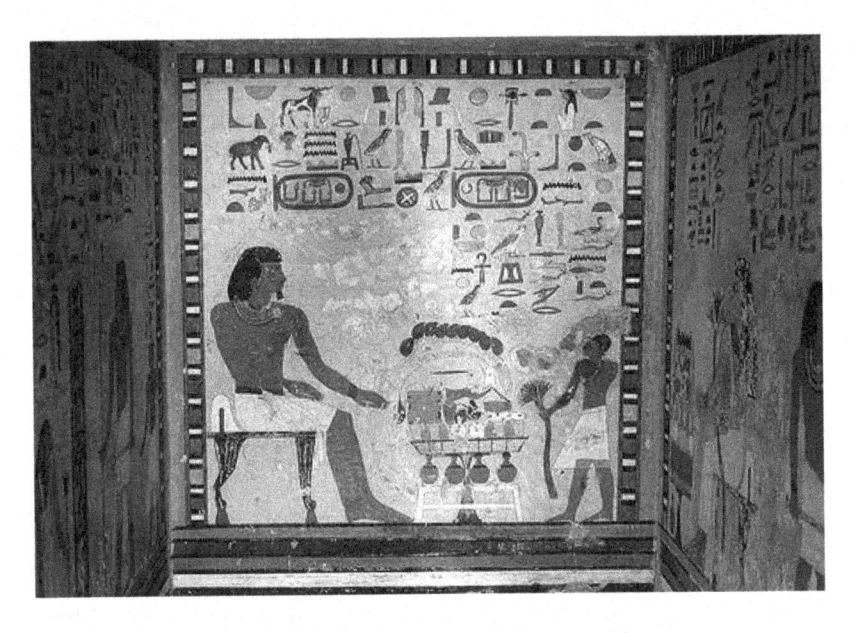

Tomb of Sarenput II Aswan, Egypt (4,500 BC)

The mythical structure shows an unperspectival 2D presentation. Although the Greeks and Romans had a prototypical perspective this did not develop fully until the 15th Century.

Mental Human (2,000 B.C. – present)

A subtle change occurred in our worldview as we moved from the earlier magical-mythical worldview, with its cyclical sense of time, toward our modern linear time. A new and heightened awareness and fear of death followed as a direct result of farming and language. Fear can only exist in linear time and stubbornly sits at the center of our modern worldview. (A great example of the Mythic structure bumping up against the Mental structure is shown in the video clip from "The Black Robe").

Early Mental Human (2,000 B.C. – A.D. 1500)

History, in the form of recorded events, began with the development of writing in this period. According to the ancient Greek scholar Bruno Shell in *The Discovery of Mind*, Homer's characters use their eyes to see or to receive optical impressions. However, they apparently took no interest in the objective essence of sight. There was no word for perspective – and as far as they were concerned it did not exist. Also the sea was port-wine-color. The color blue is only later able to be perceived. Likewise although heaven is mentioned several hundred times in the bible-the association with color blue is not.

The period of Western civilization following the collapse of the Roman Empire, from 500 to 1,500 A.D., is called the Middle or Dark Ages. As Darcy Ribeiro writes, "The history of man in these last centuries is principally the history of the expansion of Western Europe, which constituting the nucleus of a new civilization, proceeded to launch itself on all people in successive waves of violence and oppression. In this movement, the whole world was shaken up and rearranged according to European design and in conformity with European interests. Each people, even each human being, was affected and caught up in the European economic system or in the ideals of power, justice or politics inspired by it."

MENTAL STRUCTURE OF CONSCIOUSNESS

SPACE AND TIME RELATIONSHIP			
DIMENSION	PERSPECTIVE	TIME	SYMBOL
Three-dimensional	Perspectival	Spatial Abstractly Temporal (linear)	△

Late Mental Human (1,500 to present)

The beginning of the modern mental structure around 1,500 A.D. was the result of four major actions that changed the course of humankind:

- World exploration that began in the late 1400s

- The development of perspective and scientific inquiry

- The flow of inventions such as Gutenberg's movable type

- Industrial production, which began in earnest in the 1600s

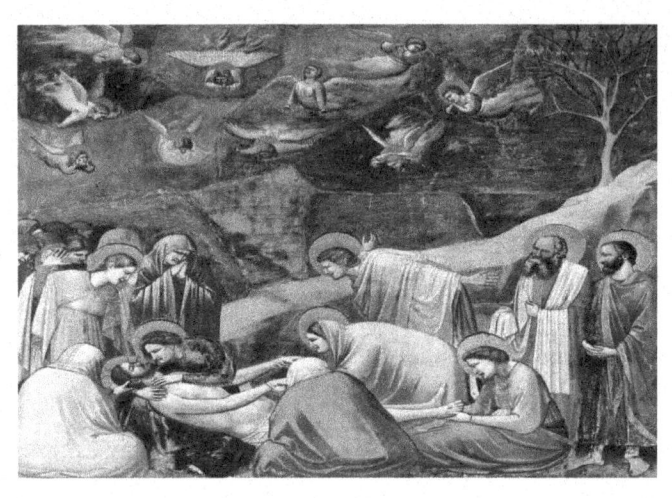

Giotto Lamentation (The Mourning of Christ (1,305 AD)

Giotto was one of the first to create a feeling of depth in his paintings by arranging his figures in relationship to each other and placing them against architectural backgrounds. This was completely revolutionary at the time and created an illusion of reality which enhanced the viewers understanding.

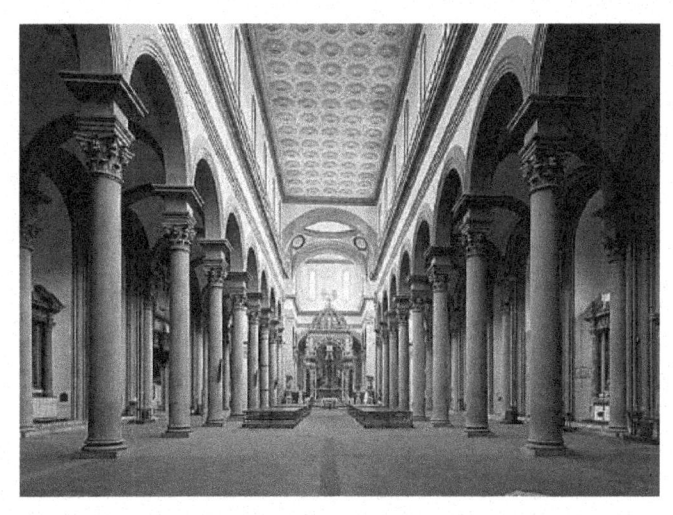

Filippo Brunelleschi Santo Spirito Florence, Italy (1436)

It was really Filippo Brunelleschi who developed perspective proper which made technical drafting possible which helped launch the industrial revolution.

(See video link: https://www.youtube.com/watch?v=bkNMM8uiMww for a great overview of the development of perspective)

The mental human relies on the eye for perceiving the world. This seeing and conceptualizing are commensurate with our mental reflective structure. How we see becomes an expression of our understanding of our world. Italian painter Giotto (circa 1267 to 1337) was the first artist of record to understand intuitively the benefits of painting a scene as if viewed from a stationary single point. The flat picture presentation, which was prevalent for a thousand years, acquired a third dimension of depth when Giotto's protoperspective placed the viewer in front of the canvas. As significant as Giotto was, Filippo Brunelleschi (1377-1446), an Italian architect, is credited with the true discovery of Western linear perspective.

Thus, in addition to the notion of linear time, the mental human is now faced with perspective and the conquering of space. Besides illuminating space, perspective lends humans a sense of their own visibility and provides a sense of distance between human and objects. The conception of the human as subject is based on the conception of world as object.

Early human's lack of spatial awareness is attended by a lack of ego. In order to objectify and qualify space, a self-conscious "I" is required that is able to stand opposite and confront space. Thus, from this time onward, humankind can be considered to have a self-consciousness rather than the simple consciousness of earlier periods. This is visible in a variety of ways: in the appearance of words expressing awareness and self-awareness in the Anglo-Saxon language, in the creation of the first novel, artists signing their works, and in the emergence of a free-floating anxiety and fear of death that so affects the modern man.

Integral Human (Our Future)

Near the close of the nineteenth century, another new appreciation of space and time emerged. Pablo Picasso (1881-1973) and Georges Braque (1882-1963) invented a new revolutionary art form called cubism at the turn of the century. Cubism, in fact, embodied the first new way to perceive space since the time of Euclid, the father of geometry, 2,200 years earlier: In the first decade of the Twentieth Century, Albert Einstein (1879-1955) overturned the foundations of classical physics with his theory of relativity, and physicists abandoned forever the notion of absolute space and time – the aperspectival worldview (space free and time free) had been born. A new "asperspectival" view is necessary for us if we are to look at the world and see it whole. Whereas the understanding of the mental structure depended on the concretion of space, our emerging INTEGRAL epoch depends on the concretion of time. Only where time emerges as pure present and is no longer divided into its three phases of past, present, and future will it be concrete.

INTEGRAL STRUCTURE OF CONSCIOUSNESS

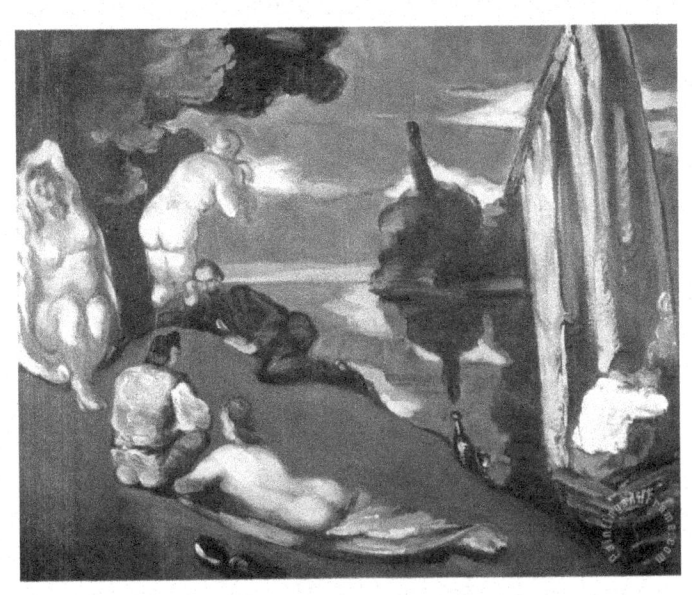

Paul Cezanne-Pastorale, France (1870)

Cezanne was the first painter to incorporate the work of art into the breadth of time. Space for Cezanne is a "continuum" – his visual field is "spherical." This aperspectival view occurred several decades before Einstein's proof and was completed toward the end of the 1880's by Van Gogh, Gaugin, Enzor and Monet. A mutation from the 3D into the 4D world.

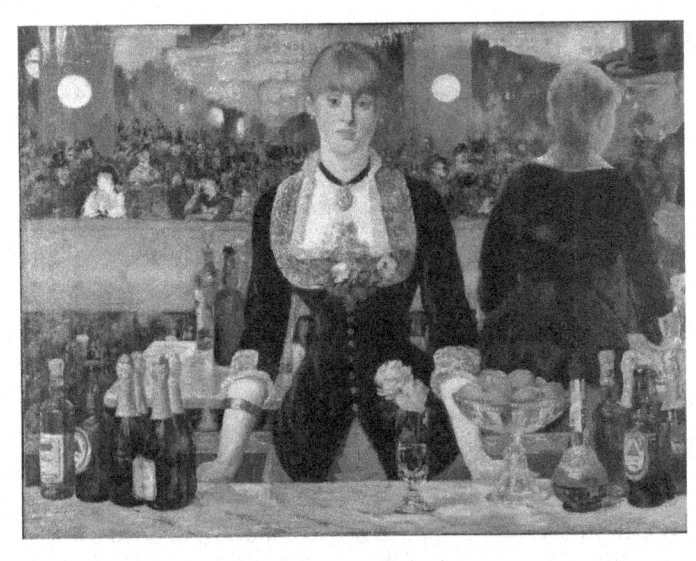

Edward Monet A Bar at the Folies Bergere France (1882)

Again the viewer here sees the reflection of the Barmaid off to the side which is an impossibility in our 3D world.

THE SUNFLOWERS, 1943

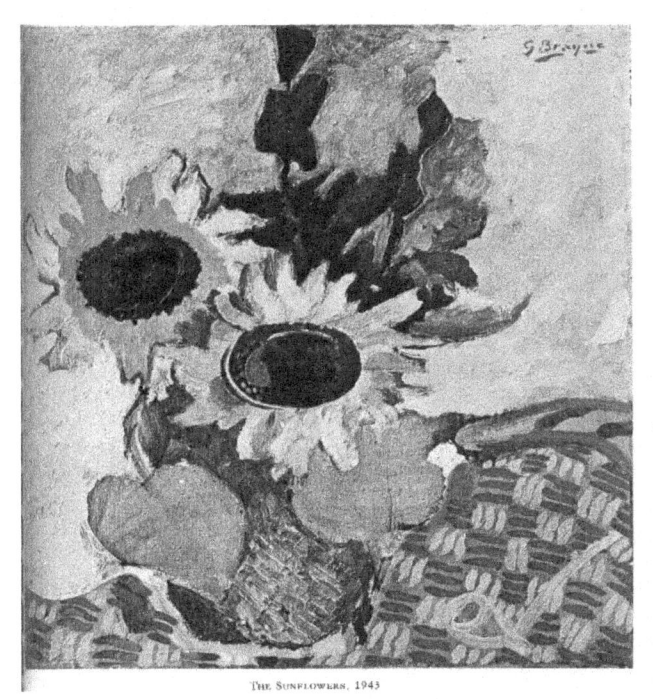

George Braque Sunflowers France (1946)

Another important cubist painting showing the predominance of curved lines clearly showing a spheroid pictorial surface of this "transparent" painting. The pictorial surface, for which the rectangular frame is inadequate, reaches into the frame which is exploded and dissolved by the pictorial structure.

We can see with this integral structure a change in how man sees himself in the world:-

MENTAL STRUCTURE (CURRENT)	INTEGRAL STRUCTURE (EMERGING)
Domination of Nature	Reverence for life
Ego fulfillment	Ego transcendence
Knowledge	Wisdom
Parts	Whole
Space fixity	Space Freedom
Obsession with time	Time Freedom
Lack of Meaning	Meaning
Boredom	Wonder
Unhappy	Happy (Joy)
Chronic Disease	Optimum Health
Isolated Minds	One Mind

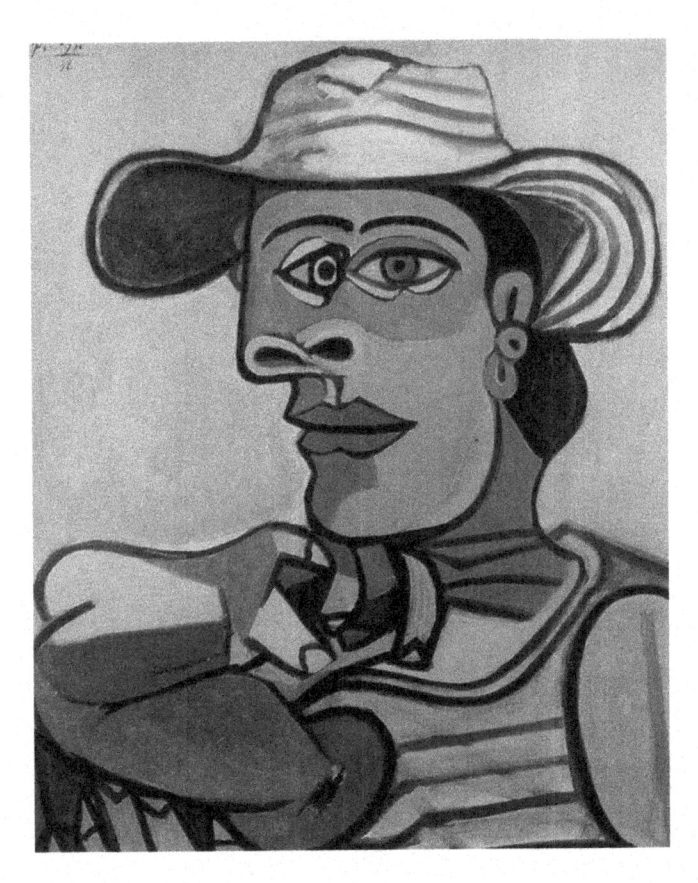

Pablo Picasso- The Sailor France (1938)

In this drawing space and time have become transparent. The "presentation" or making present evident in Picasso's painting was possible only after he was able to actualize ie bring to consciousness, all of the temporal structures of the past latent in himself (and each of us) during the course of his preceding 30 years of painting in a variety of styles. This process was unique and original with Picasso. By drawing on this primitive magic inheritance (his Negroid period), his mythical heritage (his Hellenistic-archaistic period), and his classicistic, rationally-accentuated formalist phase (his Ingres period), Picasso was able to achieve the concentration of time (or as we would like to designate this new style which he and his contemporaries introduced in painting "temporic concretion"). Such temporic concretion is not just a basic characteristic of this particular drawing, but is in fact generally valid: Only where time emerges as pure present and is no longer divided into its three phases of past, present and future, is it concrete.

CHAPTER 20: ONE MIND

Spirituality as a form of consciousness constructs the world as a systemic whole, where different parts are interconnected. Thus at the heart of spirituality lies systems thinking in one form or another. Systems thinking is a general view concerning the nature of reality – what we are, where we are going, how we know and what is of value.

As Gebser shows emergent evolution, both individual and social, would proceed beyond what we have in our current societies. Higher forms of consciousness would emerge as the relevant development requirements come into place: the overall mental and cultural evolution would not stop in the context of post-industrial consumer culture.

Larry Dossey coined the term "non-local mind" in his 1989 book Recovering the Soul to express what he believed is a spatially and temporally infinite aspect of our consciousness. Non-local mind resembled the age-old concept of the soul.

Erwin Schrodinger believed in the One Mind (as many others from very different walks of life have – See Table 1 below). As Schrodinger put it "Mind is by its very nature a "singulare tantum." I should say: the overall number of minds is just one." In his books such as My View of the World, What is Life and Mind and Matter, he painstakingly built a concept of a single mind, in which consciousness is transpersonal, universal, collective, and infinite in space and time, therefore immortal and eternal.

Examples of Different Individuals That Recognize One Mind

Christian Mystics	Theologens	Poets
Francis of Assisi (1185)	Teilhard de Chardin (1881)	William Blake (1757)
St. Theresa of Avila (1515)	Paul Tillich (1886)	Walt Whitman (1819)
St. John of the Cross (1542)	John Shelby Spong (1931)	Kahlil Gibran (1883)
Indian Mystics	**Muslim Mystics**	**Budhists**
Sri Aurobindo (1879)	Mansour Hallaj (858)	Gautama Buddha (463)
Raman Maharshi (1879)	Jalal Rumi (1207)	Tich Nhat Hanh (1926)
Yogananda (1893)	Imadaddin Nasimi (1369)	14th Dalai Lama (1935)
Philosophers	**Writers**	**Ecologists**
Franklin Merrell-Wolf (1887)	Ralph Waldo Emerson (1803)	Herbert Spencer (1820)
Paul Brunton (1898)	Henry David Thoreau (1817)	Rev. Joseph Tetlow (1930)
Jean Gebser (1905)	Herman Melville (1819)	Donella Meadows (1951)
Anthropologists	**Mathematicians**	**Artists**
Gregory Bateson (1906)	J.W.N. Sullivan (1886)	Paul Cezanne (1839)
Carlos Casteneda (1925)	Roger Penrose (1931)	Claude Monet (1840)
Richard Grossinger (1945)	Andreas Christiensen (1958)	Pablo Picasso (1881)
Biologists	**Astronomers**	**Psychologists**
Charles Darwin (1809)	John O'Keefe (1939)	Carl Jung (1875)
George Wald (1906)	Katherin Mahon (1941)	Abraham Maslow (1908)
Rupert Sheldrake (1942)	Ali Habibabad (1958)	Ken Wilber (1949)
Physicians	**Physicists**	
John Eccles (1903)	Henry Margenau (1901)	
Jonas Salk (1914)	John Wheeler (1911)	
Larry Dossey (1940)	David Bohm (1917)	
Astrophysicists	**Quantum Physicists**	
James Jeans (1877)	Albert Einstein (1879)	
Arthur Eddington (1882)	Erwin Schrodinger (1887)	
Fred Hoyle (1915)	Werner Heisenberg (1901)	

Schrodinger believed we are suffering from a consensus trance, a collective delusion, about the nature of consciousness. As he put it, "We have entirely taken to thinking of the personality of a human being... as located in the interior of the body. To learn that it cannot really be found there is so amazing that it meets with doubt and hesitation, we are very loath to admit it. We have got used to localizing the conscious personality inside a person's head – I should say an inch or two behind the midpoint of the eyes...It is very difficult for us to take stock of the fact that the localization of the personality, of the conscious mind, inside the body is only symbolic, just an aid for practical use."

Immortality for the mind was a key feature of Schrodinger's vision. He wrote, "I venture to call it (the mind) indestructible since it has a peculiar time-table, namely mind is always now. There is really no before and after for the mind. There is only now that includes memories and expectations...We may, or so I believe, assert that physical theory in its present stage strongly suggests the indestructibility of Mind by Time."

As Dossey writes: - *"The One Mind includes all individual minds. It includes thoughts, emotions, feelings, and cognition. The One Mind involves a vivid sense of connectedness and unity with all sentient life, and a profound sense of love, caring, and compassion. It is the over-arching principle that makes individual awareness possible."*

In other words, our mind is not confined to our brain or body, as we've been taught, but it extends infinitely outside them. Having no boundaries or limits, individual minds merge with all other minds to form the One Mind.

The One Mind is also a source of great wisdom and creativity, because it constitutes an infinite pool of information that we can learn to access, as many famous artists and scientists have done throughout history.

In what follows I will offer examples of how we can access One Mind and show evidence of One Mind in everyday life. As a physician I will conclude this essay demonstrating the place of One Mind in Medicine and show how people who tune in to the One Mind are more likely to be happier, healthier, more creative and wiser. This greater mind is boundless in time, therefore it is immortal and eternal. It is a cure for the greatest of all disease: the fear of total annihilation with physical death.

I too believe that their is an eternity that lies beyond the limits of my human finitude and in which I can participate in. I firmly believe that there is life after death. I believe and experience this transcending reality in the very heart of all life. I believe One Mind will finally be widely recognized and experienced apart from any religion.

Accessing One Mind

You already know the One Mind, but don't know that you know! We have forgotten this knowing and our goal is to remember and awaken to it. We just have to get out of the way so the realization comes through. This can happen in several ways.

- Some people are just born with this awareness – advanced souls who come into life knowing their larger connections.

- **Near Death Experiences (NDE's)** - unexpected events can pave the way. Over 20 million people in the USA have had NDE that often produce an unexpected knowing of how they fit in usually accompanied by a sense of joy, meaning and a new purpose in life.

- **Psychoactive Plants and Pharmaceuticals**

In many societies attempts have been made to fuse drug intoxication with God intoxication. Even in ancient Greece alcohol had its place in religion. The blissful experience of self-transcendence which alcohol makes possible has to be paid for and the price is exorbitantly high as we know today. Over the last century we have learnt about the ability of several psychoactive plants for example the Iboga root from Africa, the peyote cactus (mescaline) from Mexico and its use from writers like Carlos Casteneda and Aldous Huxley/ Mushrooms (Psilocybin) from writer Paul Stamets and LSD. John Lilly and Timothy Leary. Many individuals explaining these psychoactive methods are often searching for wholeness and a Universal identity – they are seeking One Mind. I am not advocating this method but acknowledge that an experience with these psychoactive drugs can open up one to the reality of transcendence even though not necessarily sustaining it.

A more recent Youtube video worth watching about mind beyond the brain by Graham Hancock and Rupert Sheldrake from March 3, 2022 can be found at https://tinyurl.com/2p8wy7w7

- **The Beauty of Nature** – spending time in nature often opens us up to what's really important in life and somehow resonates with that deeper part of ourselves. Many individuals have had an epiphany while immersed in nature.

- **Meditation and Contemplation**

- The One Mind favors preparation. Often this can be done while perfecting ones craft or technique.

- **Structures of Consciousness**

For most people (myself included) the realization of One Mind is not some dazzling or spectacular experience. You simply grow gradually into the realization of connectedness. It simply appears as a natural process, an awareness that is part of our psycho-historical evolution of staying alive and growing older and learning. It is here that our stories, great literature and art can help us become who we truely are best exemplified by Gebser's Structures of consciousness.

It is important to note that in all these processes they have one thing in common: the dominant sense of self, of ego, is transcended in favor of an expanded notion of who we are.

Before we can transcend the ego (self) you must develop and have one. Contrary to some Indian thought that encourages the suppression and "killing" of the ego to reach the One Mind. Paul Brunton feels that you must rather find the right relationship between your ego (self) and Over self (One Mind). This is similar to the Hindu understanding that Atman=Brahman ie the real self (soul) equals the omnipresent eternal self (One Mind) - the ultimate reality in the universe.

Franklin Merrell-Wolf in his book Philosophy of Consciousness Without An Object was convinced that the transcendent mode of consciousness could not be comprehended within the limits of our ordinary forms of knowledge. Rather it is a state wherein self-identity and the field of consciousness are blended into one indissoluble whole. This supplied the primary characteristic by which all common consciousness could be differentiated from the transcendent. The former is all of the type that may be called subject-object or relative consciousness – **consciousness without an object simply is** - this consciousness is considered original and then both subject and object becomes derivative.

Proof of One Mind

1. The recognition of One Mind is found in many religions and in different cultures:
- Zen – satori
- Yoga – samadhi
- Sufism – fana
- Hindu – tat tvam asi (thou art that)
- San Bushmen – there is "a dream dreaming us"
- Christianity – Christ Consciousness
- Taoism – Original Beginning

The experience of One Mind, however it is named involves a direct apprehension of the universe and all in it as being One. Everything is connected with everything else. Partition and separation are illusions. The experience carries with it the sense that one has apprehended Truth, the way things really are, accompanied by feelings of compassion and love. Each of us must have the courage to live and live fully to the best of our being. There are basically two types of evidence that support the idea of One Mind. One is empirical evidence which includes actual experiments. The other type of evidence is experiential and personal – the reports of thousands of individuals that affirm what the experiments are telling us. These two types of evidence reinforce each other.

I. Empirical Evidence for One Mind (Experimental)

1. Intercessory Prayer.

There are more than 40 major controlled clinical trials of distant intercessory prayer, around half of which show statistically significant results – far more than you would expect by chance.

Healing studies are also confirmed in nonhumans – plants, animals, microbes, even biochemical reactions-which show that the healing response in humans cannot possibly be attributed only to the placebo response or the power of positive thinking.

2. Presentiment Experiments

In the presentiment studies, a subject will be shown either a lovely, serene image or a violent, horrible image on a computer screen. If the violent image is going to be shown, then several seconds prior, the autonomic nervous system generates an exaggerated stress response before the randomized computer program has even selected which type of image will be shown. This is stunning evidence that we unconsciously sense the future. These results have been replicated by various scientists in dozens of studies.

3. Remote Viewing Experiments

In remote viewing studies, a distant individual is able to receive and record information that is mentally "sent" to them days before the information is sent or even selected by a randomized computer program.

Both type of experiments demonstrate the ability to know future information before it happens. These studies are important. They show that precognition, or premonitions, are not just "mere anecdotes," as skeptics charge.

The odds against a chance explanation in both cases are around a million against one.

4. Ganzfeld Experiments

A ganzfeld experiment is an assessment used by parapsychologists that they contend can test for extrasensory perception or telepathy. In these experiments, a "sender" attempts to mentally transmit an image to a "receiver" who is in a state of sensory deprivation.

5. Precognition

The definition includes the supernormal knowledge of future events, with emphasis not upon mentally causing events to occur but upon predicting those the occurrence of which the subject claims has already been determined.

In 2011, Daryl Bem published a report of nine experiments in the Journal of Personality and Social Psychology and showed precognition is scientifically valid. In 2016, Bem et al published another study of 90 experiments from 33 labs in 14 countries which yielded further positive data that exceeded "decisive evidence" in support of precognition.

6. Random Number Generator Influence

Robert Jahn, former Dean of Engineering at Princeton was well known for experiments on mind-machine interactions. In 1987, Jahn together with Brenda Dunne wrote "Margins of Reality" a result of the Princeton Engineering Anomalies Research Lab (PEAR) that Dunne ran.

Over several years, the PEAR lab built physical and electronic devices known as random event generators, designed to test whether people can influence the physical world with their thoughts. In one test, researchers dropped ball bearings through a series of channels and asked people to try to influence the outcome with their minds.

Jahn and Dunne reported in several books and numerous papers that the operators' intentions could affect results in what they said was a statistically significant deviation from chance. In other experiments, the lab reported that subjects acquired information about events with which they had no physical connection.

"We did not think we were looking at something weird or paranormal," Dunne said. "We were looking at something that was entirely normal but was anomalous."

These investigations set Jahn at odds with many colleagues, some of whom objected to any such research on campus.

Each of these 6 areas of non-local mind gives odds against chance of a billion to one or combined odds against chance that are 1054 to one!

II. **Experiential and Personal Evidence for One Mind**

1. **Saving Others**

Larry Dossey begins his book "One Mind" with the story of Wesley Autrey – who saved the life of a young man from certain death in the New York subway. What does that have to do with the One Mind?

"Wesley Autrey, 50, a black construction worker and Navy veteran, saw a young man fall onto the subway tracks in Manhattan while having a seizure in January 2007. He instantly jumped onto the tracks and tried to lift him onto the platform, but could not do so in time. As a train approached, Autrey shoved him into the slight depression between the rails and covered him with his own body. The train could not stop in time and several cars passed over the two men before it could be brought to a halt. Autrey was nearly beheaded; he had grease stains from the train's undercarriage on his cap."

A more recent example which went viral on May 26, 2018 took place in Paris where a Malian man - "Manoudou Gassama" - scaled several floors to save a child dangling from a building in minutes with no concern to himself.

Dossey himself exhibited this behavior as a battalion surgeon in Vietnam in 1969, when he rescued a helicopter pilot from a crash when everyone believed it was going to explode. After the event Dossey wondered why he or anyone else would risk their life to save a perfect stranger? He continues: -

"I eventually came across an explanation by the German philosopher Arthur Schopenhauer, described by mythologist Joseph Campbell. Schopenhauer believed that at a decisive moment the rescuer identifies so completely with the rescued person that their minds have literally fused; they have become a single mind. There mental union is so complete that the rescuer is not rescuing someone else, he is essentially rescuing himself. I felt deeply that this explanation described my own experiences in Vietnam."

In researching my book, I accumulated a number of life-saving stories. They are not just human-to-human events, but they also involve humans rescuing animals, animals rescuing humans, and animals rescuing animals – every possible combination."

Dossey felt that Schopenhauer was correct: that there is a fusion of apparently separate, individual minds into a single, collective consciousness. In these instances, something larger than individuality takes hold: the One Mind is bridging and uniting individual minds, pushing separation aside in favor of unity and oneness.

2. Telesomatic Events (Communication at a Distance)

One of Larry's favorite cases is one involving four-year old identical twin girls in Spain in the 1970's, Sylvia and Marta Landa. "When one of the little girls touched her hand to a red-hot iron, she erupted in a major second-degree burn, an actual blister, on her hand. At the same time, miles and miles away, her twin sister, who had no idea what was going on, erupted in the same way on the same hand, the same blister, the same pattern. So this is weird stuff. This is a jaw-dropping, One Mind type of phenomenon."

3. Savants

Savant is a term that originally literally means "learned one." These are people who are notorious for having low IQs. This is important because it means that most savants simply cannot learn like you and I would. They cannot acquire information by reading. But in spite of that, they have the most astonishing abilities, in music and math (doing complex calculations almost instantly) and other areas. Their knowledge is extraordinarily narrow but it is incredibly deep. For example, one savant who can't even understand that questions that he's asked about how he does all of this, can give you the zip code for any address in the United States. A lot of this knowledge is fairly useless buts it's there. And the question is: how in the world do they know this stuff? They're not teachable; they can't read.

Dossey's hypothesis is that they dip into some domain of information that's out there, that cannot be acquired by reasonable, commonsense methods of learning.

4. Dreams

Many people, lay folks and scientists have had dreams that resulted in breakthroughs for humanity. Dmitri Mendeleev's dream of the periodic table that we all studied in school was one such breakthrough.

He later reported, "I saw in a dream a table where all the elements fell into place as required. Awakening, I immediately wrote it down on a piece of paper. Only in one place did a correction later seem necessary.' As a result of this dream, the periodic table of the elements was created."

Here Larry gives us two of his favorites:

i. The Sewing Machine Dream

The sewing machine dream happened to a man named Elias Howe. He was stuck; he couldn't figure out how to make the thing work. He was trying to put the hole in the needle at the top, where he thought it logically belonged. But he had a dream one night. As he described it, he found himself before a group of savages, who told him that he had 24 hours to come up with the answer to this sewing machine problem. He couldn't do it, so he tried to run away from the savages, and in the dream he saw their spears raised above him, and they were about to stab him and kill him, when he noticed that there was a little hole in the tip-end of each spear. He woke up, went back to his laboratory and put the hole in the tip of the needle, which had never occurred to him before. That's how he got the inspiration to put the hole in the tip of the needle, where it has been ever since, through this horrific nightmare.

ii. The Founding of Organic Chemistry

Friedrich von Kekule was trying to figure out how the six carbon atoms in the benzene molecule were arranged...This was a world task in science. He dozed before the fire and in his dream he saw a snake eating its tail. And he knew in an instant that the benzene carbon atoms had to be in a circle. He did the refined experiments and found that this was indeed the pattern of the six carbon atoms. This was the founding of organic chemistry, the revelation that the benzene structure was a circle. Or as we call it now, a hexagon, but circular in any case.

5. Connections Between Animals and Humans

I met Rupert Sheldrake when my wife and I enjoyed a weekend together at Larry's house in Dallas. Rupert has written several books and is most well-known for his theory on "morphogenic fields."

Sheldrake also created a firestorm of controversy with his very subtle and rigorous experiments with dogs, who seemed to know when their owners were returning. He used a constant video stream that tracked the movement of dogs in the living room or wherever they happened to be in the house. The dogs were known by their owners, or by their caretakers who stayed home, to come to the window or the door, and stand in alert anticipation, just before their owner was about to arrive at home.

Sheldrake thought that there might be something telepathic going on between the returning owner and the animal, and he tried to fake the dogs out by having the owners return at odd times in the day, and by using different modes of travel. He tried to fool the dogs but he couldn't fool them. Statistically, this was an airtight study. The dogs tended not to make these movements when the owner wasn't coming, and they certainly did when the owner was just about to return. This seemed to be a One Mind piece of evidence showing the bridging of thoughts or feelings or something between owners and their pets.

6. Near Death Experiences (NDEs)

The concept of a higher self that often form part of the NDE is an affirmation of One Mind. It is a virtual certainty that some aspect of human consciousness is infinite in space and time, that it is indestructible and immortal. One study found that statistically everyday in the US nearly 800 people have a NDE. Many of these individuals become aware of One Mind and many are able to share their experiences.

7. Reincarnation (Past Lives)

In the field of research on past lives Ian Stevenson MD (1918-2007) professor of Psychiatry at the University of Virginia investigated thousands of children (on every continent save Antartica) who appeared to remember past lives. Typically, children will begin to speak of past lives between the ages of two and four about experiences they had in a previous life. Between the ages of five and eight, as memories fade the child ceases to speak about a remembered life. In his book, Where Reincarnation and Biology intersect, Stevenson reports 35 cases, including photographs. They show a wide spectrum of physical deformities and birthmarks that seem to be transmitted from one life to another. In addition to memories, birth defects, birthmarks, Stevenson believes that behaviors may be carried over from life to life. The most important consequence of reincarnation is the duality of mind and body. We cannot imagine reincarnation without the belief that minds are associated with bodies during our familiar life, but also at some later time becoming associated with another body. Stevenson's, "soul bearing" and Lewis Thomas (Director of Research at Memorial Sloan-Kettering Cancer Center) "biospherical nervous system" believed that consciousness did not disappear at death – both would have been comfortable with the notion of One Mind.

8. Terminal Lucidity

This phenomenon is well described by Marjorie Woollacott on YouTube. She is a neuroscientist who has been researching and teaching at the University of Oregon for 3 decades. In these cases patients who have severe Alzheimer's or people in comas will often become lucid just before they die. Roughly 5-10% of terminal Alzheimer's patients become lucid just before they pass on. Dr.Peter Fenwick did a prospective study on several hundred nursing homes and hospice centers and found that over 80% of them reported at least one or more of these occurrences each year (this was not due to removing drugs from patients at the end of life). Dr. Alexander Balthany is doing a large study the "European Study of Terminal Lucidity" - he explains this using the metaphor of an eclipse – the sun is shining brightly but the sick brain obscures the light and often terminal lucidity patients before dying the sick brain (which is just an organ of the mind) gets out of the way so that the patient can often say goodbye to love ones.

Despair seems to becoming a fixture in our modern life. The problems we face are enormous and our efforts so inadequate they often seem futile. We are paralyzed in our ability to think in rational ways. The fuse that trips the whole circuit is a sense of helplessness – how can I make any difference.

Dossey writes, "Only by realizing, at the deepest emotional level, our connections with one another and the Earth itself can we summon the courage necessary to make the tough choices that are required in order to survive. So, this is about staying alive – saving the earth and our own skin.

One Mind, its power is revealed when we realize that our combined action with it is not merely additive but exponential. In the One Mind, one plus one no longer makes two, but many. This realization diminishes the "slow-motion relentless sorrow" of individual activities. This understanding led Margaret Mead to observe,

"Never doubt that a small group of thoughtful, committed individuals can change the world. In fact, it's the only thing that ever has."

Love is a gateway to One Mind because love tempers the forces of isolation, separateness and individuality.

Similarly Alice Walker said, "Anything we love can be saved" - including, I suggest, the earth itself, ourselves, our children, and generations yet unborn. The One Mind facilitates our connectedness and oneness with all else, therefore our love for all else.

The entire universe may be suffused by love. It may even be possible to detect rudimentary expressions of love, a kind of proto-love, in the subatomic domain. As we move from there toward systems of increasing complexity, love becomes more recognizable, reaching its fullest expression in humans, with our participation in the One Mind.

Abundant evidence shows that isolation is terrible for health, happiness, and longevity. We are not designed to live apart.

A sense of being connected with all others and with all sentient life has been recognized throughout human history as a source of immense joy and fulfillment.

Unity with others has always been a highly prized goal of the great wisdom traditions.

AFTERWORD

"It seems plain and self-evident, yet it needs to be said: the isolated knowledge obtained by a group of specialists in a narrow field has in itself no value whatsoever, but only in its synthesis with all the rest of knowledge and only in as much as it really contributes in this synthesis toward answering the demand, "Who are we?"".

Erwin Schrodinger, winner of the Nobel Prize in Physics

ERA I (LB5) is important as it gives an overview of your most important biomarkers and diagnostic results to show if you have metabolic stress and insulin resistance. Using the LB5 Program you can reverse Diabesity and recover metabolic flexibility as you heal the Toxic Triad.

MEDICAL ERAS*

	ERA I	ERA II	ERA III
SPACE-TIME CHARACTERISTIC	Local	Local	Nonlocal
SYNONYM	Mechanical, material, or physical medicine	Mind-body, complementary or alternative medicine	Nonlocal medicine
DESCRIPTION	Causal, deterministic, describable by classical concepts of space-time and matter-energy. Mind not a factor; "mind" a result of brain mechanisms.	Mind a major factor in healing within the single person. Mind has causal power, is thus not fully explainable by classical concepts in physics. Includes but goes beyond Era I.	Mind a factor in healing both within and between persons. Mind not completely localized to points in space (brains or bodies) or time (present moment or single lifetimes). Mind is unbounded in space and time and thus ultimately unitary or one. Healing at a distance is possible. Not describable by classical concepts of space time or matter-energy.

EXAMPLES	Any form of therapy focusing solely on effects of things on the body are Era I approaches – including techniques such as acupuncture and homeopathy, the use of herbs, etc. Almost all forms of "modern" medicine – drugs, surgery, CPR, etc. – are included.	Any therapy emphasizing the effects of consciousness solely within the individual body is an Era II approach. Psychoimmunology, counseling, hypnosis, biofeedback, relaxation therapies, and most types of imagery based "alternative" therapies are included.	Any therapy in which effects of consciousness bridge between different persons is an Era III approach. All forms of distant healing, intercessory prayer, "psychic" and shamanic healing, "miracles," diagnosis at a distance, and non-contact therapeutic touch are included.

In **ERA II(LB100)** of the program we do an extensive longevity panel to show where on the Wellness-Illness Continuum you are. Using your methylation data, you can track your Pace of Aging and Biological Age each year. Knowing this you have the opportunity to intervene with therapies targeting each of the 10 Hallmarks of Aging to help you LB100!

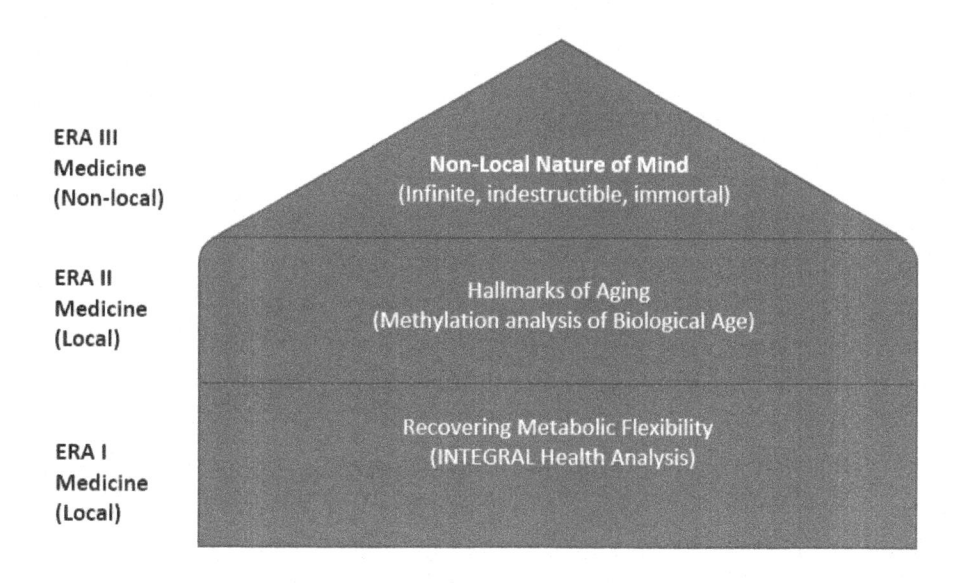

ERA III Medicine (Non-local) — **Non-Local Nature of Mind** (Infinite, indestructible, immortal)

ERA II Medicine (Local) — **Hallmarks of Aging** (Methylation analysis of Biological Age)

ERA I Medicine (Local) — **Recovering Metabolic Flexibility** (INTEGRAL Health Analysis)

It is important for you to remember the following:

1. Metabolic and Psychological Stress are the prime drivers of Aging.

2. Aging is the #1 risk factor for most chronic disease and a shorter lifespan.

3. Delaying the rate of Biological aging by just 7 years will cut your incidence of chronic disease in half.

4. Aging today is treatable and even reversible.

ERA III (One Mind) – I believe this is perhaps the most important part of the LB100 program but is only now being recognized. I believe by integrating all 3 ERAS of medicine you have "the guide to immortality."

Consciousness can be considered the ultimate non-violent approach to health and longevity when compared with the relatively violent effects of modern drugs and surgery.

One Mind includes all scientific life as shown.

SPECTRUM OF NON-LOCAL HEALING

Interacting Systems	Evidence of Interaction	Expression of Interaction
Humans and Humans	Humans interact with each other non-locally at a distance, without benefit of sensory or energy-based exchanges of information. Many controlled studies deal with distant/ intercessory prayer and other types of distant mental intent. Hundreds of telesomatic events have been reported. Numerous controlled studies have documented non-local forms of gaining or conveying information (clairvoyance or telepathy).	Love, empathy, compassion, caring, unity, collective consciousness, the Universal or One Mind, God ("God is love"), Goddess, Allah, Tao, the Absolute

Interacting Systems	Evidence of Interaction	Expression of Interaction
Humans and animals	Scores of studies involving various types of distance healing intent have been done using higher animals as "targets." These studies often involve prayer or "bio-PK" (psychokinesis). Lost pets return to owners across vast distances to places they have never been.	Love, Empathy
Humans and living organisms	Scores of controlled studies have dealt with the distance effects of prayer and other types of positive distant healing intent. In which various "lower organisms" – bacteria, fungi, yeasts – are the targets, as well as seeds, plants, and cells of various sorts.	Love, Empathy
Humans and complex machines	Humans can mentally influence the behavior of sophisticated electronic biofeedback devices – affirmed by the collective record of more than 30 years of biofeedback research in hundreds of laboratories. Humans also can mentally influence random event generators and other electronic instruments at a distance, as demonstrated in studies conducted at the Princeton Engineering Anomalies Research (PEAR) lab and many other institutions.	"Becoming one" or "falling in love" with the machine, interconnection, unity
Humans and simple machines	Humans can interact with and influence the behavior of freely swinging, pendulums, mechanical cascade devices, and other relatively simple apparatuses, at a distance – affirmed by studies conducted at the PEAR lab and elsewhere.	"Becoming one" or "falling in love" with the machine, interconnection, unity

Interacting Systems	Evidence of Interaction	Expression of Interaction
Complex physical devices/ systems	According to commonly accepted principles in physics, coupled harmonic oscillators, all common musical instruments and radio and television circuitry interact and resonate with each other. In general, all manner of physical systems-whether mechanical, electromagnetic, fluid, dynamical, quantum mechanical, or nuclear-display synergistically interactive vibrations with similar systems or with their environment.	Sympathetic or harmonic resonance
Subatomic particles	Subatomic particles such as electrons, once in contact, demonstrate simultaneous change-no matter how far apart-to the same degree. Bell's theorem, the Aspect experiment, and many other developments affirm these possibilities at the quantum mechanical level.	Non-locally correlated behavior, rudimentary or proto-love?

Adapted from Larry Dossey, MD

In conclusion, I want to point out that seven out of ten Westerners say they feel uncomfortable with death. Less than half of people over 65 have considered how they want to die.

Despite Bhutan being ranked the 134th most developed nation on earth extensive studies by Japanese researchers have found that Bhutan is among the world's 20 happiest countries. Probably what you don't know is how contemplating death contributes to their feelings of happiness. They do this by contemplating death at least 3 times each day.

I have been using a free APP called 'We Croak' for the past two years where you receive reminders (often from great writers/philosophers/poets etc.) that you are going to die.

Research from Australia found the top 3 regrets of the dying included not living in the moment, working too much and living a life they should rather than the one they truly want to.

Often when a person realizes death is imminent their long checklist and everyday concerns become irrelevant and their mind begins to center on that which makes it happy. Why not consider what will make you happy now?

The Buddha wrote , "In the end only three things matter, how much you loved, how gently you lived, and how gracefully you let go of things not meant for you."

I firmly believe a forth item is the awareness of One Mind.

Consciousness is non-local and infinite, therefore it is immortal, eternal and One. It is a fundamental principal that underlies all knowing and being.

With our recognition of this psychohistorical evolution of consciousness and the emerging integral structure of consciousness (space-free and time-free) we are able to experience One Mind – The Ever Present Origin. This is the essential ingredient for the health of humanity and the planet in the years ahead.

Find out your insulin resistance score and if you or your loved ones are at greater risk.

Take the FREE and simple online test designed by Dr Graham Simpson MD today.

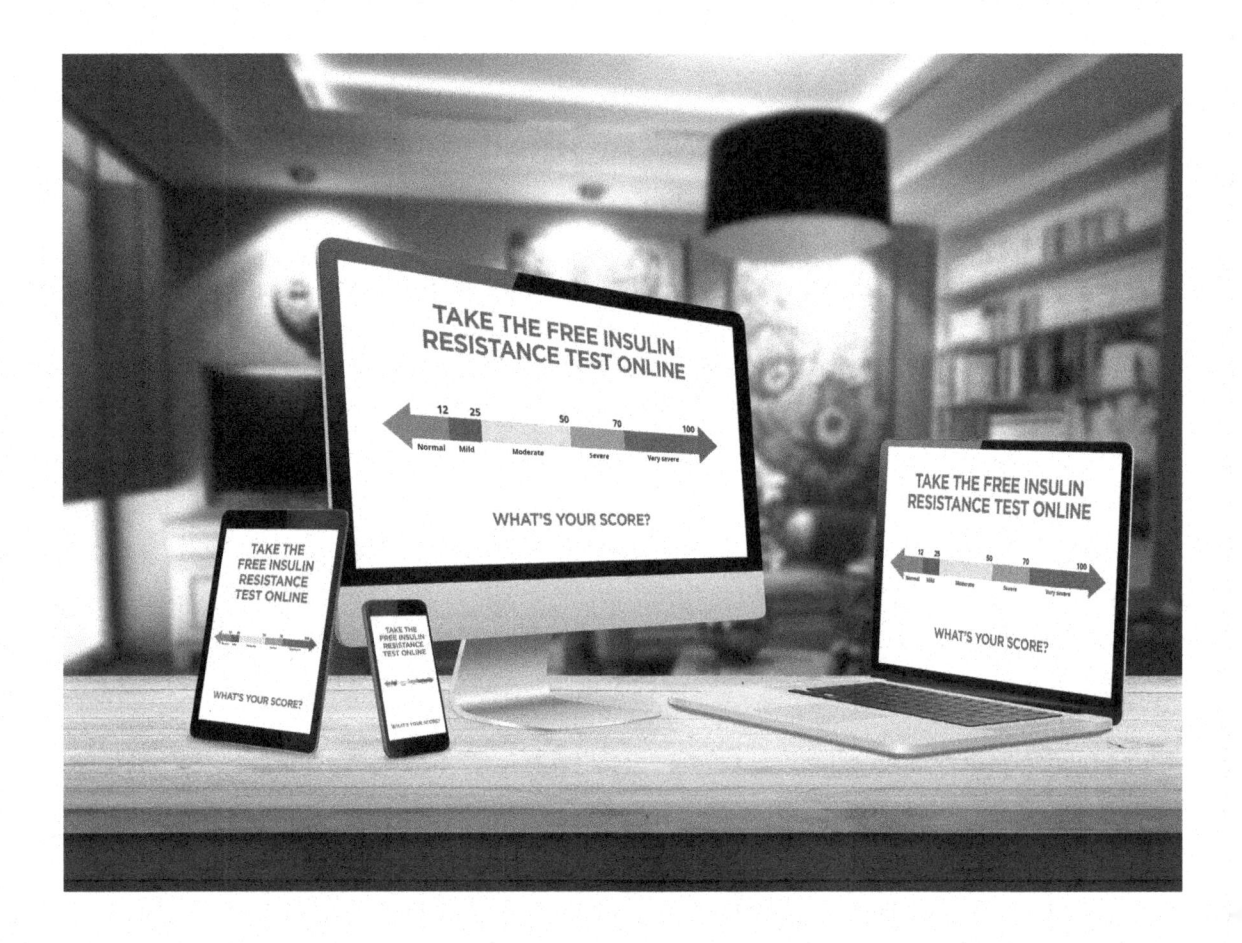

www.theinsulinresistancetest.com

REVERSE YOUR BIOLOGICAL AGE TODAY!

Did you know:
- Age is the number 1 risk for disease and death
- Metabolic and Psychological stress are the primary drivers of aging
- 88% of adults in the USA have "insulin resistance" (metabolic stress) more than 30% of adults in the USA suffer from a mental disorder
- Reversing your biological age by just 7 years will cut your risk of chronic disease by more than 50%

What we now know, the latest data and science:
- 53% of Americans have Type 2 Diabetes or Pre-Diabetes
- We can now reverse Biological age using biomarkers and epigenetic methylation data
- Nutrient sensors like MTOR and AMPK can be optimized to extend lifespan.
- The first study in humans proving that biological age could be reversed 2.5 years (in a 12 month study) used a cocktail of Growth Hormone, DHEA and Metformin and was documented using 4 Methylation Age Clocks
- By age 50, humans have lost more than 50% of the NAD vital to slow the aging process
- Diabesity is the # 1 health risk after age for the development of chronic disease and early death.
- By reversing Biological age 7 years, we can potentially reduce global chronic disease by 50+% with huge cost savings

Our Therapeutic Solution!
Live Below 5.0 to Live Beyond 100
Dr Simpsons Therapeutic Programs will help you reduce chronic disease to live a longer healthier, happier life and includes:

The Live Below 5.0 Program
You can reverse Diabesity in a few months, for some clients within weeks. Visit www.livebelow5.com

The Live Beyond 100 Program
Impacts all 10 of the 'Hallmarks of Aging' that can extend both your Healthspan and Lifespan.

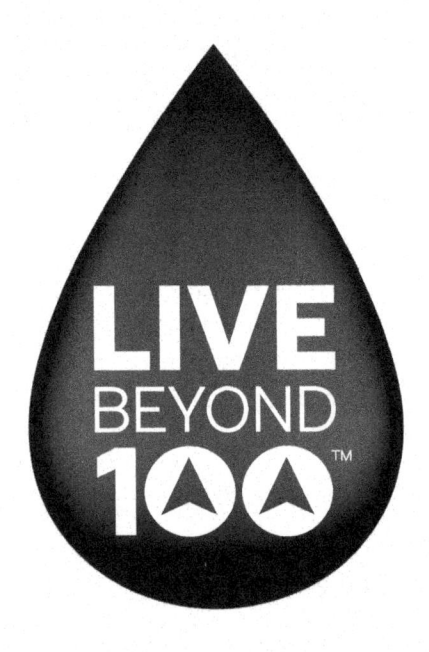

The Live Beyond 100 Program

Impacts all 10 of the 'Hallmarks of Aging' that can extend both your Healthspan and Lifespan. Depending on where you sit on the Wellness – Illness continuum both programs combined can help you reverse your biological age, reducing chronic disease to support you to living longer.

Find out:

What your key biomarkers and methylation data tell about your health today?
What do the Blue Zones tell us about longevity?

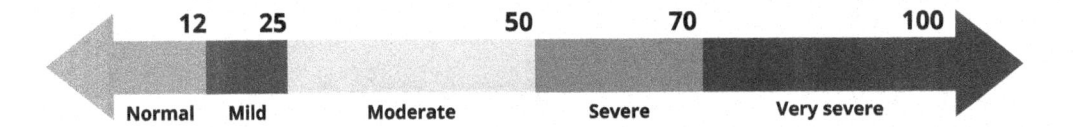

12	25		50		70		100
Normal	Mild	Moderate		Severe		Very severe	

Find out your insulin resistance score
Take the FREE online test at www.theinsulinsresistancetest.com

To learn more about how you can live beyond 100 simply visit www.livebeyond100.com

How We Deliver the 'Live Beyond 100' Solution?

- Client becomes aware of the **Live Beyond 100** programs.
- Client visits our website www.livebeyond100.com to take the FREE test.
- Client reviews the **Live Beyond 100** programs.
- Client selects the program.
- **Live Beyond 100** Health Coach makes contact to develop personalized program/answer questions before meeting with a physician.

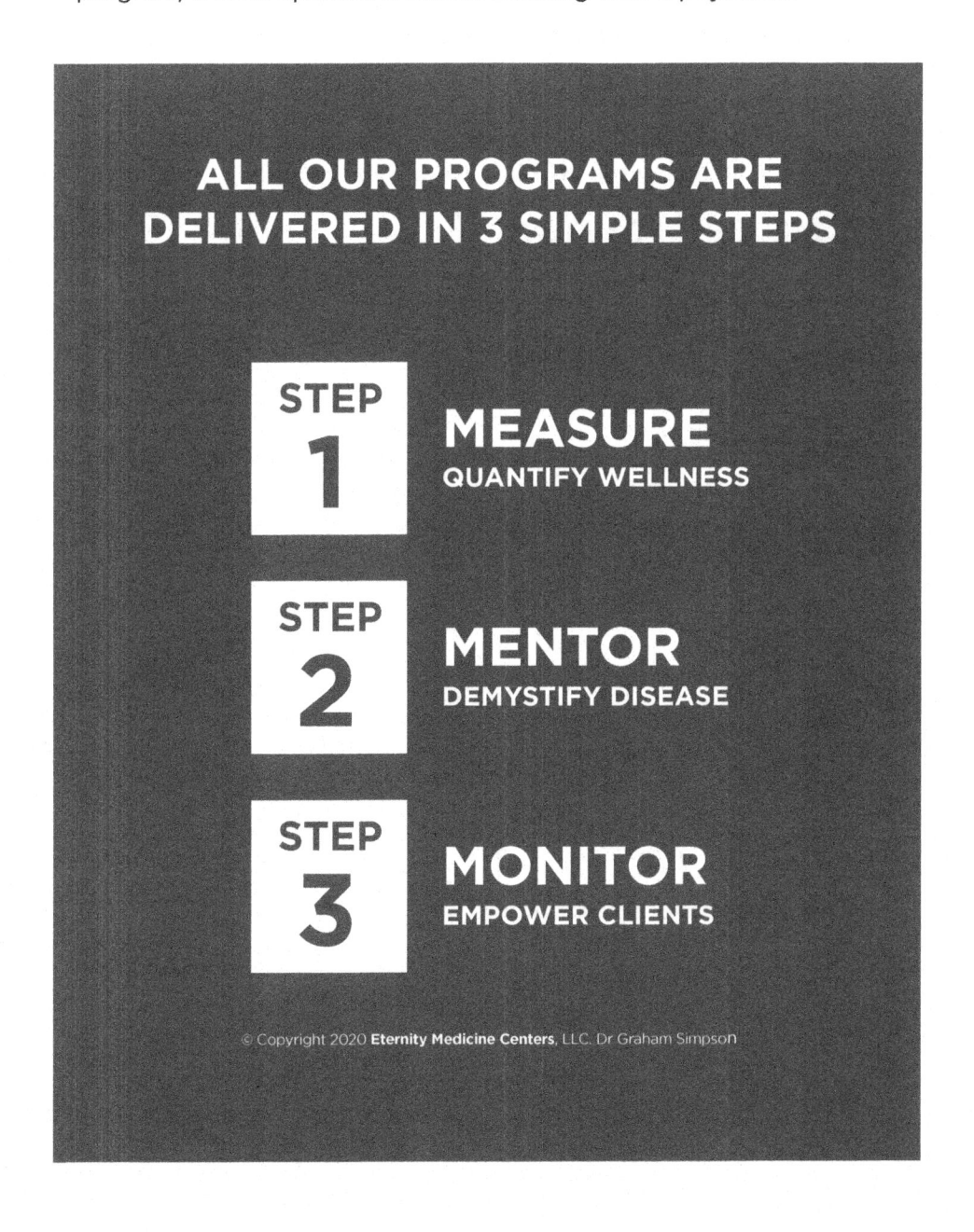

ALL OUR PROGRAMS ARE DELIVERED IN 3 SIMPLE STEPS

STEP 1 — **MEASURE**
QUANTIFY WELLNESS

STEP 2 — **MENTOR**
DEMYSTIFY DISEASE

STEP 3 — **MONITOR**
EMPOWER CLIENTS

© Copyright 2020 **Eternity Medicine Centers**, LLC. Dr Graham Simpson

STEP ONE - MEASURE

- History
- Examination
- Diagnostics

Our goal in 'Step One' is to **quantify wellness** using the Insulin Resistance Score and other critical biomarkers.

STEP TWO - MENTOR

We provide a 'whole-person' approach. Here our goal is to demystify disease by attending to all the 'root-causes' of disease especially the hallmarks of aging using the **I.N.T.E.G.R.A.L Health Model**.

STEP THREE - MONITOR

Our goal here is to empower clients. In order to do this, we employ various tools (the APP and Dashboard) together with AI and machine learning. Clients can track their biomarkers in real time to assure how well their personalized program is working and how quickly they can reverse their biological age.

Our solution is very different from the episodic and reactive disease model delivered over the last 50 years. We seek to deliver proactive health to empower clients by treating the root cause of disease with far more natural (less drug) therapies. **The Live Beyond 100 Program** contains all you need to extend your journey towards a healthy and long life.

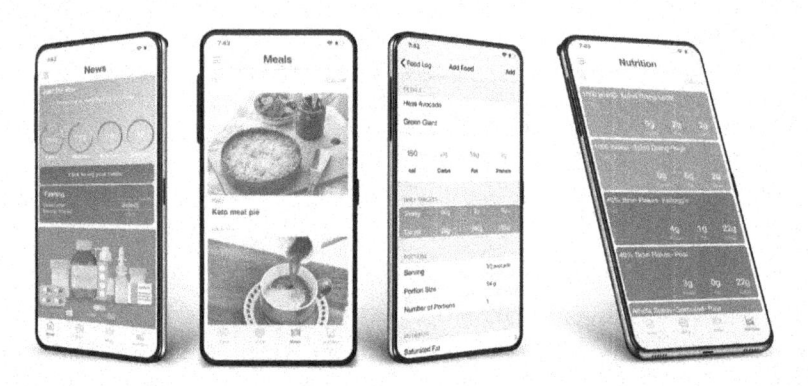

To learn more about how you can live beyond 100 simply visit www.livebeyond100.com

HOW TO DELIVER PROACTIVE HEALTHCARE

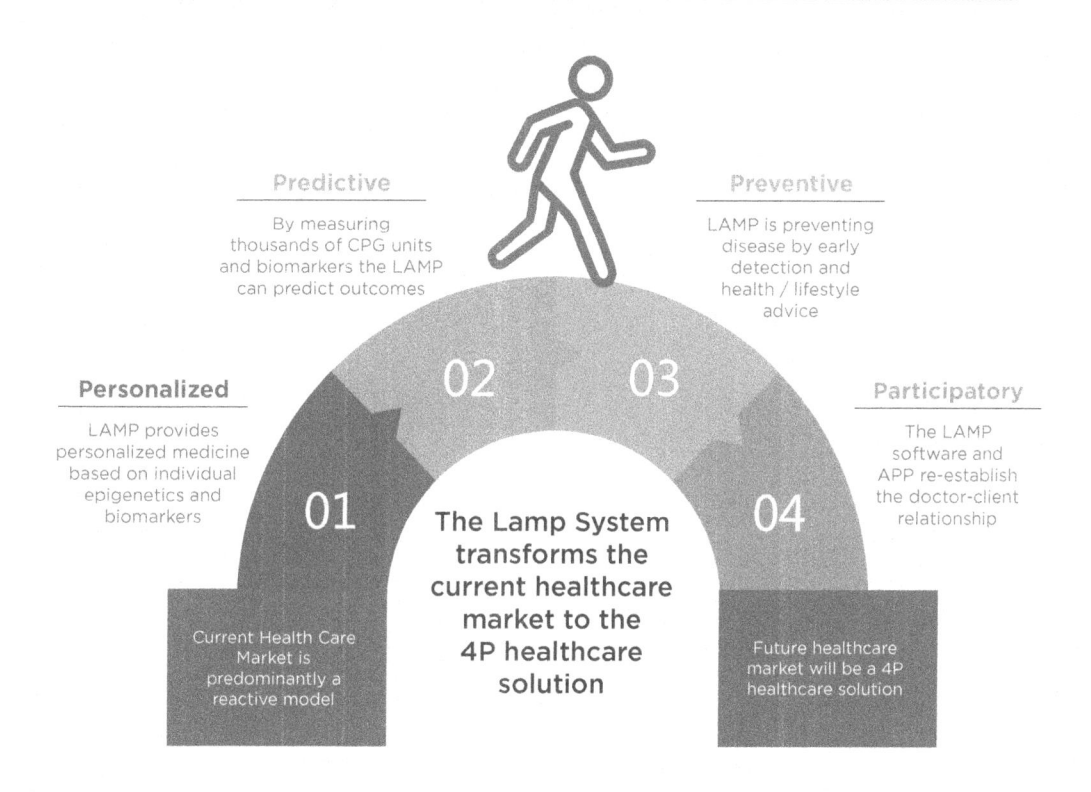

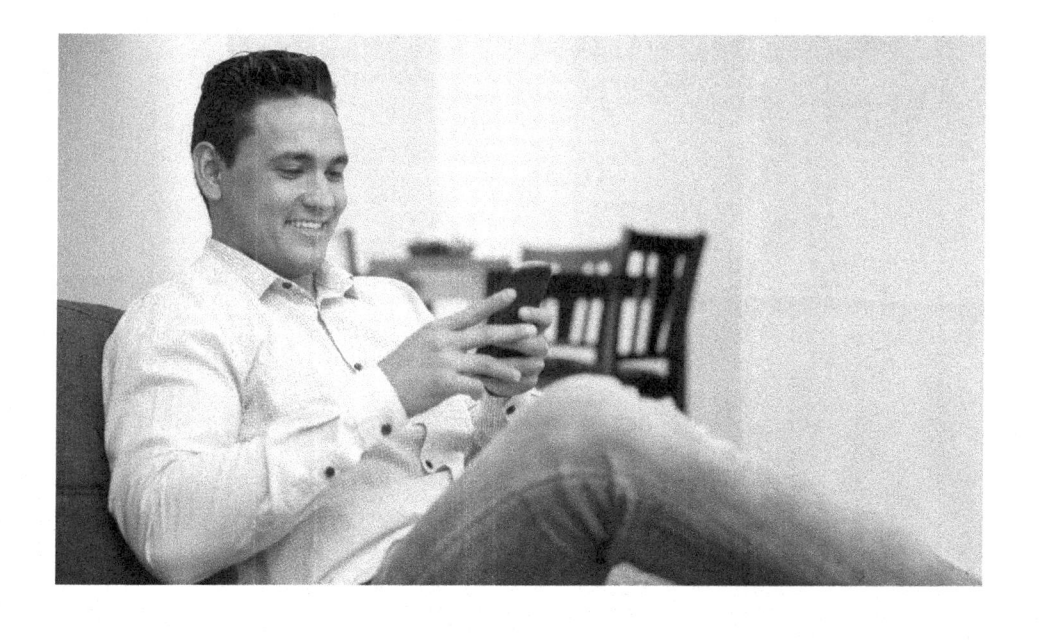

Predictive
By measuring thousands of CPG units and biomarkers the LAMP can predict outcomes

Preventive
LAMP is preventing disease by early detection and health / lifestyle advice

Personalized
LAMP provides personalized medicine based on individual epigenetics and biomarkers

Participatory
The LAMP software and APP re-establish the doctor-client relationship

01 Current Health Care Market is predominantly a reactive model

02 **03**

The Lamp System transforms the current healthcare market to the 4P healthcare solution

04 Future healthcare market will be a 4P healthcare solution

LIVE BEYOND 100 PROGRAM FEATURES

A WHOLE PERSON INTEGRAL APPROACH
That will reverse diabesity the key to Anti-Aging and address the root cause of disease.

SIMPLE 3 STEP METHODOLOGY
STEP 1 - MEASURE Quantify Wellness
STEP 2 - MENTOR Demystify Disease
STEP 3 - MONITOR Empower Yourself

CONTINUOUS MEDICAL SUPERVISION
By Our Certified Live Beyond 100 (LB100) Doctors.

YOUR OWN PERSONAL HEALTH COACH
Your own personal health coach to guide you through the program.

PERSONALISED NUTRITION
Based on your microbiome and intermittent fasting made easy.

CONTINUOUS GLUCOSE MONITORING
See how quickly a personalised diet and intermittent fasting can restore you to optimal health.

HEALTHCARE IN YOUR POCKET

LIVE BEYOND 100 RESOURCES
Menus' Blogs, Podcasts, Videos, Nutraceuticals, Articles, Keto Meals, Mobile Devices, Select Anti-aging products.

ADDITIONAL READING

ERA I

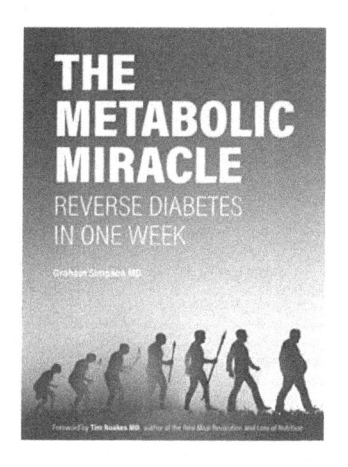

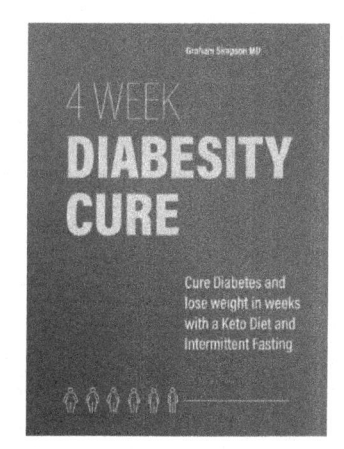

- *The Metabolic Miracle: Reverse Diabetes in One Week* — Graham Simpson MD
- *4 Week Diabesity Cure* — Graham Simpson MD
- *Good Calories, Bad Calories: Fats, Carbs, and the Controversial Science of Diet and Health* — Gary Taubes
- *The Plant Paradox Quick and Easy: The 30-Day Plan to Lose Weight, Feel Great, and Live Lectin-Free* — Steven R. Gundry, MD
- *Pure, White and Deadly: How Sugar Is Killing Us and What We Can Do to Stop It* — John Yudkin
- *Ravenous: Otto Warburg, the Nazis, and the Search for the Cancer-Diet Connection* — Sam Apple

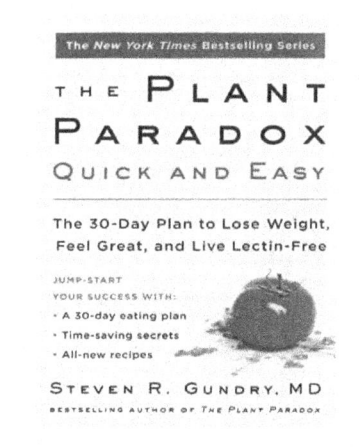

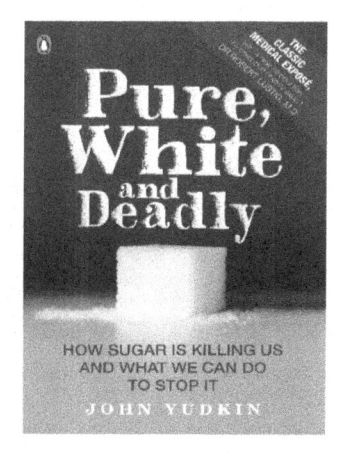

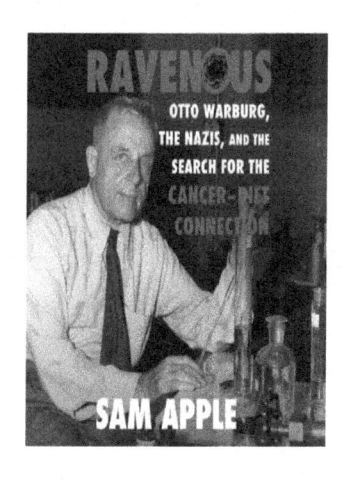

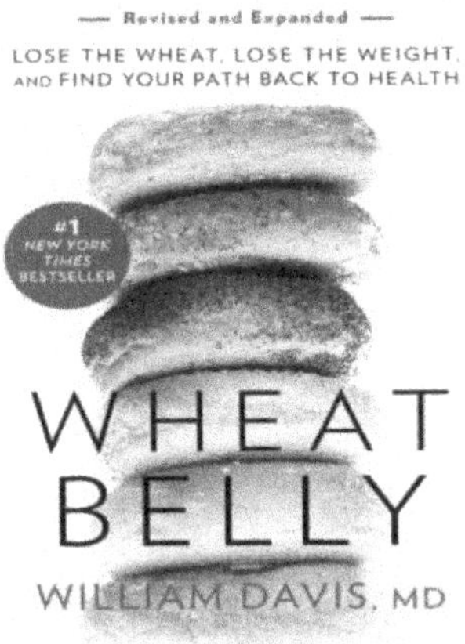
Revised and Expanded
LOSE THE WHEAT, LOSE THE WEIGHT, AND FIND YOUR PATH BACK TO HEALTH
#1 NEW YORK TIMES BESTSELLER
WHEAT BELLY
WILLIAM DAVIS, MD

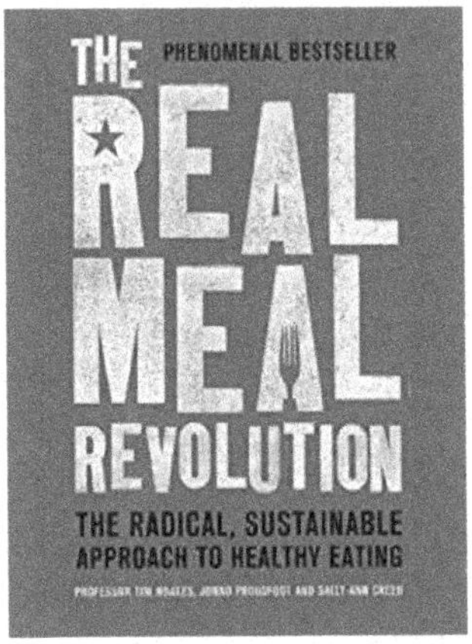
THE
PHENOMENAL BESTSELLER
REAL MEAL REVOLUTION
THE RADICAL, SUSTAINABLE APPROACH TO HEALTHY EATING

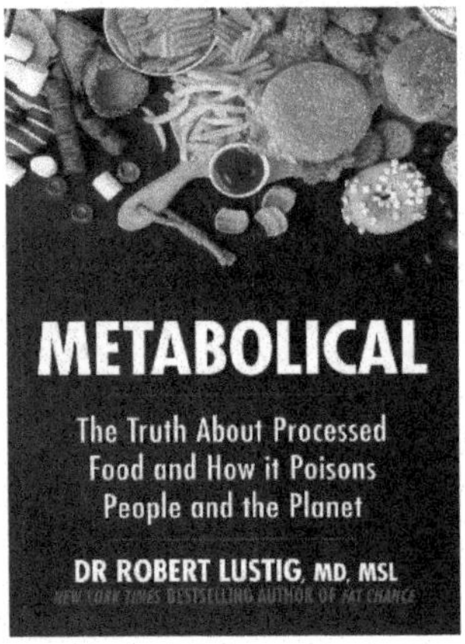
METABOLICAL
The Truth About Processed Food and How it Poisons People and the Planet
DR ROBERT LUSTIG, MD, MSL

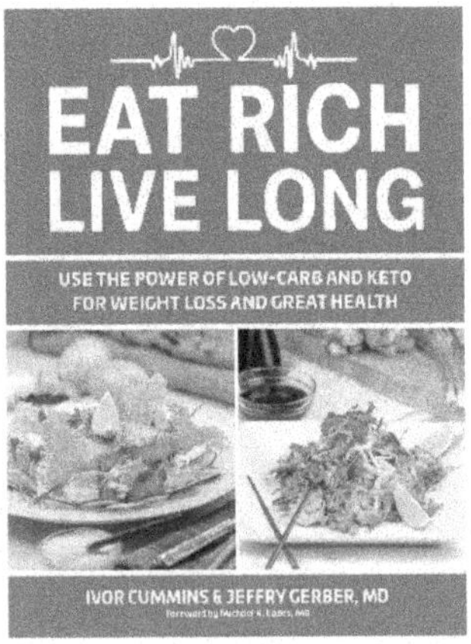
EAT RICH LIVE LONG
USE THE POWER OF LOW-CARB AND KETO FOR WEIGHT LOSS AND GREAT HEALTH
IVOR CUMMINS & JEFFRY GERBER, MD

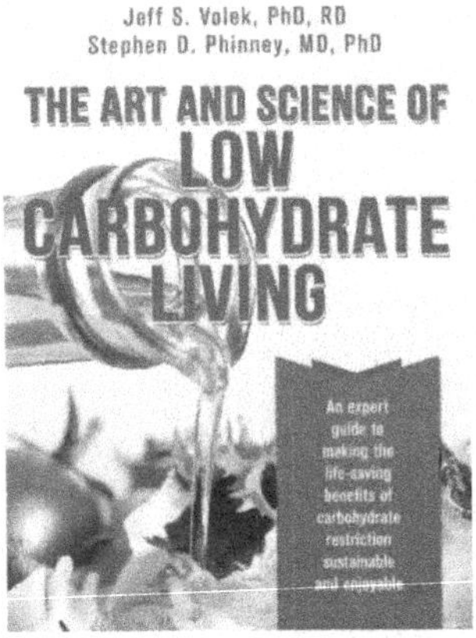
Jeff S. Volek, PhD, RD
Stephen D. Phinney, MD, PhD
THE ART AND SCIENCE OF LOW CARBOHYDRATE LIVING

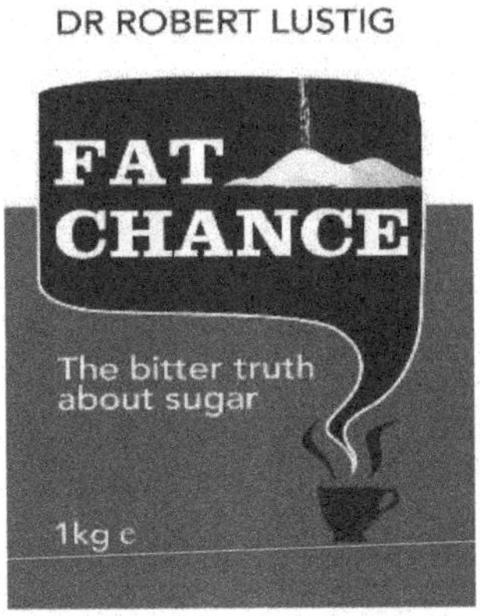
DR ROBERT LUSTIG
FAT CHANCE
The bitter truth about sugar
1kg c

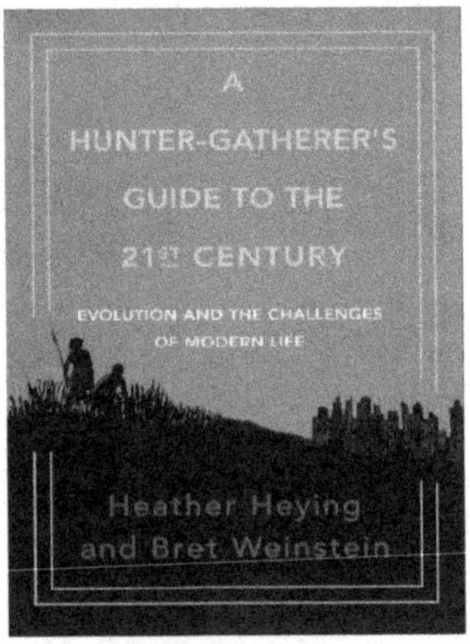
A HUNTER-GATHERER'S GUIDE TO THE 21ST CENTURY
EVOLUTION AND THE CHALLENGES OF MODERN LIFE
Heather Heying and Bret Weinstein

ERA II

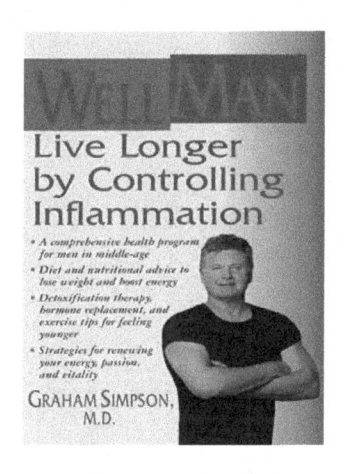

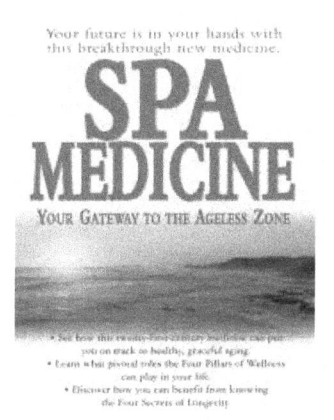

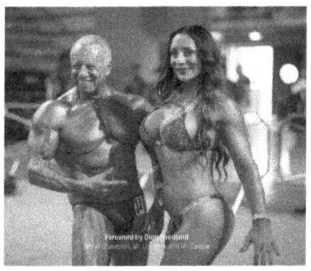

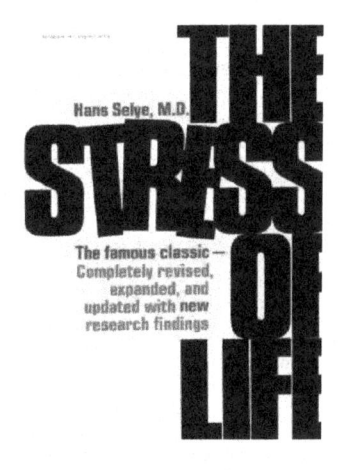

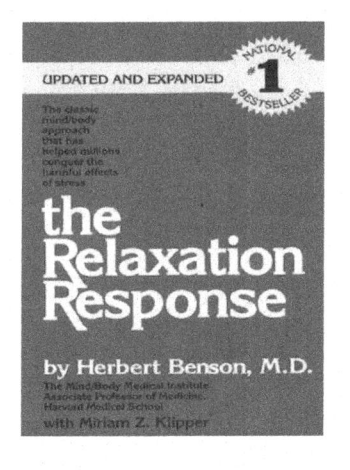

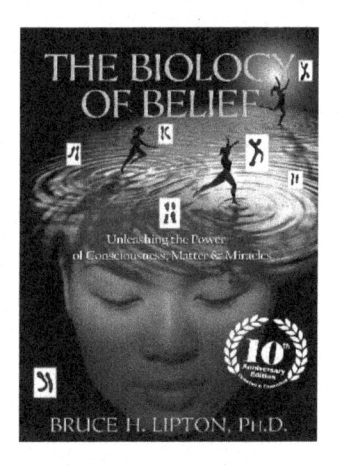

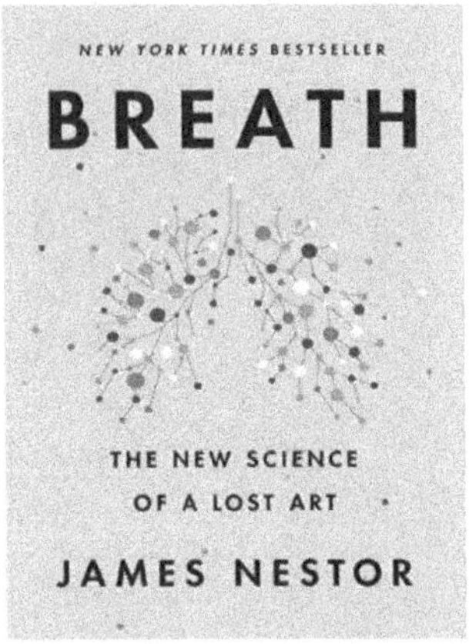
NEW YORK TIMES BESTSELLER
BREATH
THE NEW SCIENCE OF A LOST ART
JAMES NESTOR

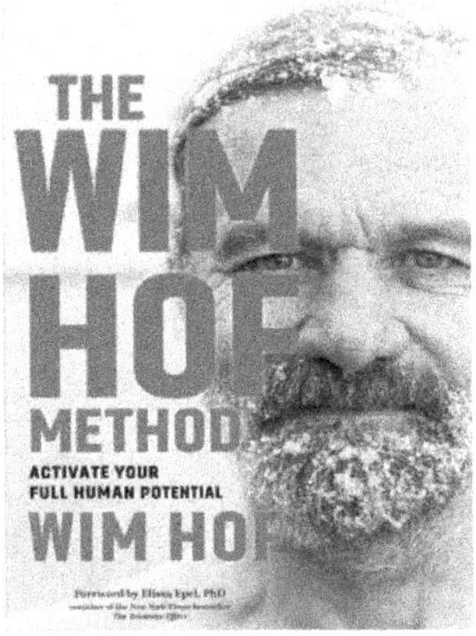
THE WIM HOF METHOD
ACTIVATE YOUR FULL HUMAN POTENTIAL
WIM HOF

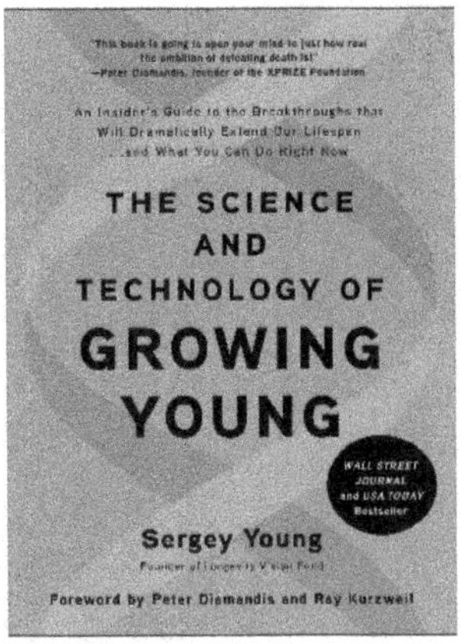
THE SCIENCE AND TECHNOLOGY OF
GROWING YOUNG
Sergey Young
Foreword by Peter Diamandis and Ray Kurzweil

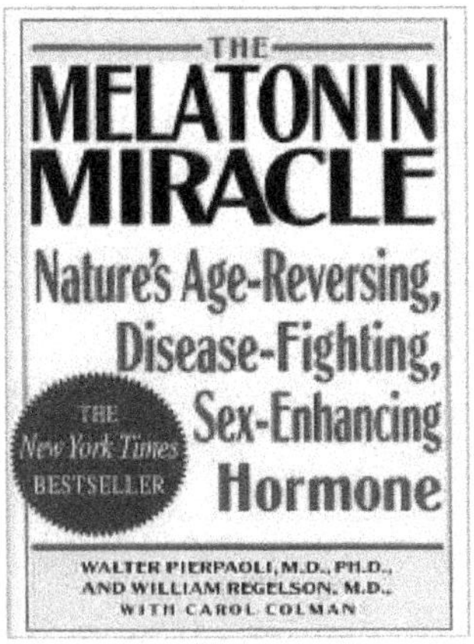
THE
MELATONIN MIRACLE
Nature's Age-Reversing, Disease-Fighting, Sex-Enhancing Hormone
THE New York Times BESTSELLER
WALTER PIERPAOLI, M.D., PH.D., AND WILLIAM REGELSON, M.D.,
WITH CAROL COLMAN

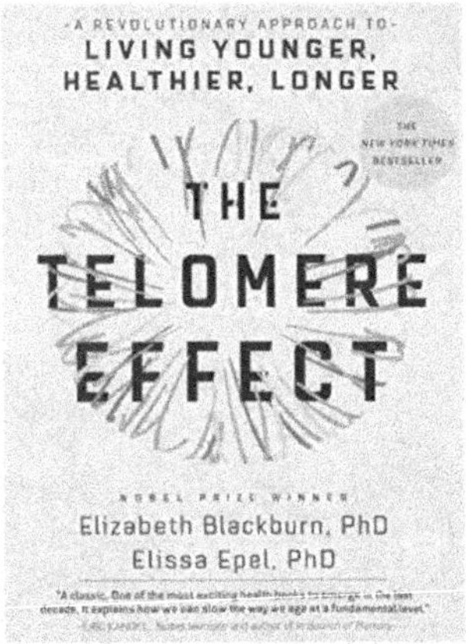
A REVOLUTIONARY APPROACH TO
LIVING YOUNGER, HEALTHIER, LONGER
THE TELOMERE EFFECT
Elizabeth Blackburn, PhD
Elissa Epel, PhD

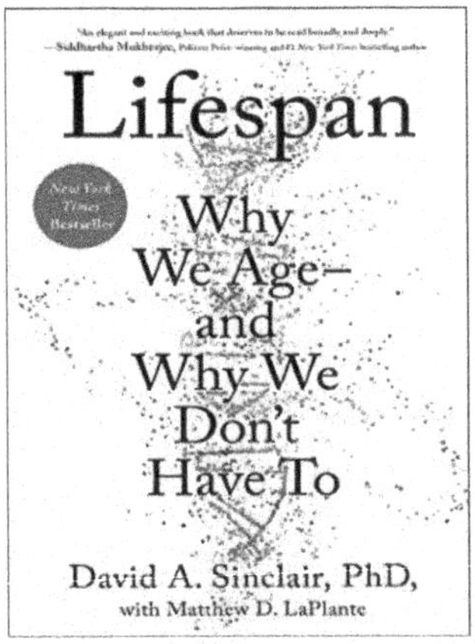
Lifespan
Why We Age—and Why We Don't Have To
David A. Sinclair, PhD,
with Matthew D. LaPlante

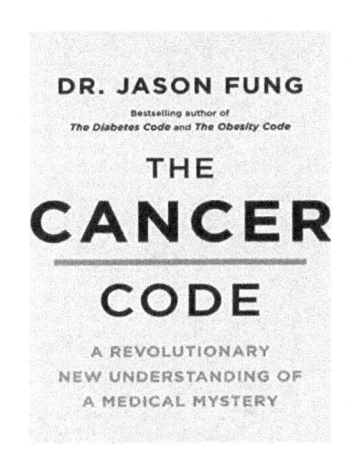

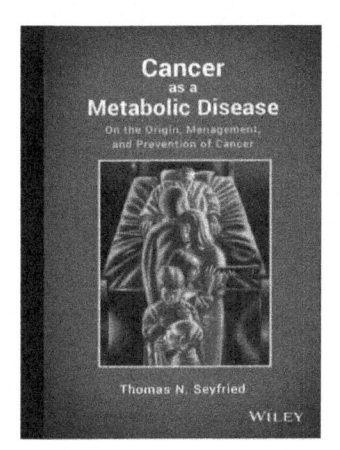

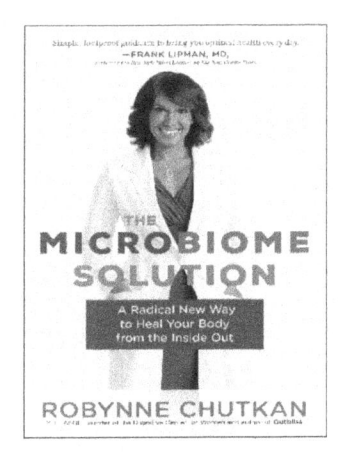

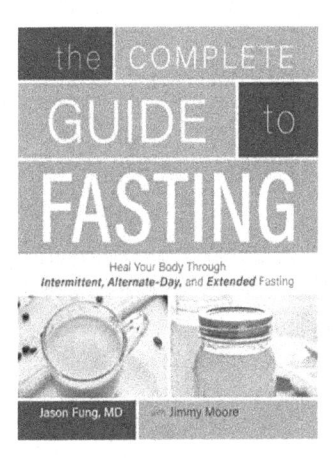

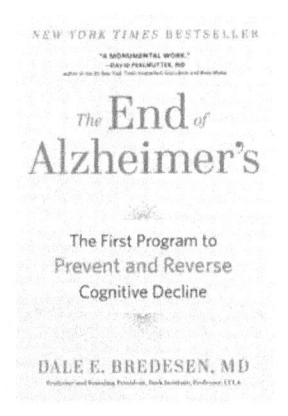

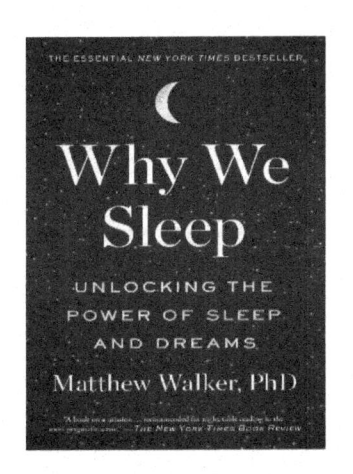

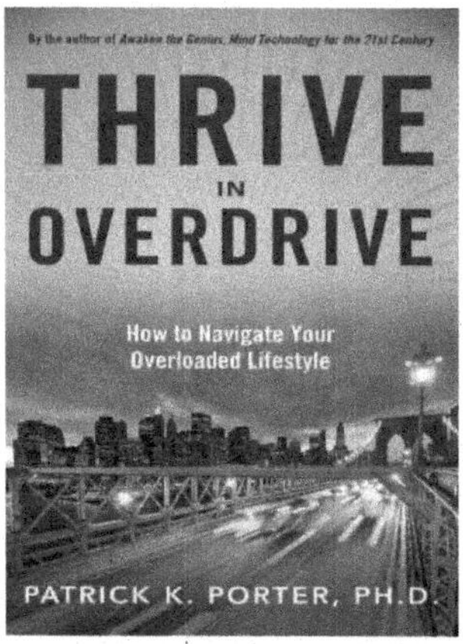
By the author of Awaken the Genius, Mind Technology for the 21st Century
THRIVE
IN
OVERDRIVE
How to Navigate Your
Overloaded Lifestyle
PATRICK K. PORTER, PH.D.

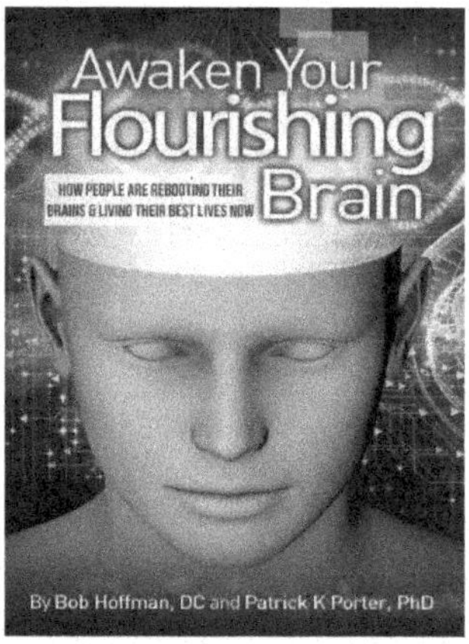
Awaken Your
Flourishing
HOW PEOPLE ARE REBOOTING THEIR BRAINS & LIVING THEIR BEST LIVES NOW
Brain
By Bob Hoffman, DC and Patrick K Porter, PhD

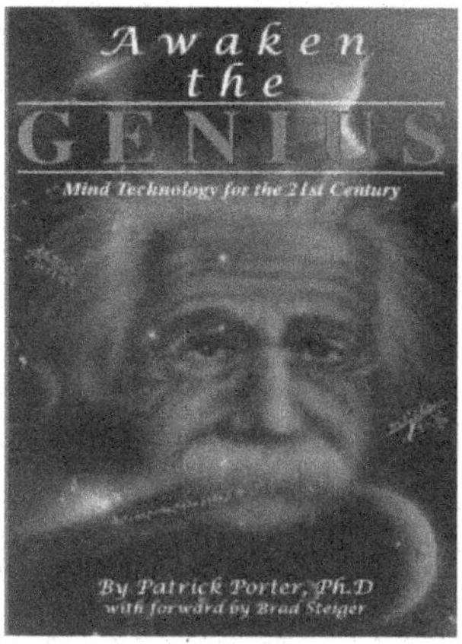
Awaken
the
GENIUS
Mind Technology for the 21st Century
By Patrick Porter, Ph.D
with forward by Brad Steiger

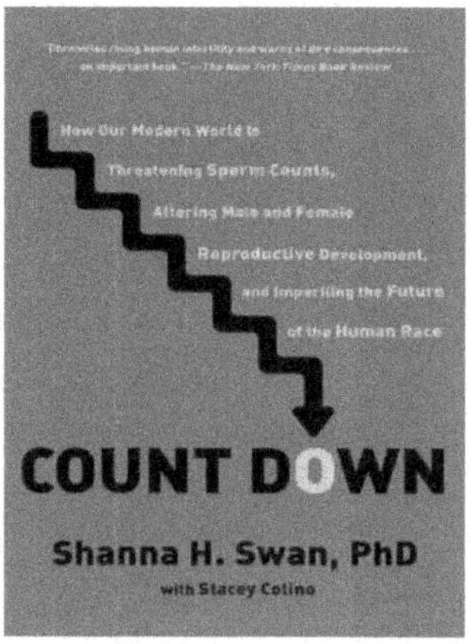
How Our Modern World Is
Threatening Sperm Counts,
Altering Male and Female
Reproductive Development,
and Imperiling the Future
of the Human Race
COUNT DOWN
Shanna H. Swan, PhD
with Stacey Colino

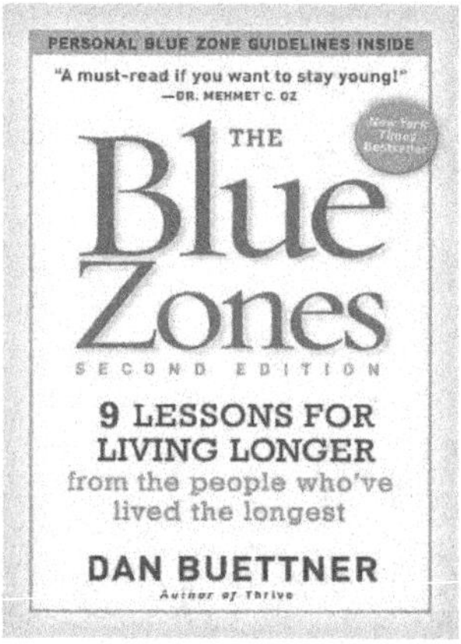
PERSONAL BLUE ZONE GUIDELINES INSIDE
"A must-read if you want to stay young!"
—DR. MEHMET C. OZ
THE
Blue
Zones
SECOND EDITION
9 LESSONS FOR
LIVING LONGER
from the people who've
lived the longest
DAN BUETTNER
Author of Thrive

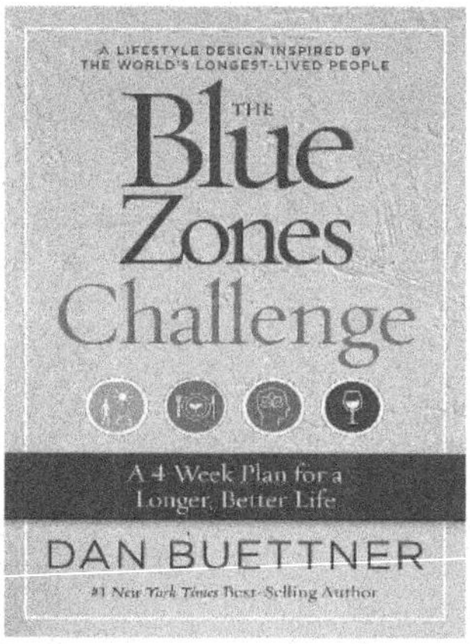
A LIFESTYLE DESIGN INSPIRED BY
THE WORLD'S LONGEST-LIVED PEOPLE
THE
Blue
Zones
Challenge
A 4 Week Plan for a
Longer, Better Life
DAN BUETTNER
#1 New York Times Best-Selling Author

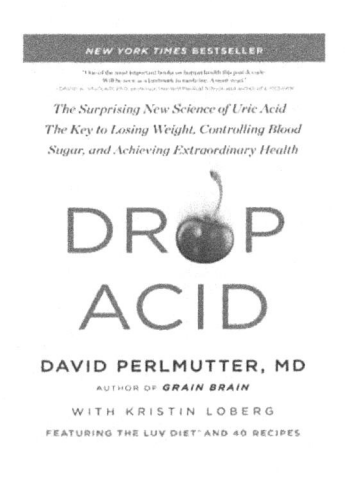

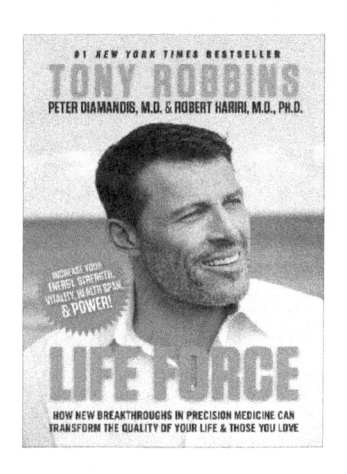

ERA III

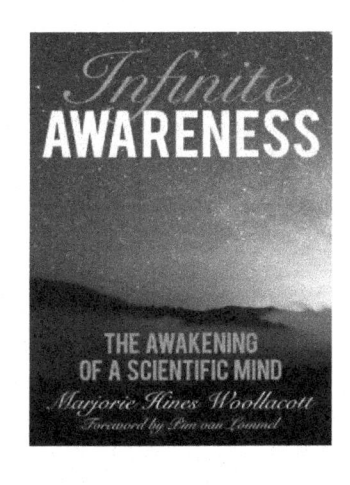

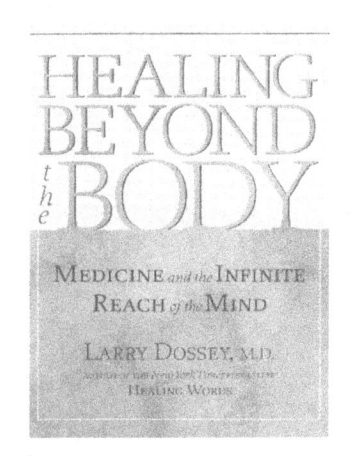

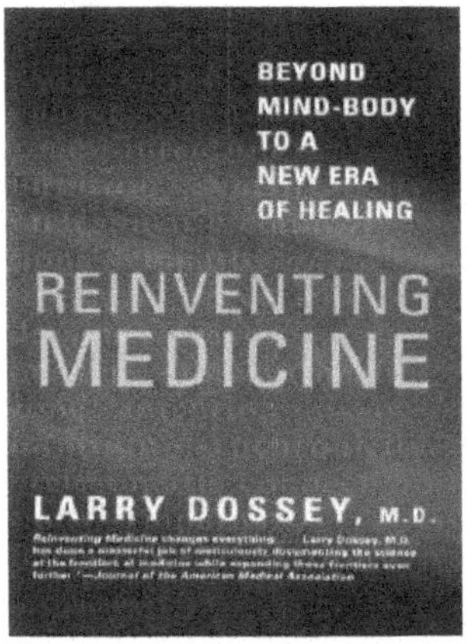
BEYOND
MIND-BODY
TO A
NEW ERA
OF HEALING
REINVENTING
MEDICINE
LARRY DOSSEY, M.D.

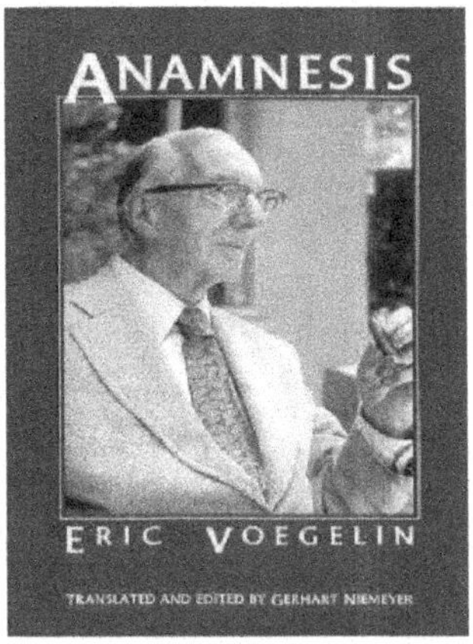
ANAMNESIS
ERIC VOEGELIN
TRANSLATED AND EDITED BY GERHART NIEMEYER

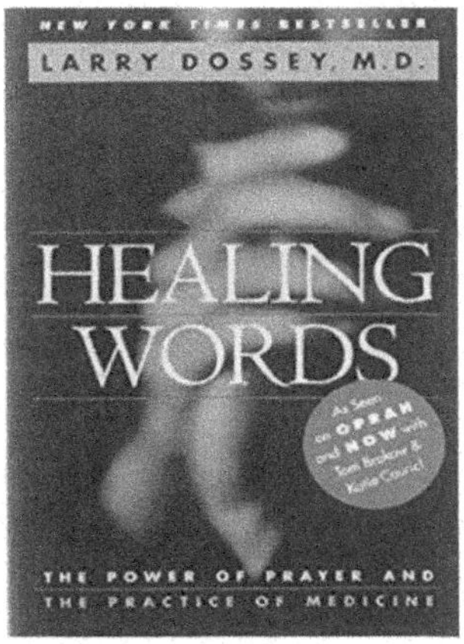
NEW YORK TIMES BESTSELLER
LARRY DOSSEY, M.D.
HEALING
WORDS
THE POWER OF PRAYER AND
THE PRACTICE OF MEDICINE

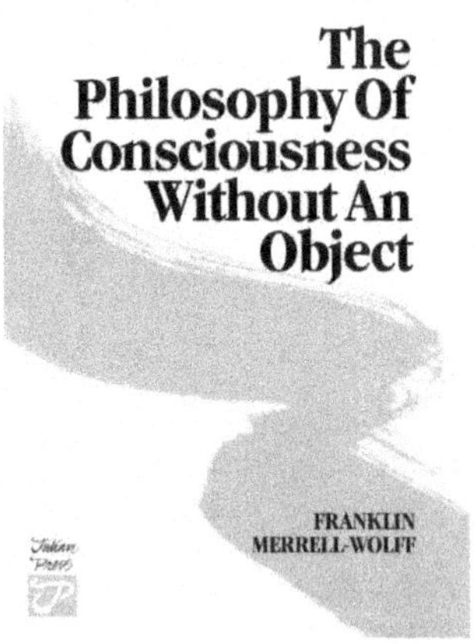
The
Philosophy Of
Consciousness
Without An
Object
FRANKLIN
MERRELL-WOLFF

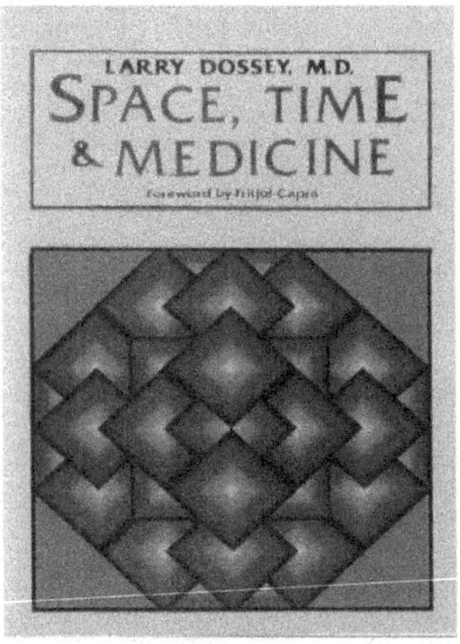
LARRY DOSSEY, M.D.
SPACE, TIME
& MEDICINE

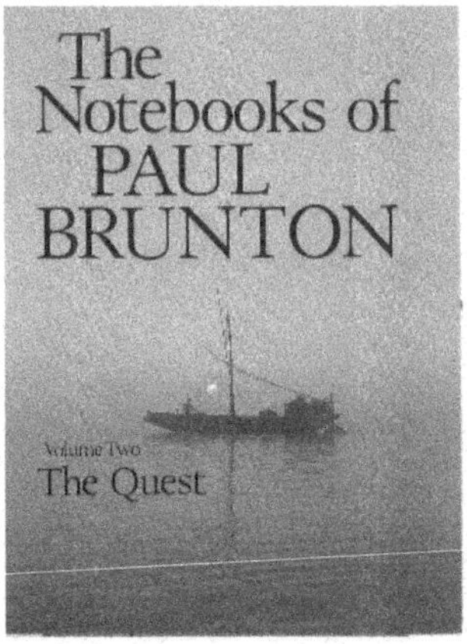
The
Notebooks of
PAUL
BRUNTON
Volume Two
The Quest

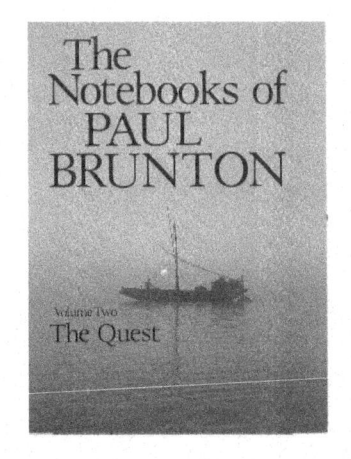

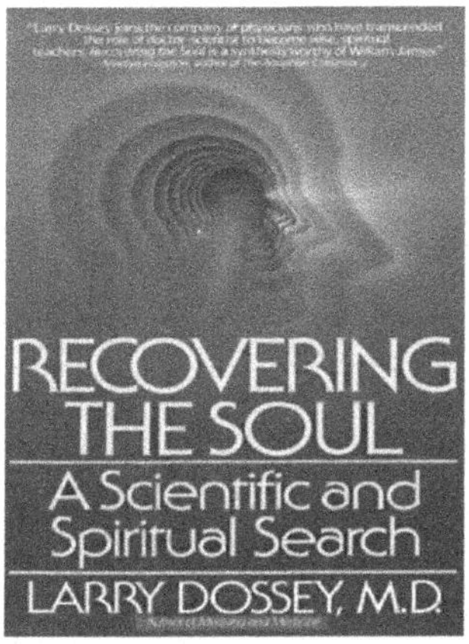
RECOVERING THE SOUL
A Scientific and Spiritual Search
LARRY DOSSEY, M.D.
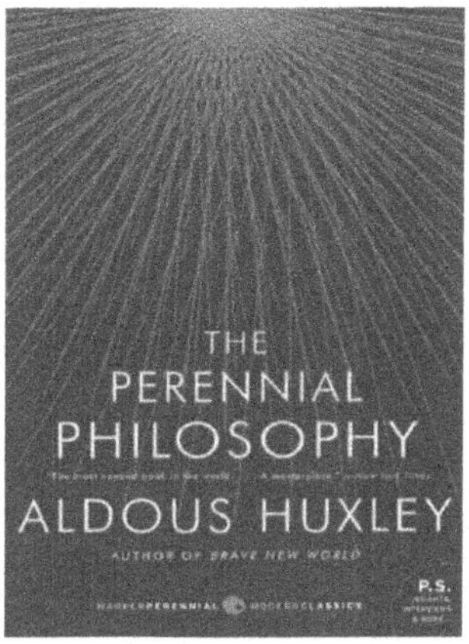
THE PERENNIAL PHILOSOPHY
ALDOUS HUXLEY
P.S.
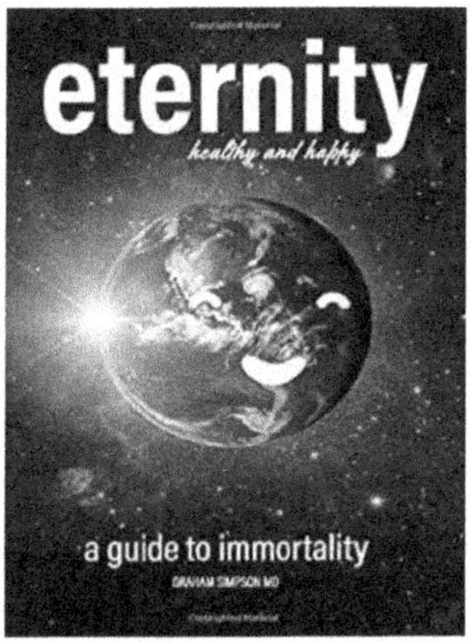
eternity
healthy and happy
a guide to immortality
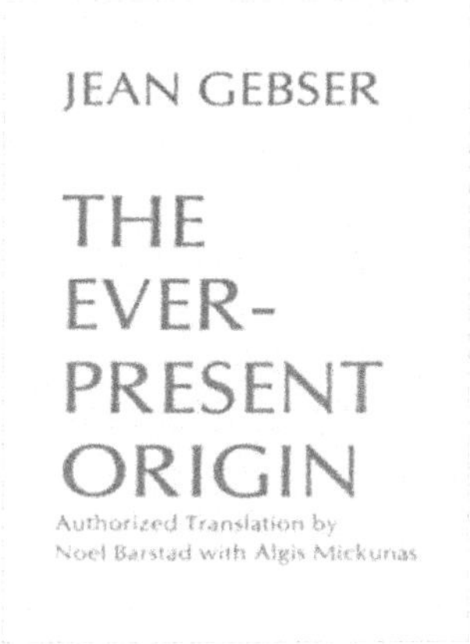
JEAN GEBSER
THE EVER-PRESENT ORIGIN
Authorized Translation by
Noel Barstad with Algis Mickunas
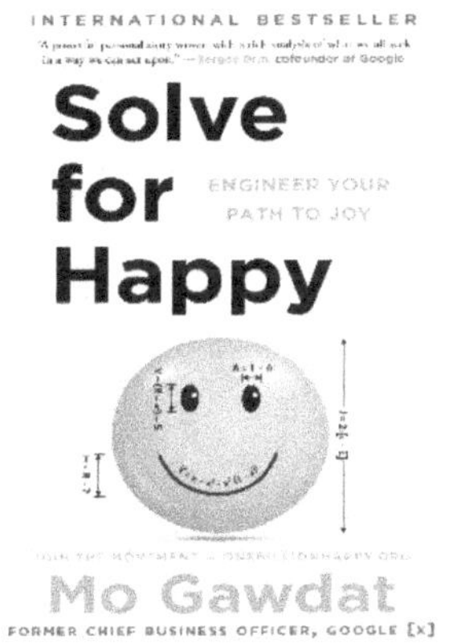
INTERNATIONAL BESTSELLER
Solve for Happy
ENGINEER YOUR PATH TO JOY
Mo Gawdat
FORMER CHIEF BUSINESS OFFICER, GOOGLE [X]
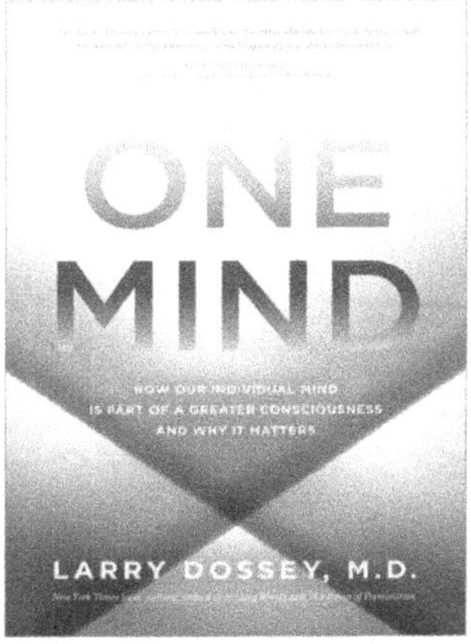
ONE MIND
HOW OUR INDIVIDUAL MIND IS PART OF A GREATER CONSCIOUSNESS AND WHY IT MATTERS
LARRY DOSSEY, M.D.

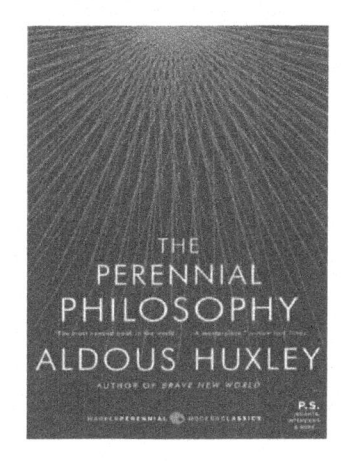

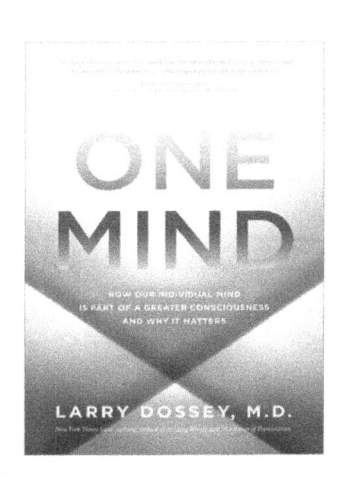

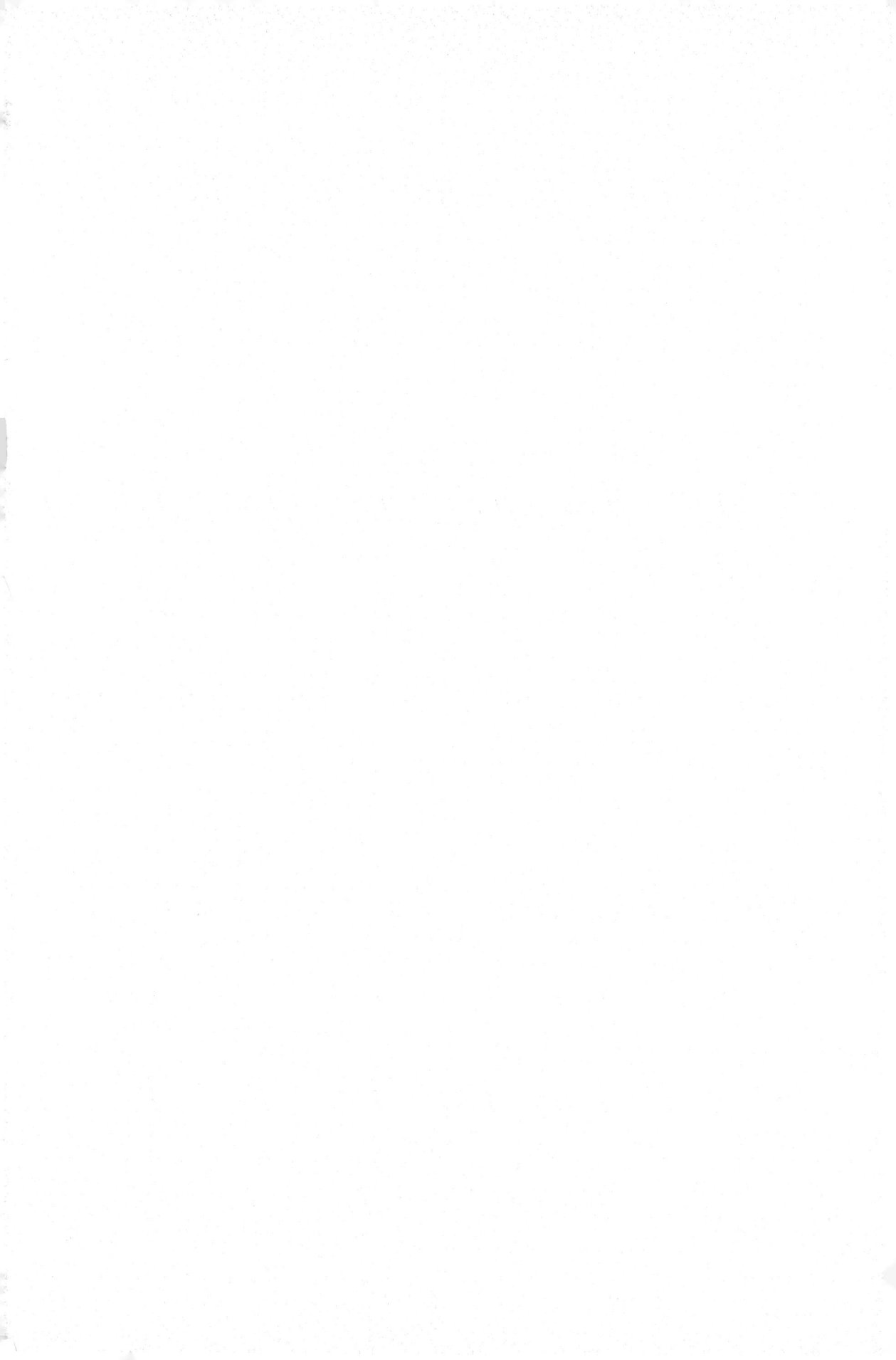